Large Animal Parasito Procedures for Veterinary Technicians

Large Animal Parasitology Procedures for Veterinary Technicians

Donald H. Bliss

MidAmerica Ag Research
3705 Sequoia Trail
Verona, WI, USA

WILEY Blackwell

Published by John Wiley & Sons, Inc., Hoboken, New Jersey.
Published simultaneously in Canada.

For general information on our other products and services or for technical support, please contact our Customer Care Department within the United States at (800) 762-2974, outside the United States at (317) 572-3993 or fax (317) 572-4002.

Wiley also publishes its books in a variety of electronic formats. Some content that appears in print may not be available in electronic formats. For more information about Wiley products, visit our web site at www.wiley.com.

Library of Congress Cataloging-in-Publication Data:

Names: Bliss, Donald, author.
Title: Introduction to large animal parasitology procedures for veterinary
    technicians / Donald Bliss.
Description: Hoboken, New Jersey : Wiley-Blackwell, [2024] | Includes
    index.
Identifiers: LCCN 2024007639 (print) | LCCN 2024007640 (ebook) | ISBN
    9780470959022 (paperback) | ISBN 9781394176267 (adobe pdf) | ISBN
    9781394176250 (epub)
Subjects: MESH: Parasitic Diseases, Animal—diagnosis |
    Parasites—pathogenicity | Livestock—parasitology | Diagnostic
    Techniques and Procedures—veterinary | Animal Technicians
Classification: LCC SF810.A3 (print) | LCC SF810.A3 (ebook) | NLM SF
    810.A3 | DDC 636.089/696—dc23/eng/20240401
LC record available at https://lccn.loc.gov/2024007639
LC ebook record available at https://lccn.loc.gov/2024007640

Cover Design: Wiley
Cover Images: © kentarus/Getty Images

Set in 9.5/12.5pt STIXTwoText by Straive, Chennai, India

Printed in Singapore
M043518_130524

Dedication and Acknowledgments

In sincere appreciation for counseling, guidance, and friendship, I dedicate this publication in honor of Professor Arlie C. Todd (1915–1984) from the University of Wisconsin, Department of Veterinary Science, located in Madison, Wisconsin (see Figure D.1). As a separate note, Dr. Todd recently received a special acknowledgement when another graduate of his department, Dr. William C. Campbell, received the Nobel Prize in 2017 for his role in the discovery and development of a parasiticide (Ivermectin) and its use to control a human parasite that causes river blindness in Africa.

Professor Todd was my mentor over a five-year span (1971–1976) during my PhD studies on "The Nature and Natural History of Worm Parasitism in Dairy Cattle." The most important lesson he taught me was how to determine the difference between "subclinical parasitism" and "clinical parasitism." He taught me that parasite detection was the single-most important determining factor that is necessary for treatment success. Leaving animals parasitized subjected those animals to increased pain and suffering, reduced growth, reduced reproduction efficiency, reduced utilization of feedstuff, and increased susceptibility to other diseases such as coccidiosis with reduced immune function. The only sure way of parasite detection in a live animal was through a sensitive and accurate fecal exam.

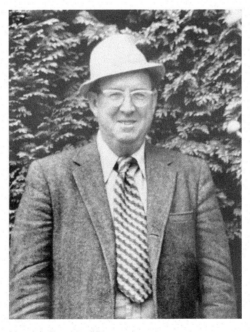

FIGURE D.1   Picture of Professor Arlie C. Todd.

Prof. Todd taught me that where parasites are present, damage is occurring. He taught me "Applied Parasitology." My job was to find these parasites cheaply and efficiently so that the cost of diagnosis did not interfere with the cost of removing these parasites. The "Modified Wisconsin Sugar Flotation Method" is that technique which provides us the most accurate and reliable way to find these parasites, identify and enumerate them whether they are found in large groups of animals, or recovered from an individual animal. If a gastrointestinal adult parasite is present within an animal but cannot be detected by the Modified Wisconsin Sugar Flotation Technique, that level of parasitism for that particular parasite is below the level necessary to cause measurable physical harm to the infected animal.

I personally have conducted fecal examinations using the "Modified Wisconsin Sugar Flotation Method" on several millions of samples during my lifetime starting with my studies at the University of Wisconsin, during an eight-year period of employment as a Senior Research scientist at Pfizer Central Research both in the United States and 14 countries in Europe plus from those thousands of samples being sent to my personal lab in Verona, Wisconsin, over the past 40 years. Furthermore, I have conducted several thousands of on-site "parasite evaluation clinics" with veterinary clinics, feed dealers, animal health stores, and on-farm clinics from across the United States and Canada examining fecal samples from swine, cattle, equine, sheep, goats, and wildlife using the "Modified Wisconsin Sugar Flotation Method."

Finally, a further acknowledgment to my entire family including my wife Sheena (see Figure D.2) who for past 40 years has received shipments of fecal samples, breaking open boxes

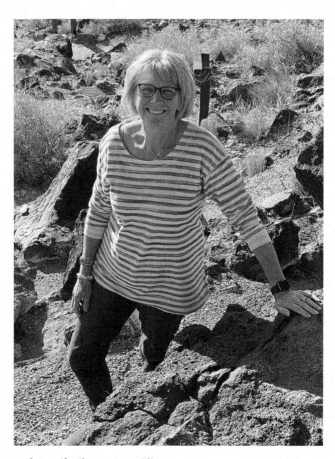

FIGURE D.2   Picture of my wife, Sheena Anne Bliss.

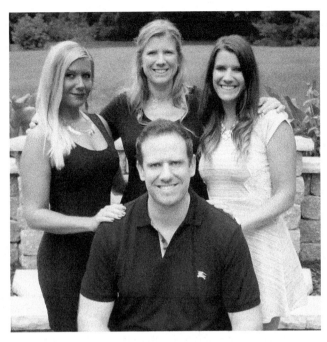

FIGURE D.3   Picture of my four children: Sheena Marie Kelter, Jonathan Bliss, Jordan Bliss, and Katrina Koenig.

daily, placing the samples in refrigerators, and to my four children including Sheena Marie (Kelter) plus her husband Patrick Kelter, Jonathan, Jordan, and Katrina (Koenig) of whom all five are well trained in the process of conducting fecal exams (see Figure D.3). Patrick Kelter is the current manager of our lab, MidAmerica Ag Research located in Verona, Wisconsin, who receives and conducts thousands of fecal samples annually coming from all across the United States (see Figure D.4) and, of course, myself (see Figure D.5) along with a picture of my grandson (one of eight grandchildren) looking the "WORMDR" Wisconsin license plate on my Ford van (Figure D.6).

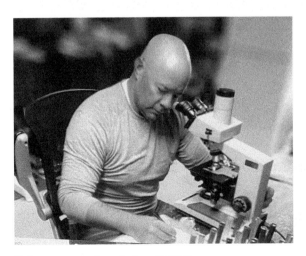

FIGURE D.4   Picture of lab manager and son-in-law: Pat Kelter.

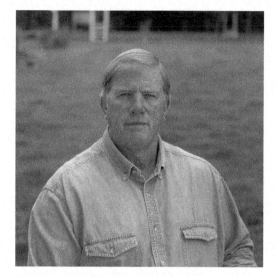

FIGURE D.5   Picture of author: Dr. Donald H. Bliss.

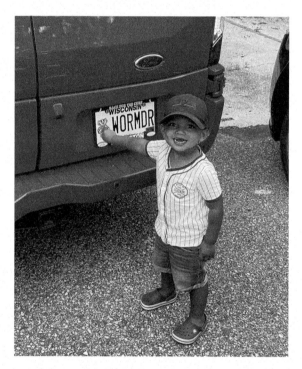

FIGURE D.6   Picture of grandson Landyn Johnson looking at my license plate (WORMDR).

Contents

4   Parasites in Dairy Cattle   171

5   Parasites in Equine   199

6 Parasites of Swine   235

Preface

Nearly all animal species found throughout the world, both domestic and wild, are exposed to internal parasites sometime during their lifetime. In many cases, exposure can be seasonal, sometimes sporadic, and other times it can be constant and severe. Overall, internal parasites present in animals today have learned to adapt to many different climatic and environmental conditions to ensure reinfection of their host animals. The situation occurs, therefore, where parasite detection through clinical observation is insufficient because it lacks the sensitivity to consistently and accurately detect the existence of a harmful parasite infection. Our primary goal is to find, identify, and remove these culprits using a simple diagnostic tool called the fecal worm egg count technique or fecal exam.

The problem that lies with current fecal exams that are taught in school and commercially available to veterinary clinics is that they are "as numerous as the sand of the seas" and mostly inaccurate, misleading, and ineffective. The fecal worm egg count technique needs to be sensitive enough to find all the worm eggs from all the gastrointestinal parasites of economic importance. Luckily, there is a fecal exam technique that accomplishes these goals and is readily available for use. It has been tested on millions of samples from all across North America and Europe over the past 50 years. This test is called the "Modified Wisconsin Sugar Flotation Method[1]" which was modified from an original method using the Sheather's solution[2] developed in the 1930s (see Figure P.1).

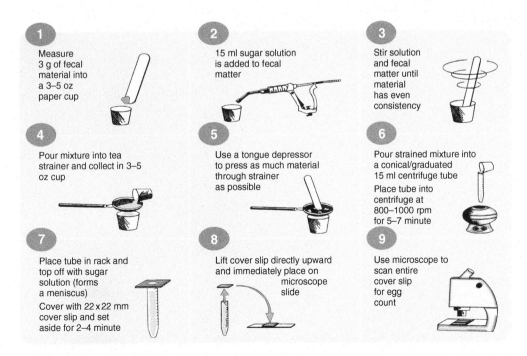

1 Measure 3 g of fecal material into a 3–5 oz paper cup

2 15 ml sugar solution is added to fecal matter

3 Stir solution and fecal matter until material has even consistency

4 Pour mixture into tea strainer and collect in 3–5 oz cup

5 Use a tongue depressor to press as much material through strainer as possible

6 Pour strained mixture into a conical/graduated 15 ml centrifuge tube

Place tube into centrifuge at 800–1000 rpm for 5–7 minute

7 Place tube in rack and top off with sugar solution (forms a meniscus)

Cover with 22 × 22 mm cover slip and set aside for 2–4 minute

8 Lift cover slip directly upward and immediately place on microscope slide

9 Use microscope to scan entire cover slip for egg count

FIGURE P.1   Wisconsin Sugar Flotation Method.

This technique was promoted since the early 1950s by Professor Arlie Todd at the University of Wisconsin, originally called the "Wisconsin Double Centrifugal Flotation Method.[3]" The modifications made for the original techniques are important because this technique can now be used by veterinary clinics and diagnostic laboratories quickly, cheaply, and with great accuracy. I have personally read over two million samples using this test, and currently our lab in Wisconsin conducts between 60,000 and 80,000 samples each year.

The Modified Wisconsin Sugar Flotation Method is very sensitive, very accurate, and the kind of specific laboratory test simple enough to apply to mass screening of parasitism. Having the ability to detect the presence of parasitism and then being able to identify the type of parasite(s) (genus and/or species) present can provide the necessary science needed by veterinarians and their staff to initiate treatment and to stop or prevent physical harm from occurring in the host animal. In many cases, this diagnosis may even save the animal's life (see Figure P.2).

In the case of gastrointestinal nematode parasites of veterinary importance, when detected early in the "parasite-to-host life cycle," this diagnosis is an extremely valuable tool. Not only does early detection allow timely treatment to help prevent suffering of the parasitized animals but also gives the veterinarian the necessary information to develop a strategy to prevent more problems later due to the continuing development and possible increased environmental contamination by the parasite(s) found. With livestock, early detection can often help to prevent economic loss for the producer where timing of treatment is often very important for successful control. It is very common for parasitic infections to become progressively more severe as time goes on, so early detection is very important.

The first goal of the veterinary technician on a fecal worm egg count should be able to obtain accurate scientific information on exactly whether or not the animal(s) in question is parasitized. This is also true when checking large groups of animals. If the animal or animals harbor parasites, they then need to be able identify the specific type of parasite or parasites that are causing the problem. The goal of the current book is to provide veterinarians and veterinary technicians the best technique to accomplish this goal. With the proper technique, all a technician needs in

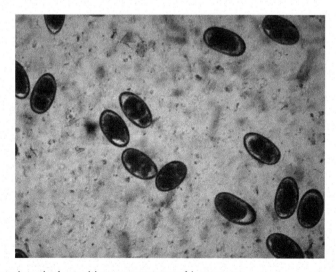

FIGURE P.2 Gastrointestinal parasitic worm eggs passed in manure.

order to be successful is a small amount of fresh (or refrigerated fresh) feces from the animal or animals in question. Knowing the answer provides the science needed for the consulting veterinarian to prescribe to their clients the best possible information or treatment to help solve the problem scientifically. Having this information provides the veterinarian the necessary knowledge and best opportunity to control the parasites correctly.

Most often, this information can also be used to design treatment protocols that will help control or even prevent parasite problems from occurring in the future. The degree of science that accurate parasite diagnosis provides is hard to quantify, but by simply having the ability to accurately detect parasites in their clients' animals separate this clinic and their technicians from all other clinics or technicians that are not using proper scientific methods to determine accurate parasite diagnosis to aid in prescribing the proper treatment.

At the current time, most veterinary clinics routinely run fecal exams only on dogs and cats. Why not other species? This question seems to have several answers. The first answer is that conducting fecal exams for livestock on a routine basis is currently not taught in most veterinary schools. Second, the fecal worm egg recovery techniques taught in most veterinary schools and schools training veterinary technicians are not sufficiently accurate to be used for routine examination of stool samples from large animals with high fecal output such as brood cows, feeder cattle, or lactating dairy cows. The third answer is that the conventional price charged by most clinics for individual fecal exams are often too high for livestock owners to justify requesting fecal checks as a routine practice since the fecal exam itself is often priced considerably higher than the cost of most dewormers available on the market.

What does an accurate fecal worm egg count mean to a producer? Let us answer this question in reverse. Without a fecal, no one knows if a dewormer is needed, if the dewormers are working properly, what type of parasites are present, or how many worm eggs are being excreted back in the environment recontaminating the environment of the animals shedding the eggs. Having a low-cost, highly efficient, but yet a very accurate fecal exam that is easy to conduct provides the answer. Whether there is only one animal that needs a fecal check or 1000 animals, knowing the parasite status at key times of the year can be an extremely valuable information to the client. I was recently riding with a rancher observing his animals. He was very often with his yearling bulls, noticing manure on their back sides. I suggested we pull fecals and check for parasites. He mentioned to me that he felt that having a pasty rear end on his bulls was a good thing indicating high protein intake (see Figure P.3). The fecals demonstrated that *Nematodirus* present in fairly high numbers was probably a serious detriment to the growth and health of his bulls.

Diagnosing parasitism is not a stand-alone science. It is a complicated marriage between detecting and identifying the parasites with an astute understanding of their individual life cycles, understanding their individual transmission patterns, knowing what pathological or detrimental effects they have on the host animal, knowing what veterinary pharmaceutical products provide the best level of control, and then knowing how to control or prevent future infections. The technicians can be confident that no parasite species is left undetected.

By bringing all these things together in a single manual, we feel we can provide a more complete picture in the quest for simple but accurate detection and identification of all economically important parasites in domesticated and wild animals that veterinarian technicians might encounter during a fecal exam. It is the primary goal of the authors of this textbook to provide the best available diagnostic procedures and to provide as many parasite identification photos as possible to help veterinary clinics and diagnostic laboratories know whether a specific parasite or type of parasites exist in a particular animal or groups of animals at any given time.

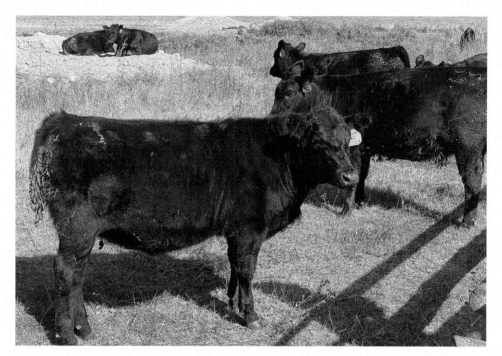

FIGURE P.3   Young bulls from Idaho subclinically infected with *Nematodirus*.

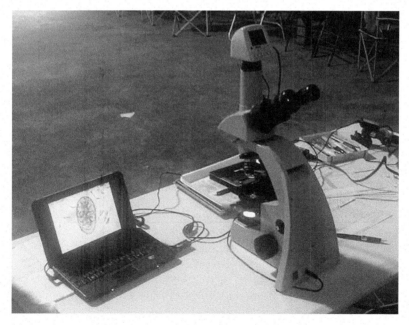

FIGURE P.4   Microscope provides an accurate visual assessment.

New and improved techniques will appear and replace some techniques outlined here. Occasionally, one technique will work better than another technique for a particular parasite. For simplicity, however, we have chosen the best overall fecal worm egg count technique for use in testing all fecal samples from all animal species coming into the laboratory and then for a particular parasite such as liver flukes, lungworms, or *Giardia*, a second or subsequent test(s) may be employed. The microscope provided an accurate visual parasite assessment for an individual animal (see Figure P.4).

Once parasite diagnosis becomes a part of a practice, many clinicians and diagnosticians may find it necessary to change their views from what they were taught regarding the physical presence and economical importance of gastrointestinal parasitisms in all species of animal. Change is never easy but it is always better to err on the side where scientific proof exists versus erring on the side where theoretical information currently being taught as fact exists without empirical proof thereof. The microscope never lies as long as the fecal examination technique is sensitive enough to find the parasites.

DONALD H. BLISS

MidAmerica Ag Research, 3705 Sequoia Trail, Verona, WI 53593, USA

Introduction to Large Animal Parasitology Procedures for Veterinary Technicians

What is Parasitism? Parasitism is defined as the condition of life that is both normal and necessary such that one organism can live on or within another host organism and that it nourishes itself at the expense of this host organism. The host organism is always a different species than the parasite and is almost always much larger than the parasitizing species. Since it is not in the best interest for a parasite to rapidly destroy its host as a predator does its prey, the parasite simply inflicts some degree of injury, negatively affecting the welfare of its host while gaining the benefit of life. The characteristic of this parasite–host ecosystem is that parasites contribute nothing beneficial to this system, but rather always cause harm to the host, which results from the activities of the parasites in their effort to survive and reproduce. Parasites often attach themselves to the gastric wall and absorb blood and nutrients (see Figure 1.1).

The survival of the parasite depends upon its ability to withstand the efforts of the host to destroy it. How harmful this relationship is dependent upon the species of parasites involved, the location of the parasite in the host, the number of parasites present, the virulence of the parasites,

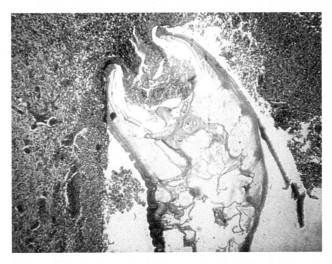

FIGURE 1.1   Strongyle nematode parasite attached to the gut wall of a horse [1].

Large Animal Parasitology Procedures for Veterinary Technicians, First Edition. Donald H. Bliss.
© 2024 John Wiley & Sons, Inc. Published 2024 by John Wiley & Sons, Inc.

the age of the host, the genetic susceptibility of the hosts to the parasites, and the previous experiences of the host with these invading parasites. Seasonality and the stage of lactation or gestation for the host animal can also influence the amount of damage caused by parasites.

Parasites have learned to adapt to the conditions of their host. Cattle in southwest Texas grazing arid range country may have less parasite exposure than cattle grazing lush pastures in Wisconsin. Twenty-five goats raised on 75 acres of land will have significantly less "parasite pressure" or parasite exposure than the same 25 goats grazing 1 acre of land. When cattle are raised under semiarid conditions, parasite pressure can be low; however, damage to the animal may be high if nutrition is inadequate (see Figure 1.2).

A few years back, I conducted a "parasite evaluation clinic" with a veterinary clinic near the town of Houston in northern British Columbia, 674 mi north of Vancouver (see Figures 1.3 and 1.4). The very first set of cattle fecal samples we checked during the clinic were loaded with *Nematodirus* eggs (see Figure 1.5). The owner said they had lost three calves over the past few days. Clinical parasitism, therefore, can occur almost anywhere animals are raised. Parasitism and production losses due to parasitism are not based solely on what part of the country the animals are located in, but rather they are based more on grazing pressure or stocking rates, climatic conditions during the season, whether or not water irrigation is used, whether there are any ponds or water source on the pasture, what the parasite contamination levels were at the beginning of the season, whether or not the animals placed on a pasture were currently carrying a heavy worm burden, where any deworming treatments used during the season, if used when were the deworming treatments administered, and what deworming products were used.

By definition, parasites always cause harm to their host while obtaining their livelihood. Furthermore, this host–parasite relationship exists because of a complex relationship whereby the parasites can contaminate the environment of their host with offspring (either eggs or larvae) to continue

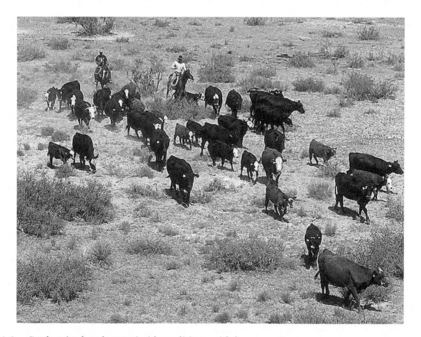

FIGURE 1.2   Cattle raised under semiarid conditions with low parasite pressure.
Source: United States Department of Agriculture/Wikimedia Commons/Public Domain.

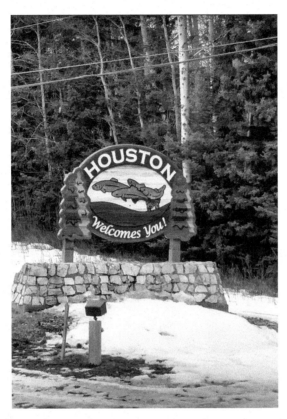

FIGURE 1.3   Location of the "parasite evaluation clinic" near Houston, British Columbia.

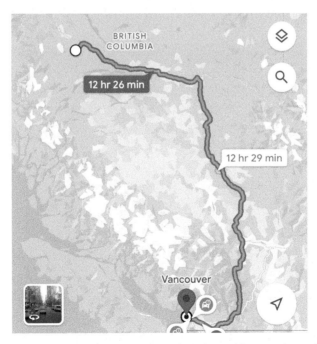

FIGURE 1.4   Distance north of Canadian border where clinical parasitism was detected (647 mi north of Vancouver).

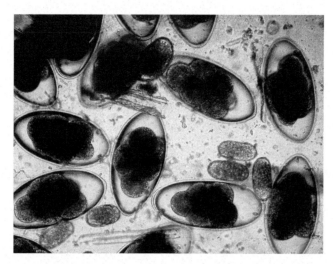

FIGURE 1.5 Microscopic picture of *Nematodirus* eggs from clinically infected calves examined in Northern British Columbia.

their relationship and to maintain their species. Whenever a parasite cannot complete their complete life cycle, they die off and disappear. A great example would be when an American traveler becomes infected through food contamination with a gastrointestinal parasite(s) when traveling abroad (especially in a country with poor hygienic conditions) but when they return home, the parasite cannot propagate because sanitary conditions in the United States are not conducive for reinfection to take place. Once this parasite is removed from the traveler (or it dies off), recontamination will not occur. Another example with domestic animals could be found when replacement dairy heifers are moved off pasture into a totally confined dairy facility where they calve and produce milk, but are now confined on concrete floors with no access to dirt lots or grass pasture areas (see Figure 1.6).

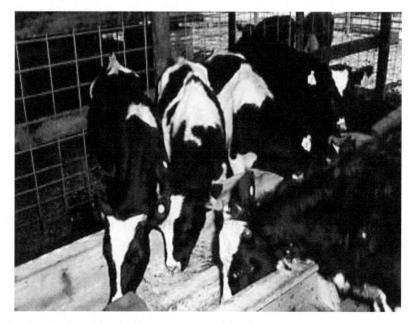

FIGURE 1.6 Young dairy cattle raised in confinement with no access to pasture.

Since these heifers are now no longer exposed to parasitic larval contamination found on pastures, their existing infections will eventually die off and since they are not replaced, they become parasite-free.

The universal existence of internal parasitism in domestic and wild animals requires the occurrence of encounters whereby the parasites can successfully establish host–parasite systems. The host–parasite relationship involves the accessibility of the host to the arrival and continued presence of the parasites. This parasitic relationship is called parasitism and the study of this relationship in domestic livestock and wild animals which are of interest to animal health is called "Veterinary Parasitology."

Veterinary parasitologists are exposed to many life-cycle variations of parasitism in animals. Cattle tapeworm (*Moniezia*) eggs, for example, simply pass through an intermediate host (Oribatid mites) while developing into an infective-stage embryophore, whereas cattle liver flukes undergo a complete development process while passing through an immediate snail host (*Lymnaea* snail), then back on vegetation to complete the life cycle once eaten by cattle. With liver flukes, they can also infect an alternate host (deer). These life-cycle variations are covered in detail in many books and research journals on veterinary parasitology.

Basically, with minor exceptions, most of the parasites of economic significance in domestic livestock and hoofed wildlife follow a simple direct life cycle. The cycle begins with the adult female and male parasites residing in the animals where they mate, following which the female worm then lays fertile eggs which pass out of the animal with the feces. Since these infections are unseen, this is the only point in the life cycle when a worm egg test can be conducted to detect the presence or absence of a mature infection. The standard, most efficacious, and simplest fecal worm egg count test I recommend is "The Modified Wisconsin Sugar Flotation Method" which will be covered in detail in the following chapter [2].

The typical life cycle of gastrointestinal parasites starts when each passed egg develops into a first-stage larva that hatches in the manure, provided that conducive (warm and moist) conditions persist. This first-stage larva then develops into a second-stage larva and then finally into an infective third stage, also called a L_3 larva. The infective L_3 larva is mobile and randomly moves away from the fecal matter onto vegetation. These infective larvae are subsequently ingested by the animal grazing this area and become re-established within the host where this life cycle continues (see Figure 1.7). Minor variations occur with nearly every parasite.

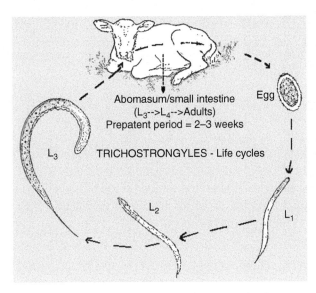

FIGURE 1.7   Typical life cycle of gastrointestinal parasites in grazing animals.

It is an essential feature of parasitic nematodes (roundworms), cestodes (tapeworms), and trematodes (flukes) that they can reproduce within a host, but then each new generation must undergo some development in the outside world before re-entering a host and adopting a parasitic way of life. The reproductive forms of these parasitisms are mostly ova (eggs), larvae, cysts, oocysts, or trophozoites, which pass out in the feces and redistributed into the environment of the host animal. This recontamination of the environment surrounding the host animals is paramount to the overall survival of the parasite because it ensures that future infections and/or re-infections occur, so the propagation of parasitic life continues. Internal parasites, therefore, have two basic goals in life: one is to live off their host animals that they invade, and the other is to reproduce back into the environment of host animal to ensure continuation of their species.

To the average person, the thought of having parasitic worms living in their own stomach, intestinal tract, or lungs is almost too much to bear. Yet, nearly all animals are exposed to parasitism sometime in their life, especially those parasitisms that invade and live in the gastrointestinal tract. Many animals become heavily infected on an annual basis depending upon environmental contamination levels and whether any means are taken to reduce their exposure level. It is not uncommon for horses, sheep, or goats to have fecal worm egg counts well over 1000 eggs/sample during the summer grazing season. This high level of worm egg shedding from a 3 g fecal sample can mean that a horse, for example, would be shedding 150,000 eggs per pound ($3 g \times 150 = 454 g$ or 1.0 lb, so multiply 150×1000 eggs) of manure or as many as 9 million eggs per horse per day should this animal be producing approximately 60 pounds of manure per day. As one can imagine, in just a short time, the pasture would become heavily contaminated by just one horse such that an animal grazing this pasture later in the year could be ingesting hundreds and even thousands of infective larvae every day. These larvae follow moisture trails moving up on the vegetation with the morning dew or with moisture from rainfall (see Figure 1.8).

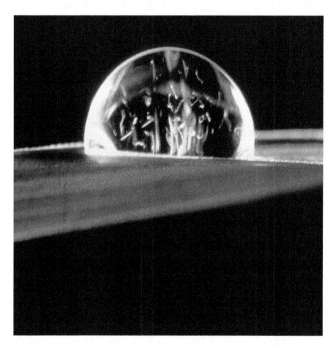

FIGURE 1.8   Famous picture of a dew drop with infective larvae on a blade of grass.

I believe there is a role humans must play to help prevent animals from suffering due to parasitic infections. I often see animals standing in fields all around the country looking heavily parasitized. I feel like it is our role as humans to help spread the word to owners and caretakers that these animals should not have to suffer. "Ivory tower" parasitologists often tell me, we cannot do anything because it will cause parasite resistance! My argument is that the correct treatment given at the correct time will help clean up the environmental contamination and thereby prevent parasite resistance. Allowing parasitism to reach very high levels makes the task of the dewormer much hard and provides a greater chance for leaving exposed parasites without killing 100% of their parasitic burdens. A dewormer with a 98% efficacy will leave 20 worms out of 1000 or 20,000 worms out of a million. So for a dewormer, it is also better treat when parasite burdens are low and prevent clinical parasitism, then wait until worm burdens have become extremely high. Remember, once the worm burdens are high in the animals, they are also high in the environment; so, treating heavily infected animals and then returning them to their heavily contaminated environment is a foolish waste of time and effort plus it greatly increases the chance for parasite resistance to occur. The correct deworming strategy, therefore, is to not only treat the animals but also to time the deworming to clean up the pasture environment, reducing the overall exposure to parasitism. This concept will be explained in detail later in this chapter.

Parasitism can be broken into two main stages or clinical conditions: The first stage is called "subclinical parasitism" while the second stage is called "clinical parasitism." Subclinical parasitism is often compared to an iceberg where the major portion of the iceberg is unseen being below the surface of the water (see Figure 1.9).

Therefore, with subclinical parasitism, the damage caused may not be readily visible to the owner or producer. Parasitism is most often first visibly evident in livestock through observing rough hair coats or animals showing "pasty rear ends" (see Figure 1.10). The largest part of the iceberg lies unnoticed under the sea and thus the greatest damage from subclinical parasite infections often occurs without being noticed by the owners, producers, or their veterinarians such as a drop in dry matter intake, reduced feed efficiency, lower weight gains, reduced milk production, reduced breeding efficiency, reduced body condition scores, and reduced immune function [3–8]. Subclinical infections may lead to "hard to observe" changes in behavior such as animals showing

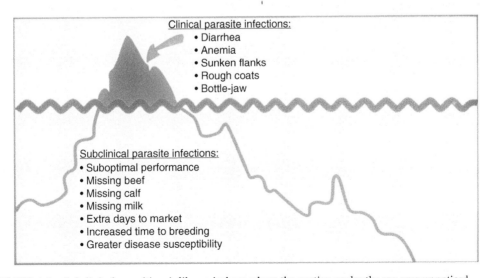

Clinical parasite infections:
- Diarrhea
- Anemia
- Sunken flanks
- Rough coats
- Bottle-jaw

Subclinical parasite infections:
- Suboptimal performance
- Missing beef
- Missing calf
- Missing milk
- Extra days to market
- Increased time to breeding
- Greater disease susceptibility

FIGURE 1.9   Subclinical parasitism is like an iceberg where the portion under the sea goes unnoticed.

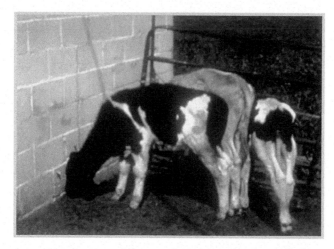

FIGURE 1.10   Three Holstein dairy calves with clinical signs of *Nematodirus* infection.

reduced grazing time with longer periods of standing or lying around. Based on years of research conducted throughout the world, there is no question that gastrointestinal parasitisms even at subclinical levels are a major deterrent to efficient production. Parasitism commonly found in livestock follows an age pattern depending upon housing location and access to pasture (see Figure 1.11).

Clinical parasitism is simply the stage where physical effects of the infection are visible evidence in the physical condition of the animals infected. Sometimes the evidence is as simple as checking mucous membranes such as eyelids for sign of anemia (a pale membrane caused by the loss of red bloods cells), which is a common practice used with sheep and goat owners to detect heavy *Haemonchus* (barber's pole worm) infections. Even baby calves can become clinically infected with threadworms (Strongyloides) where larvae can pass in the mothers' milk as well as a direct infection acquired from the bedding (see Figure 1.12).

Common Dairy Parasites

Commonly Found Parasites

Production Group	Giardia	Coccidia	Threadworm	Whipworm	Hookworm	Nematodirus	Tapeworm	Stomach Worms	Cooperia	Nodular Worm	Lungworm
Pre-Weaned Calves	X	X	X	X							
Weaning - 3 mo. old		X	X	X	X	X					
3 mo. - 11 mo.		X	X	X	X	X	X	X	X	X	X
Yearlings/Breeding age heifers						X	X	X	X	X	X
Bred Heifers						X	X	X	X	X	X
Fresh Cows							X	X	X	X	X
Lactating Cows							X	X	X	X	X
Dry Cows							X	X	X	X	X

Barnyard Infections - Heavier bedding increases risk (eg. Manure pack)
Both - These parasites can be transmitted in bedding and on grass
Pasture - These parasites usually require grass for transmission.

FIGURE 1.11   Parasites commonly found by various age groups.

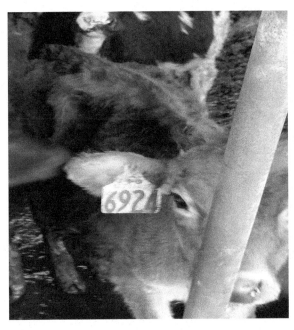

FIGURE 1.12   Picture of baby calves showing clinical parasitism due to a heavy threadworm (*Strongyloides*) infection.

Since gastrointestinal parasites live unseen within an animal, they can go unnoticed until at which time they can build up to high and often dangerous levels before visible signs become evident. It has been stated that clinical parasitism occurs when insufficiently resistant animals are exposed to an excessive rate of infection. This situation may arise when susceptible animals graze a heavily contaminated pasture (see Figure 1.13). Once it has been decided that treatment is necessary, we find little success in treating heavily infected animals and then returning them back to the

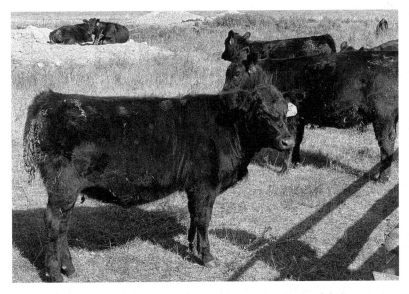

FIGURE 1.13   Idaho yearling bulls with *Nematodirus* infections showing rough hair coats.

same contaminated environment. The contaminated pasture this animal or animals are grazing should be vacated at this time, with a better deworming strategy to be developed for the following year. Ignoring the presence of parasites means animals are unnecessarily being exposed to pain and suffering plus resulting in production losses for the owner.

Even when parasite infections reach a level when clinical signs are present, positive confirmation is best completed using a fecal exam. Furthermore, if one waits until clinical signs are present before treating, considerable damage may already have occurred in the animals. Although sometimes it is possible to "feed past a parasitism" with considerable feed loss, but remember "the parasites" always get their "bite first." There is a definitive clinical process of an infection in cattle as follows:

1. The first signs of parasitism are usually the development of a rough and scruffy hair coat. Some young animals will also develop a "pot belly" along with the rough hair coat (see Figure 1.14).

2. Lack of weight gain or loss of weight during the grazing season, especially in younger animals.

3. Reduced reproduction efficiency in animals of breeding age.

4. Reduced milk production in lactating animals.

5. Reduced digestion and poor fetal development.

6. Reduced immune function. Coccidia outbreaks become common here.

7. Body and survival maintenance affected, which will soon lead to death if not treated.

As worm burdens build and clinical parasitism develops, immediate treatment may be needed to save the life of the animal. Being able to detect, treat, and/or prevent parasitic problems before clinical signs appear should be the goal of every veterinary hospital or clinic in the world. This is exactly where a quick and accurate fecal exam can play a very important role in preventing production losses or in alleviating unnecessary pain for the animals in question. A fecal worm egg counts using the Wisconsin Sugar Flotation Method is the best way to determine the presence of subclinical parasitism (see Figure 1.15) (this method will be described in detail in Chapter 2).

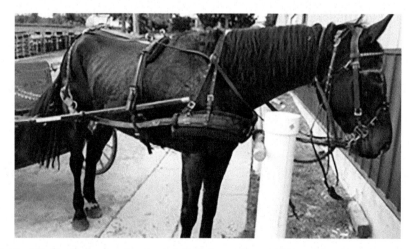

FIGURE 1.14   Working horse showing signs of clinical parasitism with an extremely high fecal worm egg count.

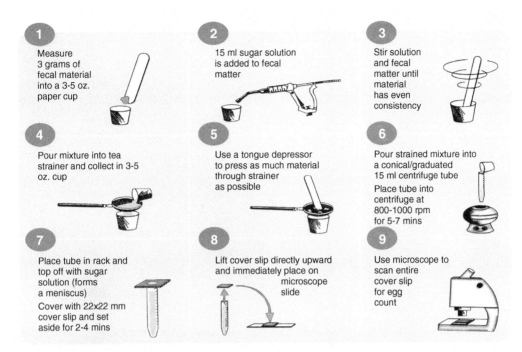

1

Measure 3 grams of fecal material into a 3-5 oz. paper cup

2

15 ml sugar solution is added to fecal matter

3

Stir solution and fecal matter until material has even consistency

4

Pour mixture into tea strainer and collect in 3-5 oz. cup

5

Use a tongue depressor to press as much material through strainer as possible

6

Pour strained mixture into a conical/graduated 15 ml centrifuge tube

Place tube into centrifuge at 800-1000 rpm for 5-7 mins

7

Place tube in rack and top off with sugar solution (forms a meniscus)

Cover with 22x22 mm cover slip and set aside for 2-4 mins

8

Lift cover slip directly upward and immediately place on microscope slide

9

Use microscope to scan entire cover slip for egg count

FIGURE 1.15   Modified Wisconsin Sugar Flotation Method.

The main question of this discussion is to ask veterinarians and their staff throughout the world why they do not use fecal exams as a routine method to monitor parasitism in livestock and what can we do to help change this. Treating without knowing whether an animal really needs treatment, treating animals at the wrong time of the year, and not knowing whether the treatment given actually works are all reasons the practicing veterinarian needs to be able to provide accurate fecal worm egg counts to all their producers. These fecal worm egg counts should be done in order to monitor fecal worm egg output with all livestock on a routine basis. We also need to convince owners on the value of fecal exams to monitor their animals.

Paying a Veterinary Service for a fecal worm egg counts on animals to know when to treat could save producers thousands of dollars for unnecessary treatment, incorrect treatment, using the wrong products, and not knowing whether the products they used were effective. Furthermore, there is now a number of FDA-approved deworming products on the US market that have become "parasite resistance." Being able to monitor these products is extremely important. Remember, products that fail to control parasites may be as bad for the animals as a failure to treat altogether causing unnecessary suffering in the animals and production losses for the owners (see Figure 1.16).

Fecal exams using the correct method can provide the science that is necessary to ensure treatment is given correctly, is given at the right time, and is effective. At the present time, very little is being done on a routine basis to monitor deworming treatments in domestic livestock. Thousands, even millions, of treatments are given annually to cattle, sheep, goats, horses, swine, and poultry, but very little is done to actually monitor infection levels or even determine whether or not treatments given are working correctly and providing the protection they were approved to do by the FDA regulatory authorities.

Over the past 38 years, I have dedicated considerable amount of my consulting time for conducting parasite evaluation clinics using the Modified Wisconsin Sugar Flotation Technique all

Trial Summary for Fecal Egg Count Reduction Tests Reported on the Merck National Data Base Conducted with FDA Approved Macrocyclic Lactone Products.

Products	No. of Trials	No. of Samples	Egg Counts/3 g*		Percent Efficacy (%)
			Pre-Rx	Post-Rx	
Injections					
Ivomec® Inj.	25	1352	70.1	37.1	47.0
Ivomec® Plus	17	823	102.6	55.7	45.7
Dectomax® Inj.	44	1791	64.1	15.4	76.0
Cydectin Inj.	12	614	36.9	5.3	85.7
Ivermectin Inj.	13	630	90.0	45.6	48.3
Ivermectin Plus	5	193	97.5	48.6	50.1
Inj. summary:	116	5403	76.8	34.6	54.9
Pour-ons					
Ivomec® PO	21	823	61.8	27.0	56.3
Ivermectin PO	81	3378	62.6	29.2	53.4
Dectomax® PO	23	941	67.9	23.7	65.1
Cydectin® PO	25	1044	60.9	14.5	76.1
Eprinex®	5	224	38.1	25.8	32.2
PO summary	155	6410	58.3	24.0	58.8
Overall summary:	271	11,813	68.4	29.8	56.4

* All samples taken at Rx and again 2 wks post-Rx. (Ivomec®, Eprinex® – Boehringer Ingelheim), (Dectomax® – Zoetis) (Cydectin® – Elanco).

FIGURE 1.16   Fecal worm egg reduction studies on commonly used endecticide deworming products.

across North America, working with the veterinary pharmaceutical industry, veterinary clinics, feed companies, feed stores, and dealer stores. Typically, I would fly into a designated location early in the week carrying a microscope equipped with a camera to conduct clinics at different chosen locations in a particular part of the country. The clinics would be set up by a pharmaceutical territory rep that would contact the desired clinic location, work with their clients by sending out invitations for the "parasite evaluation clinic." Producers would be invited to bring samples from their animals to be processed at the clinic location for a one-day free evaluation (see Figures 1.17–1.19). Our goal for each clinic is to have from 100 to 300 samples per clinic from invites sent to producers for the designated location. The centrifuge plus supplies needed to conduct the clinic would be supplied by the pharmaceutical rep.

The labs are usually set up in the morning and sample analysis would be conducted through late afternoon followed by a producer dinner meeting in the evening, where the results are shared with each individual producer and a presentation on strategic timed deworming would be given to the invited producers. Fecal samples are collected a few days ahead of the clinics (see Figures 1.20 and 1.21) and the labs are set where samples will be run throughout the day (see Figures 1.22–1.25) while training students and conducting producer meetings explaining treatment options (see Figures 1.25–1.35). For many of these clinics, individual treatment history and lab results would be entered into a national database for further evaluation, summarization, and publication. Whenever we were working with a veterinary clinic, the clinic would usually retain the results for their clients

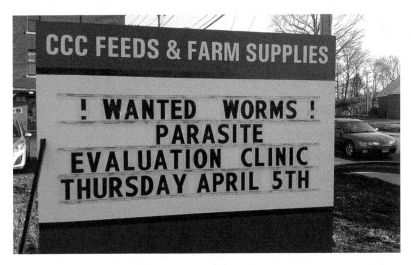

FIGURE 1.17   Sign inviting clients to bring fecal samples to "parasite evaluation clinic" (CCC feeds).

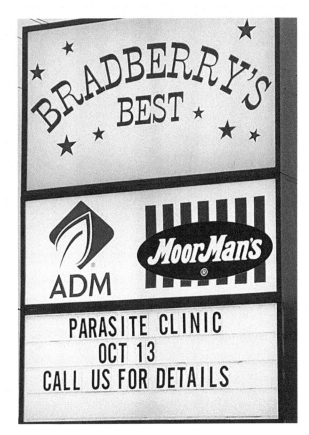

FIGURE 1.18   Sign advertizing parasite clinic with Bradberry's Best.

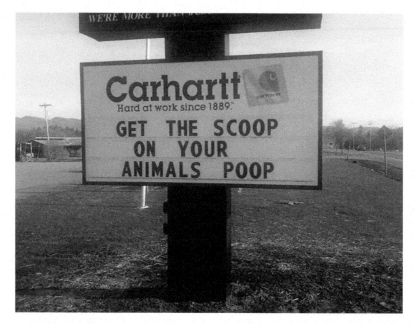

FIGURE 1.19 Sign telling animal owners to bring samples to our clinic and "get the scoop on your animal's poop."

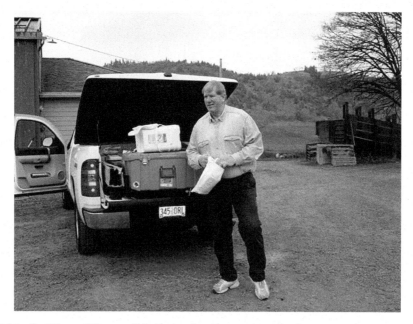

FIGURE 1.20 Dr. Bliss on K Bar ranch in Oregon heading out to get fecals.

for future treatment evaluations. Any retesting or further treatment evaluations could then be sent to our lab in Wisconsin for further evaluations.

Because parasitism is a complicated phenomenon, it is often hard to separate diagnosis from treatment in terms of to how to treat, when to treat, and what products should be used. A further question should be asked as to whether treatment can be given in such a way as to prevent

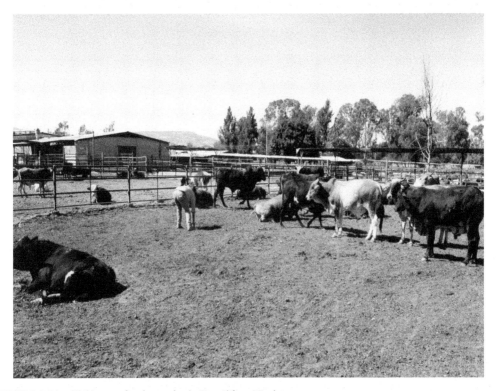

FIGURE 1.21   Picking up fecal samples in Tepatitlan, Mexico.

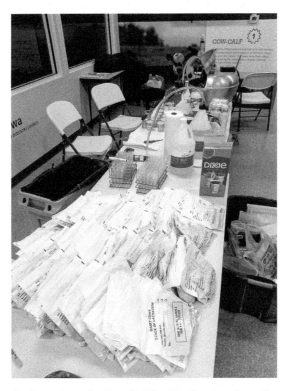

FIGURE 1.22   Lab setup for "parasite evaluation clinic" at Northeastern Iowa Community College in Calmar, Iowa.

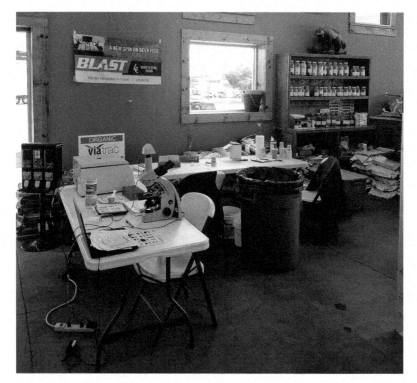

FIGURE 1.23   Parasite evaluation at feed mill in Nebraska.

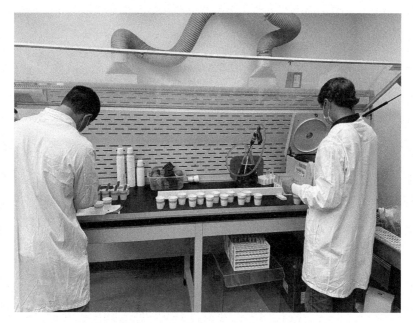

FIGURE 1.24   Lab setup conducting a large number of samples at the same time.

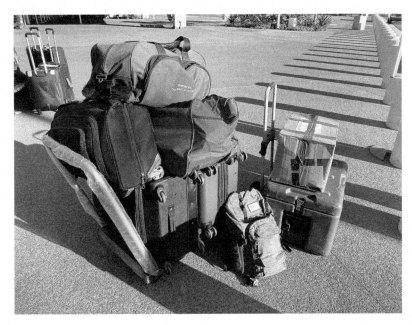

FIGURE 1.25   Shipping clinic supplies to Kona, Hawaii, for conduction of "parasite evaluation clinics."

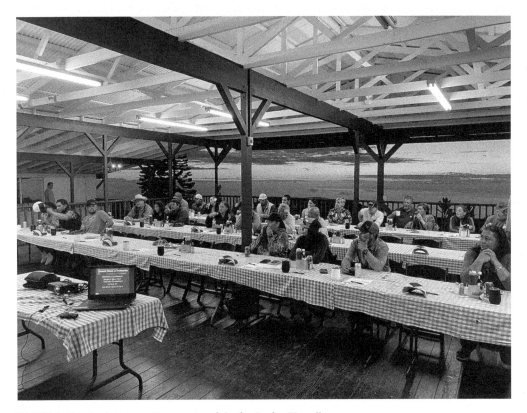

FIGURE 1.26   Producer meeting on a ranch in the Puako, Hawaii.

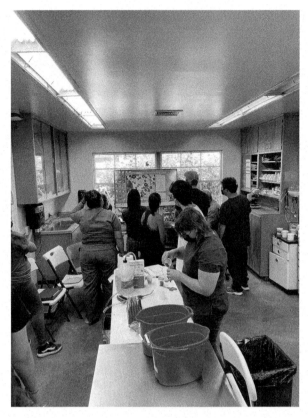

FIGURE 1.27   Training vet tech students at California Polytechnic State University.

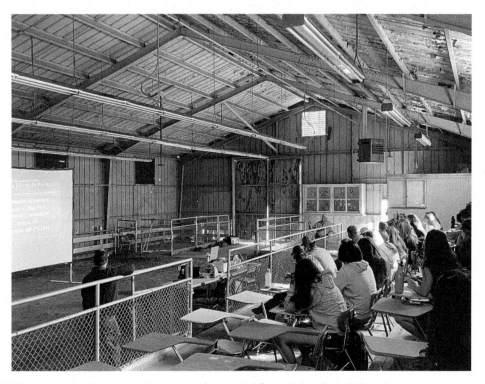

FIGURE 1.28   Parasite presentation to ag students at California Polytechnic University.

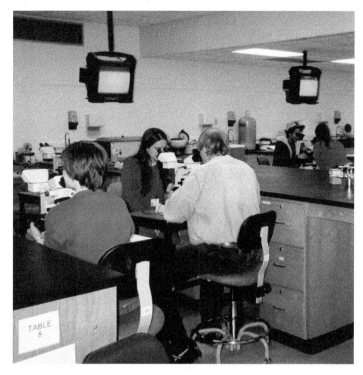

FIGURE 1.29   Scope training with vet students at University of Wisconsin School of Veterinary Medicine.

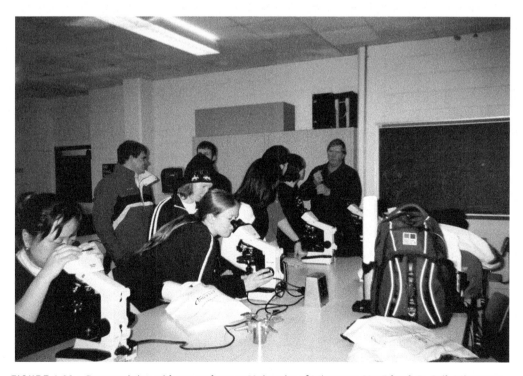

FIGURE 1.30   Scope training with vet students at University of Minnesota Vet School, St. Pail, Minnesota.

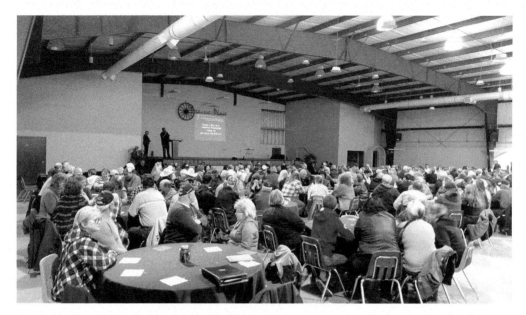

FIGURE 1.31 Large producer meeting in Saskatchewan.

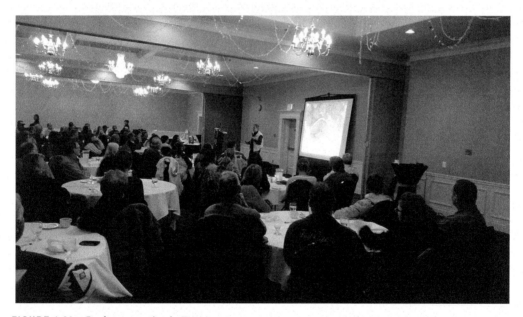

FIGURE 1.32 Producer meeting in Texas.

future infections. The most common question from producers and animal owners about parasite treatment in an animal or group of animals is how high does the worm burden need to be before treatment should be recommended? Again this question is hard for most veterinarians to answer without knowing all the facts, like which types of parasites were found, what time of the year were the samples conducted, what is the age of the infected animals, are the animals pregnant, how long since the last treatment was given, what product was last used, and are the animals living in a contaminated environment?

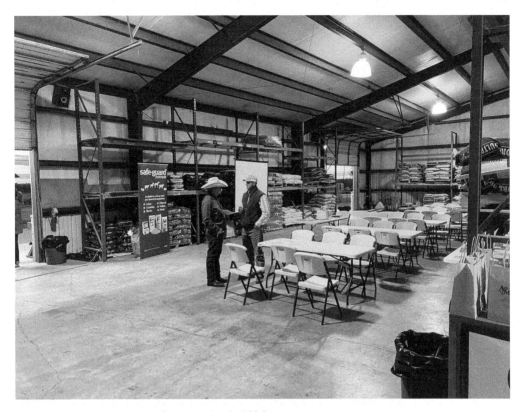

FIGURE 1.33   Setting up a producer meeting in Oklahoma.

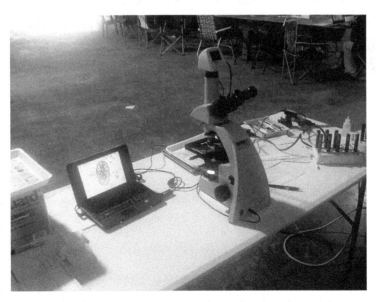

FIGURE 1.34   Camera on scope showing a parasite egg.

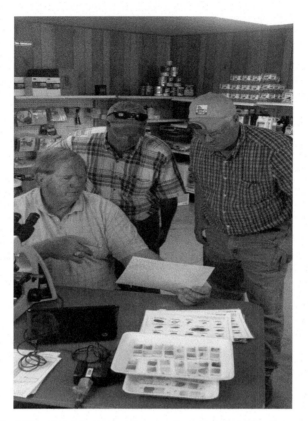

FIGURE 1.35   Dr. Bliss talking to producers and showing them their fecal results.

GASTROINTESTINAL PARASITISM CAN BE CATEGORIZED INTO FOUR DISTINCT PERIODS OF DEVELOPMENT

EARLY LARVAE DEVELOPMENT AND TRANSLATION PERIOD

It is the period of time the parasite spends outside the host. During the development phase, the parasite is dependent upon environmental conditions for its survival as it develops into the infective L_3 phase. Adult male and female parasites live in the gastrointestinal tract, mate, and lay eggs which pass out in the manure. After eggs pass in the feces, a L_1 larva quickly develops inside the egg, provided the outside temperatures are sufficiently warm. This L_1 larva will hatch in just a few hours after passing while the manure pat is still warm, and then after several days, it will begin to molt into a L_2 larva. Provided environment conditions are good, it will then continue development into a L_3 infective-stage larva in a couple of weeks. The first and second larva stages remain in the fecal pat and feed on bacteria and debris in the manure pat while the L_3 larva is very mobile and will follow moisture trail away from the manure and onto the nearby vegetation. The L_3 larvae retain their outer sheath when they molt from a L_2 to and L_3 larvae which provides the L_3 larvae additional protection form environmental conditions (see Figures 1.36 and 1.37). When viewing live L_3 larvae under the microscope, they are in constant motion.

If temperatures go below freezing for a long period of time, the eggs, and L_1 and L_2 larvae are killed. Because the third-stage larva (L_3) retains its outer sheath, it now becomes a protective

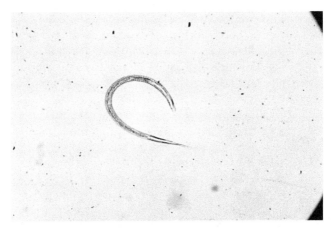

FIGURE 1.36   L$_3$ infective larva showing outer protective sheath.

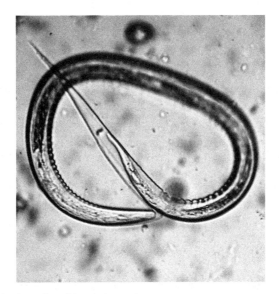

FIGURE 1.37   L$_3$ infective larva found in stool samples.

covering that helps this larva survive unfavorable weather conditions. It can also move deeper into fecal pat or into the soil to find protection. Only the L$_3$ larvae are able to survive extremely cold temperatures. These L$_3$ larvae that survive the winter are immediately infective once temperatures warm up and grazing begins [9]. Because of this, some winter-time transmission can take place on warm winter days if the temperature stays above 65–70° for several days.

Moist, warm climatic conditions provide an optimal environment for eggs and larvae. When culturing larvae from manure under controlled laboratory conditions, L$_3$ larvae recovery is usually successful between 10 and 14 days after eggs are placed in the culture. Under natural field conditions, however, embryonation from newly excreted eggs to L$_3$ larvae development in the manure will take considerably longer time depending upon moisture and temperature at the ground level. Air temperature versus soil temperatures or temperatures in the manure pat will differ greatly, but temperatures between 65 and 85 °F seem to be ideal, for larval development. Some development will occur at lower temperatures; however, development stops after temperatures fall below 50°.

Under favorable summer weather conditions, this larval development process can occur in a couple of weeks. But under cool spring temperatures or during adverse weather conditions, this development process can take as long as three to four months. What happens in a normal year is eggs that are shed in early spring may take several months to become infective larvae, whereas when summer approaches, eggs will turn into larvae more quickly. This means many eggs are maturing at the same time and thus larvae contamination of pasture will increase rapidly once summer arrives. This maturation of infective larvae all at the same time provides a midsummer rise in pasture contamination and clinical disease will occur soon after, especially with sheep and goats. For cattle, this jump in contamination often occurs just as spring calves are large enough to begin grazing (see Figure 1.38).

Since an infective L_3 larva can no longer feed because its mouth parts are covered by the protective outer sheath, it has to been eaten in a timely fashion or it will die off naturally. Numerous studies show that once the L_3 larva survives the winter and moves onto the spring grass, it must be eaten by the host animal during the first 60–90 days of the season or it will eventually disappear off the vegetation [9–11]. If, for example, no animals are present on the spring pasture until late June or July, this pasture becomes a mostly parasite-free pasture.

On the other hand, extreme dry conditions can destroy L_3 infective larvae. Also, cool or cold weather may not be totally lethal but will retard larval development. Direct sunlight also can kill infective larvae. This is why eggs and larvae do not survive well under feedlot conditions or in concrete barn lots where there is no vegetation for the larvae to hide under in order to escape high temperatures or direct UV sunlight. Larvae that survive the winter from one season to another are protected in the manure pat as a L_3 infective larva. Spring rains break these pats apart and as temperatures begin to warm up, the surviving larvae move onto the vegetation as spring green-up begins. When conditions are right for spring grass growth, conditions are as right for parasite development and translation onto the vegetation for the infection process to start again.

The translation phase is the time after the larvae become infective. Infective larvae are very active moving away the fecal pat onto the vegetation in order for transmission to be completed. This is greatly facilitated by rainfall and dew. Other mechanical means such as insects, birds, and cattle feet also help the distribution of larvae on the pastures. The feet of cattle stepping on fecal pats become especially important when fecal pats become hard and crusty without rain and the larvae become trapped inside of the pat. Once rain breaks up this pat, parasitic gastroenteritis can follow soon after, especially if it has been dry for a long period of time and large numbers of infective larvae can move onto the vegetation at the same time.

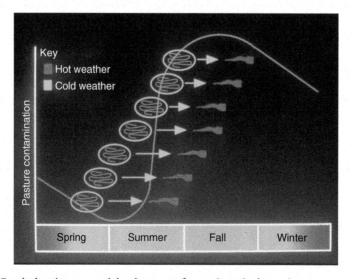

FIGURE 1.38 Graph showing seasonal development of gastrointestinal parasites on pasture.

Cattle going onto spring pastures shedding a high level of parasitic worm eggs will immediately begin contamination of the pasture (see Figure 1.39). Once the larvae escape the fecal pat, they move to and survive on the vegetative material surrounding the pat, contaminating the pastures just like weed seeds (see Figure 1.40) waiting to be ingested by grazing animals. The best time for transmission is usually in the morning when there is dew or a light rain providing the necessary

Beef Cattle Parasite Evaluation Form PEC: Mail In:

Date Samples Collected: 8-10-10

Ranch or Farm:

Producer's Name:

Address:

City: Newberry State: SC Zip:

Phone: E-mail: Fax:

Laboratory Consultant:

Sponsor:

Sponsor Contact:

Address:

City: State: Zip:

Phone: E-mail: Fax:

Representative Name: Fax:

Page of

Animal ID		Sample ID	Total Count (eggs/3 gm sample)
1	Str	67	184
2	"	68	159
3	"	69	212
4	"	70	289
5	"	71	230
6	"	72	172
7	"	73	13
8	"	74	102
9	"	75	167
10	"	76	85
1	Hfr	77	144
2	"	78	180
3	"	79	203
4	"	80	88
5	"	81	74
6	"	82	80
7	"	83	146
8	"	84	152
9	"	85	119
10	"	86	132

(X 150) =

Average eggs/gram X 150 = Eggs Shed/Pound of Manure

COMMENTS: UNTREATED

Copies: White–Database • Yellow–Sponsor • Pink–Producer Part # 66500R12-15-MAC 02/09 ©2009 Intervet/Schering-Plough Animal Health

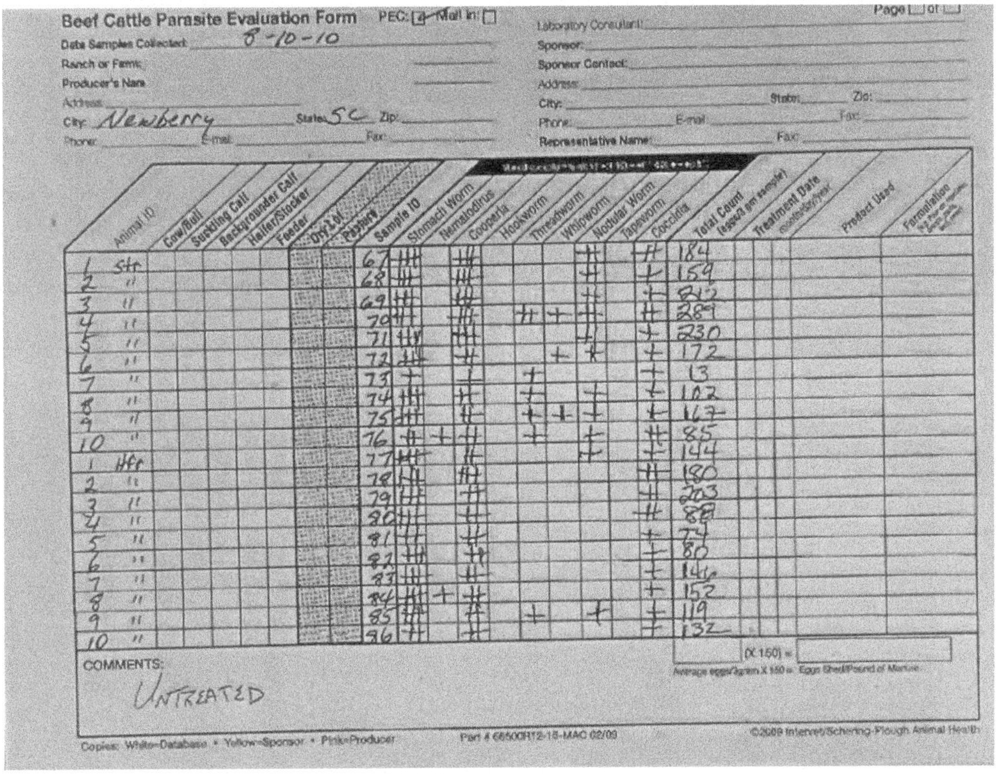

FIGURE 1.39 Fecal worm egg counts from heavily infected beef calves.

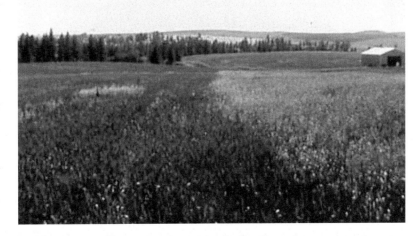

FIGURE 1.40 Worm eggs are like weed seeds recontaminating the pastures.

moisture to allow the parasitic larvae to move up on the vegetation in order to reach the animals when they are grazing. When the sun comes out and the moisture dries off, the larvae move back to the base of the vegetation. There is constant movement by the larvae in order to be consumed by the grazing animals. The survival of gastrointestinal parasites, therefore, depends on an encounter by the infective larvae with the host animal.

Worm eggs that are shed on the pasture in the spring of the first year have the propensity to survive until the spring of the following year. Larval contamination of spring pastures, therefore, comes from two sources: the first source is from the larvae that survive the winter from the previous season. The second source of larvae contamination is from the worm eggs that are shed on spring pastures after the grass has begun to grow and that have developed to infective L_3 larvae over the spring into early summer.

Due to temperature, the worm eggs that go down in early spring will take longer to develop into third-stage infective larvae than those eggs that are excreted later when temperatures are warmer. Hence, eggs shed in early spring will take longer to develop into infective larvae than eggs shed in midsummer when temperatures are the warmest (see Figure 1.41). If temperatures are perfect for development and moisture is lacking, egg development will stop. The inside of the fecal pat will stay moist much longer than outside conditions when the grass turns brown. If you step on a cow patty in the hot summer and it is still moist inside, larvae development will continue but translation to the grass may not occur until the rains come and break the manure pat open and allow the larvae to move onto the vegetation.

Eggs shed in late fall will stop development when temperatures reach freezing conditions. Eggs that make full development into infective L_3 larvae in the fall have a 15–20% chance to make it through the winter. Remember, since these larvae are infective as soon as conditions are right for grass growth, conditions are right for larvae movement onto the vegetation. Animals grazing these spring pastures can therefore become infected immediately. These larvae must be eaten or they die off since they can no longer feed on debris and bacteria in the manure. Data indicate that the larvae that survive the winter will disappear off the pasture within the first 60–90 days after first grass growth, if they are not eaten.

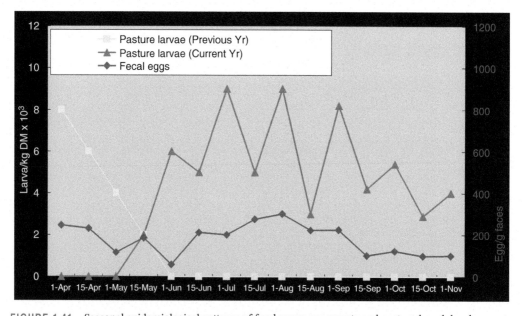

FIGURE 1.41   Seasonal epidemiological patterns of fecal worm egg counts and pasture larval development.

A comprehensive field study on the epidemiology of parasite gastroenteritis was conducted at 10 separate geographical locations across the United States and Canada [9]. The trial locations were Gainesville, Florida, Orono, Maine, West Lafayette, Indiana, Viroqua, Wisconsin, Oxford, Mississippi, Griffin, Georgia, Fayetteville, Arkansas, Moscow, Idaho, Eugene, Oregon, and Richmond, Quebec, Canada. The study demonstrated that the number of larvae present on the fall pastures (at the end of the grazing season) was five times higher than the numbers of larvae found on the spring pasture at the beginning of the grazing season. The number of worms recovered from tracer calves that grazed for two weeks prior to the end of the season from 10 separate locations across North America averaged 34,091 gastrointestinal nematodes of mixed infections. The number worms recovered the following spring on the same pastures from tracer calves that grazed for the first two weeks at the beginning of the spring season was 5731 parasites indicating that less than 17% of the parasite found on the pastures in the fall survived until the following spring season. These data indicated that approximately 83% reductions in the numbers of worms that were available to animals in the spring compared to those found in the calves that grazed for the same amount of time at the end of the previous grazing season. This reduction demonstrated that approximately 17% of the infective larvae on the pasture in late fall were able survive through the winter to be present on the spring pastures.

The second part of this comprehensive field study demonstrated that if the larvae picked during the first 90 days of the grazing were eliminated, the cumulative worm burdens in the cattle grazing these pasture for the entire summer grazing season were reduced by an average of 91% reduction. The cumulative worm burden from non-treated cattle at all 10 locations was 61,040 parasites per animal. The cumulative worm burden from cattle treated to prevent recontamination of the pastures was 10,963 parasites per animal for an 82% reduction in total worm burden per treated animal for the entire grazing season.

If the cattle are worm-free during the winter months, this is the first step to pasture control since they are not shedding eggs on the spring pasture. The first step in controlling parasites for an entire grazing season is to first stop reseeding the pasture with worm eggs during the early part of the season which reduces the number of worm eggs seeding the pasture in the spring, thus reducing the parasite challenge for the entire season (see Figure 1.42). The second step is to allow the cattle to graze the spring pasture and work like a vacuum cleaner picking up the infective larvae that survived the winter. As these larvae begin to mature in the cattle's gastrointestinal tract, the goal is to deworm the cattle strategically to kill the developing parasites before they have a chance to lay eggs and recontaminate the pasture. The prepatent period (period of time between the ingestion of infective larvae until an egg-laying adult worm is present for adult cows) is approximately 40–45 days for mature cows and bulls while for yearling cattle it is approximately 25–30 days [3].

When adult cows grazing the spring pasture are treated between 40 and 45 days or approximately 6 weeks into the grazing season to remove the larvae they have consumed during the first 6-week period, the new larvae they consume following treatment will take another 6 weeks before mature infections are actively laying eggs back onto the pastures. Thus, the mid-spring treatment will terminate the infections accumulated during the first six weeks of grazing, and then it will be another five to six weeks before eggs shedding begins again. This means that there is no major shedding of worm eggs for a total of 12 weeks or for the first 3 months of the grazing season. This means, since no new worm eggs have been shed on the pasture and providing the larvae from the previous season can either die off or been consumed by the animals grazing this pasture and no new worm eggs contamination has occurred, these pasture are now relatively parasite-free. In the northern more temperate areas of the United States, the holidays of Thanksgiving for the late fall deworming usually works and in the spring, we suggest more deworming should be completed before 4 July (see Figures 1.43 and 1.44). In the southern parts of the United States where spring

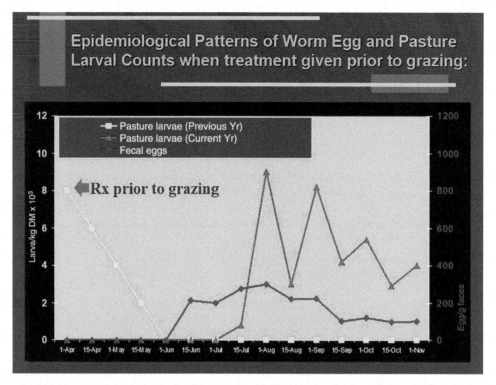

FIGURE 1.42   Epidemiological patterns of worm egg and pasture larval counts follow treatment given prior to grazing.

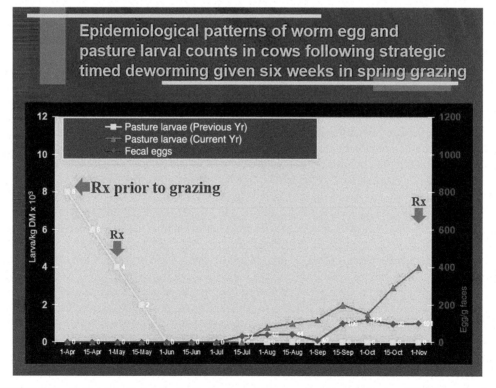

FIGURE 1.43   Epidemiological patterns of worm egg and pasture larval counts in cows following strategic timed deworming given six weeks into the spring grazing season.

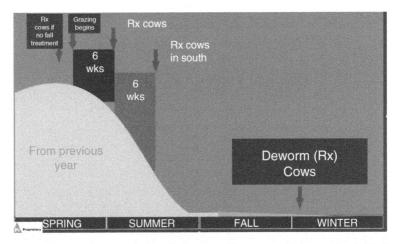

FIGURE 1.44   Graph showing fall and spring deworming effect on pasture contamination in brood cows.

begins and grass growth begins around 1 March, we use tax time (15 April), Memorial Day (late May), and Thanksgiving Day (late November) as the key suggested (approximate) treatment times.

The idea of seasonal control of parasites on pastures is to time the treatment to coincide with larval development and to treat just prior to when the maturing worms would begin laying eggs back on the spring pasture. This strategy prevents recontamination of the spring pasture since the cows are treated before their worm burdens have a chance to shed eggs. During this period, the larvae from the previous season are dying off naturally or are being eaten by the grazing cattle, which are then treated before they can shed eggs on the pasture. This is called strategic timed deworming to clean up the pastures and prevent parasite contamination from infective larvae.

In summary, fecal worm egg counts demonstrate that the egg shedding for cows on a parasite-contaminated pasture occurs approximately six weeks after ingestion of L_3 larvae. The mid-spring treatment is timed to treat the animals six weeks into the spring just before worm egg shedding should occur and then this treatment will provide a 6-week protection period following treatment for a total of 12 weeks (84 days) with no egg shedding [9–11]. This single mid-spring treatment in cows will therefore provide season-long control because if the parasites in the spring are killed and no new parasite eggs are shed on these pastures, the pasture will remain relatively free of infective larvae for the rest of the season. The goal is to reduce the level of parasite contamination on the pasture below the level that will interfere with efficient production. The data demonstrated an 80% reduction in parasite contamination for an entire grazing can be achieved. In the Deep South, a second treatment six weeks following the first treatment may be necessary to achieve the same result because of a longer growing season [12, 13].

For yearling cattle, replacement heifers, and stockers, since the prepatent period is shorter (approx. 25–30 days) compared with mature cattle, a second mid-spring treatment is recommended at a 4-week interval called a 0–4–8 week treatment period is recommended (see Figure 1.45). Treatment is given at Day 0 only if the cattle in question are determined to be parasitized to start the grazing period. These younger animals will begin shedding worm eggs approximately 25–30 days after exposure and, therefore, two treatments are recommended given four weeks apart beginning 4 weeks after grazing begins. The second treatment (given four weeks after the first treatment), means these cattle will not be shedding parasitic worm eggs for another 4 weeks for a combination of 12 weeks with no eggs shed during for the first 12 weeks of the grazing period. This recommended interval for small ruminants is only 3 weeks (see Chapter 7).

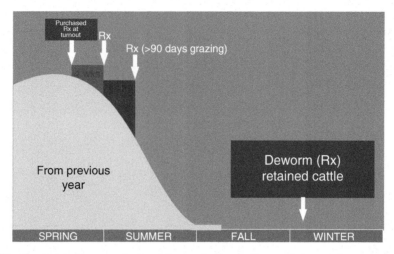

FIGURE 1.45 Graph showing strategic timed deworming in yearling cattle (two spring treatments given four weeks apart).

THE INGESTION AND INFECTIVE PREPATENT PERIOD

It is the time from when infective larvae are ingested until they have developed into mature egg-laying adult worms. Ingested infective *Ostertagia* larvae, for example, lose their protective covering in the first stomach (rumen) and then move down to the abomasum where they penetrate and encyst themselves in an existing gastric gland. The L_3 larva moves into the gland and then begins development into the fourth stage (L_4) in the gland in approximately four to five days. A mucus plug covers the opening of the gland and the larva begins to destroy the gland by stopping stomach acid (HCL) production. Usually by the end of the second week of infection, the larva has molted into an early fifth-stage larva (L_5), also categorized as a young or early adult worm (see Figure 1.46).

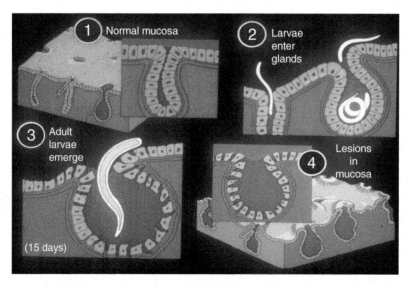

FIGURE 1.46 Exsheath L_3 larvae penetrating gastric glands and developing to a late L_4-stage larvae when it remerges on to the surface of the abomasum.

If conditions are right in the gut track, a few days following this molt, these worms then emerge, forcing their way out of the gland onto the surface of the gastric mucosa where they attach to the wall of the abomasum, mature, mate, and begin to reproduce eggs which pass down the gastrointestinal tract into the environment where the development process begins again. This prepatent period is influenced by the immune state of the infected animal and the pH level of the abomasal fluid. For young cattle, the prepatent period is usually three weeks, whereas for mature cattle, it often takes four to five weeks before an egg-laying adult worm develops and eggs appear in their feces following ingestion of infective larvae.

THE INHIBITION OR ARRESTED DEVELOPMENT PHASE

It is the period when arrested development or the inhibition of larval development can occur. During this period of time which occurs soon after infection, the developing larva stops the maturation process and becomes dormant for an extended period of time. The reemergence of these larvae usually occurs during a period when parasitism is not expected to be a problem just after prolonged drought period or during the middle of a winter season. For the northern half of the United States and Canada, the best time to check fecals for parasite eggs in horses and small ruminants is in late March or April just prior to the beginning of the grazing season. It is not uncommon to find very high eggs at this time of the year despite having been treated in late fall. The reason for this is that heavily infected animals coming into the fall and early winter period are carrying heavy worm burdens and often high levels of inhibited larvae in the abomasal glands. As the animals go into the winter period, they are no longer ingesting infective larvae and as the old worms die off, the condition of the gut improves thus communicating to the inhibited larvae that conditions are conducive for redevelopment. Of course, as the inhibited larvae begin to maturate, it is just the right time to begin seeding the spring pasture with a new crop of parasite eggs (see Figure 1.47).

Inhibition is a phenomenon that reportedly can occur in most parasites but is most common with the Brown Stomach Worm (*Ostertagia*) in cattle, the Small Strongyles (Cyathostomins) in equine, and the barber's pole worm (*Haemonchus*) in small ruminants. Inhibition appears to be a somewhat continual process that only occurs starting when worm burdens are at their highest point. There are numerous reports, however, when animals are reportedly dying from parasitism in March when it seems least highly unlikely since the pastures are dormant. The reason is that

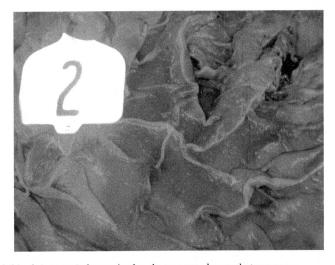

FIGURE 1.47   Inhibited *Ostertagia* larvae in the abomasum observed at necropsy.

in many cases, the inhibited larvae all maturate at the same time causing clinical disease. This is called Type II disease.

Considerable controversy exists among scientists on why and how inhibition occurs. Data from Louisiana indicate that inhibition in the south begins in May whereas northern inhibition occurs later in August much like the European model [11]. Necropsy shows that when some larvae are simply slow to develop where other larvae turn into a state of complete inhibition. (Necropsy shows that some larvae continue to slowly develop in the adult stage while other larvae remain in a state of complete inhibition.) These inhibited larvae usually stay in an inhibited state until winter time when transmission stops, the gut begins to improve and then these inhibited larvae begin to return to normal and emerge into the gut tract. The same phenomenon occurs in the southern United States but triggered by drought conditions rather than winter conditions (see Figure 1.48). As parasite burdens build in the gut, the physiology of the abomasum changes. As more and more gastric glands are invaded by newly ingested and acid production stops, the pH in the gut starts to rise. The ideal pH at the surface of the abomasum is between a pH 2 and pH 3. As the abomasum pH rises too high, an increasing number of gastric glands are shut down, digestion slows and eventually stops altogether, and the animal dies.

If a developing larva in the gland realizes that the condition of the gut is no longer conducive for development (as the pH raises in the lumen of the abomasa), the larva stops developing and undergoes arrested development and becomes inhibited. Once the conditions of the abomasa improve, development resumes. It is not in the best interest for the parasitized animals to die because they also die. Inhibition is therefore a protective mechanism to prevent overwhelming their host. Two key periods cause a redevelopment of these larvae: a prolonged drought and natural winter conditions. So, as cattle undergo a severe drought or winter condition, they are no longer exposed to infective larvae. As winter or drought conditions persist, the old worms gradually die off and conditions in the gut improve, triggering the inhibited larvae to begin maturation again.

The inhibited or arrested state of developing larvae occurs when the invading larvae stop development in the host animal and remain in a stage of arrested development only to begin development later in the year such as during the middle of winter when external conditions are better. The cattle parasite that is most well known for becoming inhibited is *Ostertagia* (also known as the Brown Stomach worm); however, *Haemonchus* (also known as the barber's pole worm) for sheep and goats and small strongyles in horses undergo an inhibited period in their development from

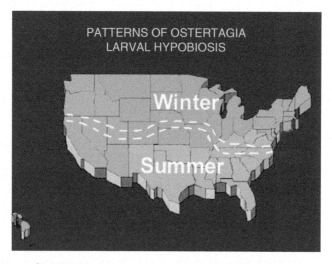

FIGURE 1.48   Patterns of inhibited larvae, northern versus southern climate.

infective larvae to an egg-laying adult parasite. This inhibition state occurs primarily in weaned calves and yearling cattle. Inhibition is almost always found later in the season starting mostly in mid-summer lasting until the end of the season.

The speed with which larvae develop in the gastric glands and emerge into the abomasum as an early adult worm varies from 10 days to 6 months depending upon the level of worm burden present and conditions of the gastrointestinal tract at the time of larval ingestion. The triggering mechanism that tells the inhibited larva is the pH of the abomasum. If it is in the normal range of pH 2–pH 3, larval development is normal. During inhibition, infective exsheathed third-stage larvae move into the gastric glands and molt, but instead of continuing to develop, these early fourth-stage larvae remain in a dormant state. During this period of inhibition, larval metabolism is thought to be minimal. This phenomenon of arrested development is also referred to as hypobiosis and can last for several weeks or even months. These larvae often emerge at a time of the year when parasitism is not suspected such as during the winter.

The true cause for this inhibition is not fully known; however, it appears to be tied to total worm burden. When an animal becomes heavily infected, physiological conditions of the gastrointestinal tract changes making conditions such as high pH affecting conditions such that conditions are no longer right for larval development, and development stops following which new incoming larvae begin to undergo arrested development. As pasture conditions change such as during a pasture "brownout" caused by a hot dry summer or when cattle are removed from pasture during the winter, larval intake stops; as worms mature and older worms die off, the gastrointestinal conditions begin to improve. Previously inhibited larvae now begin to develop, emerge, and mature to adult egg-laying worms.

The buildup of parasitic infections on pasture probably accounts for most of the variations found as to when inhibition is reported to take place in different parts of the country. In southern regions of the country, inhibition is reportedly most common in late spring or early summer. The reason for this is that favorable grazing conditions develop early in the year and parasite larval development can begin as early as late February or early March in very southern regions. Pasture contamination, therefore, can occur as soon as late April or early May with inhibition occurring in late May through August. Under northern conditions where cattle may only begin to graze in May and early June, pasture buildup does not occur until late August or early September with inhibition occurring from September onward, which coincides with the northern inhibition period. A very important point to consider when talking about pasture contamination is to keep in mind, the condition of the pasture in terms of rainfall (or irrigation) and stocking rate has more influence on parasite population and reinfection rate for the animals grazing that pasture than geographical location of the pasture (see Figures 1.49 and 1.50).

The normal process is for these inhibited larvae to emerge slowly over a long period of time; however, if the inhibited larvae in a heavily infected animal emerge all at once, disease characterized is broken down into two separate types: Type I and Type II disease.

Type I disease is caused by a heavy infection during the grazing season for horses, cattle, sheep, and goats. This disease outbreak is defined as parasitic gastroenteritis, which is caused by a heavy infection of adult worms and is easily diagnosed since it occurs during the middle of grazing season. Type I disease is a due to a buildup of larval contamination on the pasture and occurs in late spring/early summer in southern regions of the country and in mid to late summer in the more temperate regions of the country. Type I disease is most common in non-treated, heavily infected, poorly managed animals on a low plane of nutrition. Often, only several animals out of a group will first show symptoms for Type I disease. With sheep and goats, Type I disease usually occurs where the stocking rate is high and parasite contamination becomes overwhelming for the animals. Fecal worm egg counts are a great indicator whether parasite worm burdens are reaching a clinical threshold (see Figure 1.51).

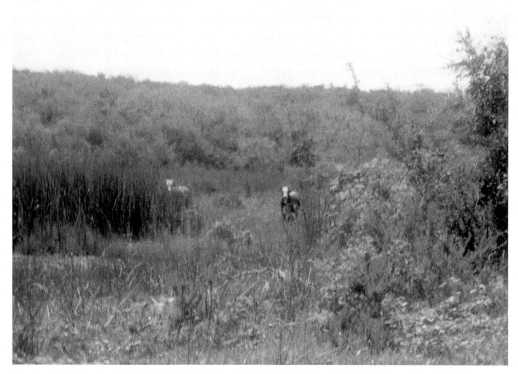

FIGURE 1.49   Low stocking rate (in West Texas) means less parasite exposure.

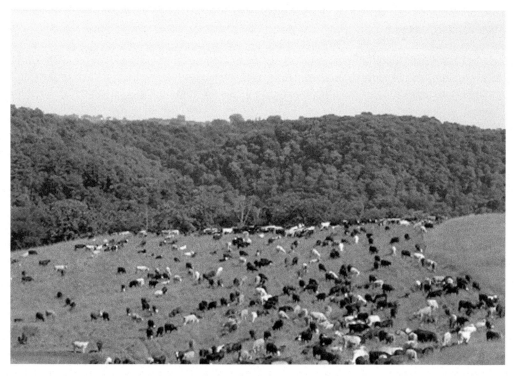

FIGURE 1.50   High grazing density in rotational grazing setup.

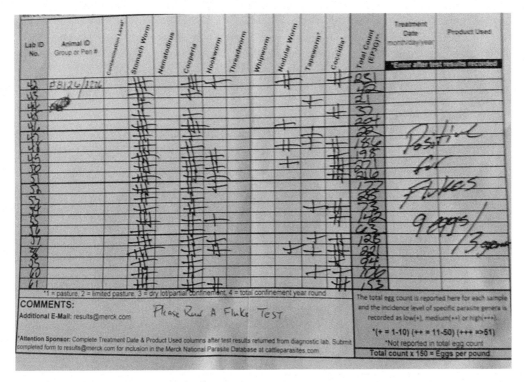

FIGURE 1.51   Texas cattle showing high worm egg counts.

Type II disease may occur when most unexpected, even several months after the animals have been removed from pasture and is caused by a large number of inhibited larvae emerging into the lumen of the gut at the same time. Type II disease can also occur in the south during hot dry summers when contamination of the pastures are low parasite transmission due to poor grass or "brown out" conditions. The mechanism, which causes this sudden emergence of larvae, is not fully understood but is often associated with poor nutrition or other stress-related conditions. Type II disease, therefore, usually occurs either in the middle of the winter when animals are housed in crowded conditions being fed poor quality of hay and feed or during the summer during "brown out" conditions in Southern United States.

The inhibited phase is a survival mechanism that gastrointestinal parasites have to help maintain a continued life process, enabling parasites to survive unfavorable pasture or weather conditions. It also helps parasite survival by preventing the parasites from overwhelming and killing the host. When an animal becomes heavily infected, if some of the infecting larvae stop development and remain inhibited, both the parasite and its host have a better chance for long-term survival. Some veterinary parasitologists have compared this inhibition mechanism to the diapause phenomenon in insects which works like a biological clock, which programs the larvae to cease development until a more favorable environment is present.

THE PATENT PERIOD

It is the survival and reproduction time of adult worms (both female and male worms are required) in its host animal. This the reproductive phase of parasitism. Each female worm can lay thousands of eggs during her adult life, which may be as short as a few weeks and as long as several years. Some parasites such as *Trichuris* have been reported to live in an animal for several years. Basically, the entire infection process is a dynamic process where larvae are constantly being ingested as old parasites are dying off and passing out in the feces. Winter or dormant pastures change this process when new larval ingestion slows down or stops; this is the time of the year when inhibited larvae begin development and emerge, keeping the parasite life cycle going.

Worm egg shedding can vary from animal to animal. Equine seem to mix their manure better internally, so repeated worm egg counts from one animal is often very similar, whereas with cattle you can take five divots from the same paddock and get five different answers. Multiple fecals are often required to get a reliable result; therefore, 5–10% of each animal grouping should be random sampled. Biostatisticians tell us 20 samples are the maximum number of samples needed regardless the size of the group sample [14].

The patent period is the period when the worm parasites lay eggs and the fecal count becomes positive and then the first question is how many eggs do I need to find to make treatment worthwhile? From a parasitologist standpoint, this can be frustrating or it can be the golden moment when people begin to understand the economics of parasitism.

How do all the different gastrointestinal parasites ensure survival? Parasites survive by contaminating the environment of the host animal to ensure propagation of their species. Mostly, all animal species are infected by more than one species of parasite at any given time. In grazing cattle, it is very common to find eight or nine different species present upon necropsy. Monospecific infections are rare and usually only seen with young animals infected with what is called "barnyard infections." Most problematic parasites such a *Haemonchus* in goats or small strongyles in horses survive because of the high degree of fecundity by these parasites and their ability to lay thousands of eggs keeping the environment of these animals heavily contaminated, especially in late summer.

It is not uncommon for equine to shed over 500,000 eggs per animal per day back in their environment. There are parasites, like the whipworm, which are noted for being low-egg shedding parasites, however, because their eggs can survive in the environment for many years and they too have very good survivability of their species. The whipworm larvae remain protected in the egg shell until it is eaten or the infective larvae is released from the shell. Each parasite seems to have found its niche in being able to survive. Another factor that helps survivability is the ability of these parasitic larvae to accumulate or buildup in the animal's environment over a summer grazing season.

During the parasite life cycle, pastures are contaminated by infective larvae, which develop from worm eggs passed in the feces of infected cattle. This is a very important part of the transmission cycle. Worm eggs must hatch and develop into infective larvae for this parasite cycle to continue. Worm eggs need favorable weather conditions to develop. Ideal conditions are plenty of moisture and warm temperatures. When these conditions are present, worm eggs can develop into infective larvae in just a few days. If the temperatures are cool, it will take longer for development to occur; it may take weeks or even months for the development to take place. If the temperatures are too cold, the development process stops altogether. Since a female worm can lay thousands of eggs in its lifetime, and the parasite's life cycle in a young calf can take as little as three weeks for infective larvae to develop into an egg-laying adult parasite, one worm and her progeny can produce several million eggs over a summer grazing season. So, if only a few worms survive the winter or a dry period, the pastures can still become heavily contaminated in a very short period of time.

Factors that affect the level of pasture contamination include:

1. The level of worm egg excretion and total number of eggs passed in the manure.

2. The stocking rate or density of grazing animals. The more animals present, the greater possible number of eggs being shed on the pasture.

3. The survival rate of different worm eggs and hatched larvae.

4. The survival rate of infective larvae. Larvae that remain in the manure in late fall have the greatest chance of surviving until the following spring.

5. Pasture management variations. Number of trees or shaded area of the pasture, whether or not harrowing of the pasture is practiced, and whether pastures are grazed down completely can all affect the infection rate.

6. Anthelmintic treatment, the brand of dewormer used, and time of treatment can all affect pasture contamination level or control thereof.

Most parasitic larvae can survive for one year on pasture. This means that parasite eggs shed in the spring can survive on pasture until the following spring. One parasite species, *Nematodirus*, has been reported to survive for several years under Canadian winter conditions. Parasitic larvae that survive the winter have a limited life, however, and will only survive for (at best) several months into the spring. Parasites that get caught on pasture herbage when severely cold or dry conditions develop soon die without moisture; those larvae in the pat and soil, however, usually have sufficient moisture to survive even under very dry or very cold conditions.

Worm egg development on the pastures follow a cyclic pattern with peak contamination rates occurring at various times of the years depending on the weather, the grazing pattern or pasture management used, and the type of animal grazing these pastures. Egg development in the spring is slow while the weather is cool, but as the temperature becomes warmer, the time for egg development decreases. In this way, a large number of worm eggs can reach maturation almost simultaneously, resulting in a large increase in pasture contamination. This sudden increase in pasture contamination is called "spring or mid-summer rise."

What is the meaning of positive fecal worm egg counts in beef cattle? The first step in conducting fecal worm egg counts is to determine the types and prevalence of various parasites in a particular area to help establish product and treatment times necessary. The first step in developing treatment strategies is to determine the presence of parasitism under natural field conditions.

A total of 17,973 non-treated cattle were examined using the "Modified Wisconsin Sugar Flotation Method" fecal exam from nearly 2000 cattle operations (see Figures 1.52–1.57). Results indicated the prevalence of a number of parasites such as tapeworm (*Moniezia*), *Nematodirus*, and whipworm (*Trichuris*) was considerably higher than expected. Results demonstrated that up to 71.4% of the operations with nursing/weaned calves were positive for *Nematodirus*. Feedlot

Prevalence of Parasites found in 5981 Non-Treated Beef Cows from 427 Beef Operations:

Parasites	Number of Farms	Number of Cattle	Percent of Farms Infected (%)
• All parasites	427	5981	N/A
• Stomach worms	377	3765	88.3
• *Nematodirus* spp.	47	101	11.0
• Threadworm	27	96	6.3
• *Cooperia* spp.	292	2178	68.4
• Hookworm	14	18	3.3
• Whipworm	10	22	2.3
• Nodular worm	104	361	24.4
• Tapeworm	135	274	31.6
• Coccidia	268	1674	68.4

FIGURE 1.52   Prevalence of gastrointestinal parasites in non-treated beef cows.

Prevalence of Gastrointestinal Parasites found in 1102 Non-Treated Nursing Calves from 101 Separate Midwest Ranch Operations:

Parasites	Number of Farms	Number of Cattle	Percent of Farms Infected (%)
All parasites	101	1102	N/A
Stomach worms	82	796	81.2
Nematodirus spp.	53	240	52.5
Threadworm	8	33	7.9
Cooperia spp.	72	625	71.3
Hookworm	0	0	0
Whipworm	12	45	11.9
Nodular worm	10	39	9.9
Tapeworm	34	129	33.7
Coccidia	72	535	76.3

FIGURE 1.53 Prevalence of gastrointestinal parasites in non-treated nursing calves.

Prevalence of Parasites found in 1,773 Non-Treated weaned "backgrounder" Calves on 105 Ranches:

Parasites	Number of Farms	Number of Cattle	Percent of Farms Infected (%)
All parasites	105	1773	N/A
Stomach worms	96	1292	91.4
Nematodirus spp.	75	479	71.4
Threadworm	13	71	11.9
Cooperia spp.	93	1245	88.6
Hookworm	6	8	5.7
Whipworm	31	77	29.5
Nodular worm	24	168	22.9
Tapeworm	54	215	54.4
Coccidia	87	986	82.9

FIGURE 1.54 Prevalence of gastrointestinal parasites in non-treated weaned calves.

cattle operations were 60.3% positive for *Nematodirus*, 22.2% positive for whipworms, and 47.6% were showing tapeworms. Many of the dewormers used today lack efficacy for parasites such as whipworms, *Nematodirus,* and tapeworms, so producers are actually selecting these parasites to become more prevalent and, of course, become more of an undetected economic problem.

The fecal worm egg count is really a predicable value because it determines what the future infection of the animals that are sampled is going to be. The following are the key points to the question on the true meaning of fecal worm egg counts in beef cattle:

1. The first step is to determine the shedding rate in terms of fecal worm egg output on a daily basis, for example, cows averaging 10 eggs/3 g sample × 150 1500 eggs/lb of manure × 60 lb per day equals = 90,000 eggs/day/cow.

2. The second step is to determine if the animal has been treated in the previous 14 days while on pasture to determine if dewormer last used was effective (positive worm egg counts should not be seen for at least 14 days following treatment in any aged animal). Also, if the animal is in confinement or is on a winter pasture since the last treatment, the previous treatment

Prevalence of Parasites found in 3447 Non-Treated Replacement Heifers and Stockers from 213 Operations:

Parasites	Number of Farms	Number of Cattle	Percent of Farms Infected (%)
All parasites	213	3447	N/A
Stomach worms	194	2633	91.1
Nematodirus spp.	90	459	42.3
Threadworm	18	39	8.5
Cooperia spp.	160	1902	75.1
Hookworm	11	40	5.2
Whipworm	31	88	14.6
Nodular worm	54	496	25.4
Tapeworm	72	269	33.8
Coccidia	160	1677	75.1

FIGURE 1.55   Prevalence of gastrointestinal parasites in non-treated yearling cattle and stockers.

Prevalence of Parasites found in 2835 Non-Treated Feeder Cattle from 126 Operations:

Parasites	Number of Farms	Number of Cattle	Percent of Farms Infected (%)
All parasites	126	2835	N/A
Stomach worms	122	2056	96.8
Nematodirus spp.	76	482	60.3
Threadworm	6	18	4.8
Cooperia spp.	119	2055	94.4
Hookworm	1	1	0.8
Whipworm	28	66	22.2
Nodular worm	27	167	21.4
Tapeworm	60	252	47.6
Coccidia	112	1589	88.9

FIGURE 1.56   Prevalence of gastrointestinal parasites in non-treated feedlot cattle.

still should be effective and fecal worm egg counts should remain negative until the treated animals are moved to an infective pasture.

3. The third step is evaluating the egg count based on the season of the year.
    A. **Wintertime:** There is no need for cattle to harbor parasites through the winter. The first reason is that winter often has the highest maintenance cost for cattle and so why have parasites increased this cost and, second, wormy cattle during the winter will shed eggs on the spring pasture re-establishing the infection level of this pasture.
    B. **Springtime:** Any shedding in the spring is bad because it re-established the infectivity of the pasture. The goal of strategic deworming is to keep the animals worm-free during the winter and the first six weeks of spring grazing. If the cattle are worm-free from Thanksgiving to 4 July, then they are basically free of parasite problems for the rest of the year.
    C. **Summertime or early fall:** There are no worries here because parasite level will be low if winter/spring control strategy is successful.

Combined Summary of Gastrointestinal Parasites Recovered from 17,973 Non-treated Midwestern Cattle – all age groups:

Parasites	Number of Farms	Number of Cattle	Percent of Farms Infected (%)
All parasites	969	17,973	N/A
Stomach worms	903	16,733	93.1
Nematodirus spp.	450	3177	46.4
Threadworm	93	336	9.5
Cooperia spp.	810	13,593	83.5
Hookworm	52	127	5.3
Whipworm	154	426	15.8
Nodular worm	289	2487	29.8
Tapeworm	450	1957	46.4
Coccidia	764	9929	78.8

FIGURE 1.57   Prevalence of gastrointestinal parasites – all age cattle summary.

1.   What category of animal is the count from: cows, calves, stockers, heifers, bull, or feeder cattle?

2.   What time of the year is it in terms of each season of the year: winter, spring, summer, or fall?

3.   Are the animals in confinement or on permanent pasture, do they go to mountain pasture, high desert pasture, an irrigated pasture, or are they rotationally grazed?

4.   When were the animals last treated?

5.   What product was used for the animals' last treatment?

See: Chapter 2 on strategic deworming strategies for beef cattle.

What is the meaning of positive fecal worm egg counts in dairy cattle? An important first question for dairy cattle is: are the milk cows, dry cows, replacement heifers, or calves on pasture or have exposure to pasture?

1.   Milk cows and heifers not on pasture for over six months do not need treatment.

2.   Positive Dry Cows should be treated prior to or at the time of freshening to reduce stress at calving and help keep cow in best shape for the start of producing milk.

3.   All positive calves and yearling cattle on pasture should be dewormed strategically.

4.   Baby calves of up to three to four months old should be checked for "barnyard infections."

5.   Milk cows with exposure to pasture should be checked annually during the first trimester to make sure parasites are now interfering with milk product and reproductive efficiency.

Parasites reduce dry matter intake and reduce gastric gland function, so any milk cows with positive counts should be treated during the first trimester of milk production.

See Chapter 3 for more information on deworming dairy cattle.

What is the meaning of fecal worm counts in horses? There is nothing good about gastrointestinal parasites in horses. Horse owners with small numbers of horses can eradicate parasites in their horse altogether. First of all, worm-free animals on worm-free pasture stay worm-free. Horses made worm-free are then brought on to a farm where horses have never resided will stay, that way providing no new horses are brought on to the location. Any horse leaving the property has a chance to bring parasites back to property. Routine fecal exam will prevent this from happening. Horses less than six months of age should be checked with a fecal exam and may need monthly treatment to remove any threadworm (*Strongyloides*), strongyles, or roundworms (*Parascaris*) if any of these worm eggs are found from a fecal examination.

See Chapter 4 for detailed information on deworming horses.

What is the meaning of fecal worm egg counts in swine? All sows should be worm-free at the time of or just prior to farrowing. Sows that are not worm-free at the time of farrowing will immediately infect their baby piglets. Purchased grower pigs should always receive a fecal worm egg count to make sure they are worm-free. A second fecal worm egg count should be conducted when the grower pigs are around 100 lb. Show pigs should be routinely checked because parasitized swine are harder to maintain good outward appearances for showing.

See Chapter 5 for more deworming information on parasite control in swine.

What is the meaning of fecal worm egg counts in small ruminants and hoofed wildlife? Small ruminants are relatively new to the deworming scene. Never move a parasitized animal. If you are buying or selling, always make sure a fecal worm egg count is conducted. Over the past 30 years, thousands of people bought "wormy" goats and brought them home to where goats have never lived and within 2 to 3 years, they have dead goats from heavy Haemonchus infections and now they are living with a nightmare of seasonal Haemonchosis but during the summer (Type I disease) and during winter early spring (Type II disease).

See Chapters 6 and 7 for more deworming information and deworming strategies for small ruminants and hoofed wildlife.

Summary on why gastrointestinal parasitism is so important for food animal production as well as for companion animals? A parasitized disease state can be a resultant condition occurring either from or during the establishment process of a parasitism. The condition may be prevalent whether the endpoint or the encounter results in rejection or death of the parasite or in the concession of accommodations to it by the host. The situation occurs where clinical detection is insufficient because it lacks the sensitivity to detect the existence of harmful parasitic infections unless this infection has progressed to the state where clinical signs are present. The parasite encounter, therefore, often remains undetected by humans unless a specific and sensitive laboratory test is available. In many cases the presence of parasitism means economic loss to a producer or owner, but in other cases where companion animals harbor parasites, the concern may strictly be due to the ability of the owner to know whether or not parasites are present and then being able to remove the parasites and improve the animal's health and well-being.

Parasitism can masquerade in many forms and cause extensive losses directly or indirectly. The extreme of parasitism may result in intestinal irritation with diarrhea, anemia, severe loss of general condition, and eventually death. Parasites have often been described as ubiquitous, unseen, and of great variety and abundance, and because of their effects are generally not apparent, they undermine the health of countless thousands of animals and a constant hazard to efficient profitable production for food animals. Parasites can cause damage to the animal and loss to their owner by:

1. Reduced yield and depreciation of animal products such as milk, eggs, hides, and wool.

2. Condemnation of animal parts such as liver, intestines used for casings, and meat carcass to federal meat inspections. Value of hides can also be reduced with cutouts due to parasite damage.

3. Waste of feeds, labor, and space to bring animals to mature productivity or market.

4. Interference with breeding, reduced reproduction efficiency, diminished fertility, reduced litter size, and lower egg-laying or poultry.

5. Reduced quality of animal – lower grades of market stock and reduced sale.

6. Lowered efficiency or work animals such as horses and mules. Reduced longevity in animals used for labor in third-world countries.

7. Depreciation of capital items – breeder animals, farm properties, and abandonment of properties. Cost of plowing down parasite-contaminated pastures and reseeding.

8. Inefficient utilization of pastures, barns, and pens by unproductive stock.

9. Lower resistance of infected stock to other diseases and parasites such as coccidiosis. Reduced efficiency of vaccines in heavily parasite-infected animals.

10. Death, suffering, and anxieties imposed on humans by parasites transmitted from domestic animals or by disease carried by parasite that are primarily animal rather than humans.

11. Reduced performance by "competition animals" such as race horses, hunters, jumpers, rodeo animals, and negative impact on physical appearance by show animals.

12. Expenditures for worthless or inefficient drugs, and related treatments and equipment. Cost of failure to control parasites because of using "dewormers" at the wrong time of the year.

13. Pain and suffering by the parasite-infected or parasite-infested animal themselves.

Animals suffer daily from parasites, especially by those parasites that infect the gastrointestinal tract that can only be controlled through treatment with an anthelmintic or dewormer. Oftentimes, the longer an animal goes untreated, the greater the infection becomes with increased pain and suffering.

The economic importance of parasitism is changing as animal production becomes more efficient due to continued improvements in genetics, nutrition, implant technologies, and disease control measures. A recent study from Iowa State University identified parasite control as the single-most import factor in producing beef efficiently. This study identified parasites as a primary detriment to efficient production and that gastrointestinal parasites are responsible for adding as much as $190.00 per animal to the cost of raising beef cattle from birth to slaughter. A second comprehensive study by Dr. Judith Capper was conducted on the environmental and economic impact of withdrawing parasite control (fenbendazole) from the US beef production. The summary study from published field studies reported 10% better pregnancy rates, 8.5% better weaning weights (+46.2 lb), 11.8% lower feed cost (−187 lb), 15.4% better land and water utilization, 17.1% less fossil fuel used, 13.3% less greenhouse gas emission, and an over 15.4% better land and water utilization [15, 16]. A third comprehensive study was conducted monitoring deworming treatments given to grazing cattle versus only treating cattle upon arrival in the feedyard. There was a clear statically significant advantage in deworming cattle on pasture versus only treating after arrival in the feedyard in terms of both better gain and feed efficiency but also in terms of significantly better health data (stronger immune function). The economics of parasitism calculated for this analysis came from the effects of parasitism upon reproductive efficiency, rate of gain, feed efficiency, carcass quality, milk production, and the immune system through reduced mortality and morbidity.

These measurable parameters most importantly do not consider the amount of pain and suffering that can take place within infected animals (which also goes unnoticed) during the early phase of infection. Parasite-infected animals are often seen standing around or lying down rather than up grazing, this is because they do not feel well even though the signs of an infection is not yet visible when looking at the physical condition of the animals in question. Leaving parasitized animals untreated or allowing them to become heavily infected before giving treatment can, therefore, sometimes become an issue of concern regarding animal welfare. The harmful effect on the animals themselves can be seen in the following photo (see Figure 1.58).

The parasite-infected cattle are on the greenest pastures showing less grazing due to appetite suppression caused by the parasites. The pastures grazed by the treated cattle are grazed down

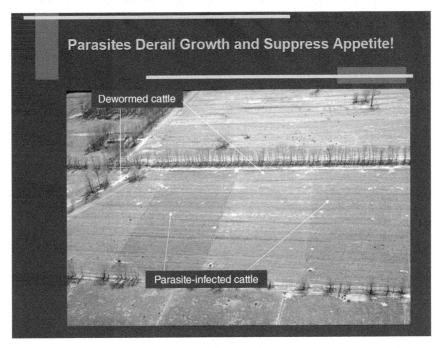

FIGURE 1.58   Pasture view showing the effect of parasites on appetite.
Source: Gasbarre [17] with permission from ELSEVIER.

because the cattle feel well and, therefore, are eating well. The cattle on the grazed pasture averaged +60 lb heavier than their herd mates grazing the parasitized pastures.

A popular theory prevailing in the United States is that treatment for parasites should only occur or be recommended for treatment after infections level reach a high point [18]. This is touted as a way to prevent parasite resistance from occurring. This theory is simply a theory not proven by research data of any kind, instead it is quickly seen as a very harmful theory for the animals themselves endure pain and suffering caused by the parasite before treatment is instituted. Parasitism is a process by which one organism invades and lives off another organism and thereby causes harm throughout this invasion process. The damage usually begins immediately upon contact with the parasite or parasitic stage that is involved with the invasion and continues throughout the life cycle of that organism. There is nothing good about parasites and the process of parasitisms, the animal under attack most often suffers damage long before the presence of the parasite is diagnosed.

Internal parasite can also adversely affect the immune system. Recent data indicate that gastrointestinal parasites have a strong effect on the animal's immune system [19–21]. One benefit to deworming that is often overlooked is its impact on the effectiveness of vaccinations. Cows that are infected by parasites have compromised immune systems caused by the negative nutritional impact gastrointestinal parasites have on the immune system. In addition to this indirect effect, some parasites have a direct effect on the immune system through mechanical damage they cause to the animal itself.

Immunosuppression occurs when parasites actively hinder one or more of the host's defense mechanism. Because the *Ostertagia* larvae damage the glands of the abomasum during the development, they disrupt metabolism and are thought to affect development of immunity simply by reducing the necessary substances such as protein and trace minerals. It has been shown that some parasites in cows create immune cells that shut down the production of antibodies and macrophages, key components in a functioning immune system. Such measures ensure that the parasite will survive and be able to reproduce in the cow. These immune-suppressive tactics that protect the parasite leave the cow susceptible to other invaders such as bacteria or viruses. As noted previously, immunosuppression interferes with the host's ability to respond to a vaccination, our most effective tool for preventing infectious diseases [19, 20].

Cooperia spp. has now become of one the most prevalent parasite species in US cow/calf operations as observed by our data (see Figures 1.52–1.57). This is at least in part due to the widespread use of endecticides that have minimal activity against these parasites. The effects of *Cooperia* spp. on cattle productivity has not been studied until recently [22]. This study demonstrated the *Cooperia* has a deleterious effect on both appetite and nutrient uptake or utilization. Mesenteric lymph nodes were increased in size and the small intestinal mucosa was thickened with an increased amount of mucus. The most prominent histological changes in the small intestine involved mild to moderate numbers of intraepithelial lymphocytes and globule leukocytes as well as aggregates of eosinophils within the lower lamina propria (see Figures 1.59 and 1.60).

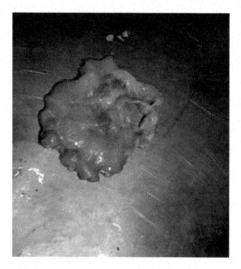

FIGURE 1.59 Normal small intestines from "parasite-free" calf.

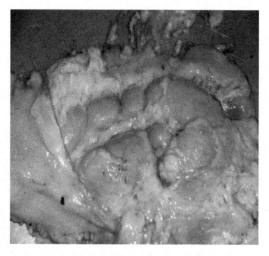

FIGURE 1.60 Enlarged lymph nodes in small intestine from artificially induced *Cooperia* infection in young calf.

What are the goals for parasite control? The monetary cost of parasite control depends upon the economic benefit achieved minus the cost of treatment. With pets and companion animals, swine, or cattle in total confinement and, in many cases, horses that are isolated from other horses, eradication of the parasites is possible. This eradication effort can be coupled with key strategies. Another area where eradication of parasites would be excellent is with the expansion of the goat market, producers that had never had goats on their operation before, have the opportunity to thoroughly deworm every animal before arrival, preventing these animals from contaminating the new place.

The eradication of parasites of grazing animals is not a practical proposition. Strategic deworming is designed to reduce parasite contamination throughout the grazing season. Fecal worm egg count monitoring is excellent here to help devise the correct treatment timing. Fecal checks during the winter months are an excellent time to make sure all animals are parasite-free. Fecal check during this spring is conducted to make sure animals are not shedding eggs during the early part of the grazing season. Fecal checks during the summer and fall are designed to provide information on whether the parasites are being controlled. A high worm egg count during this period indicates treatment failure and that a re-evaluation of what deworming product was used and when the treatment was given are both necessary.

Veterinarians routinely perform fecal examinations for cats and dogs but not for other species. Why not? Providing companion animal and food animal clients with up-to-date practical advice that will help them keep their animals healthy and improve the efficiency of their operations is the key to a successful practice. Conducting fecal examinations is a professional value-added service that provides scientific basis for diagnosis or treatment recommendations and can determine whether a particular treatment was successful. The service fecal exams provide separates the veterinarian advice from layman's suggestions. The veterinarian can help protect clients' profits and minimize their losses from parasite infections by building a long-term parasite-control strategy. An accurate and simple fecal examination(s) will help accomplish this goal.

Internal parasites are most small organisms that live, for at least part of their life, within a larger host animal, maintaining their survival at the expense of their host. Internal parasites have two main functions of life; one is to survive by finding and living off the host, while the second is to reproduce by excreting ova (eggs), cysts, oocysts, trophozoites, or larvae, which pass out of the host contaminating the host's environment which is necessary to sustain future generations of these parasites. Since detecting live parasites from within a host animal would require killing the host animal to recover and identify the parasites, the best way to detect parasitic infections is accomplished by finding eggs, oocysts, or larvae in the feces, urine, blood, or mucus of the infected animals. An adage that states "where there's smoke there's fire" is the same for internal parasites where it can be said that "when parasite eggs are found, adult parasites must be present."

What is the importance of parasite diagnosis? There are many reasons why providing an accurate parasite detection service has become very important to the veterinary field. One of the first reasons is that many of the pharmaceutical companies bringing new products or supporting existing products are spending millions of dollars on advertisements, thus creating an increased awareness to the producers or animal owners about the importance of controlling parasitic diseases. This awareness raises concerns by producers and pet owners about potential parasite problems in their animals and they are turning to the veterinary profession for help and advice. Secondly, the economic importance of treating internal parasites in domestic animals has gained increased emphasize in recent years as products to remove these infections have become highly efficient and the negative economic effects of parasitism has become more clearly established.

Improved production parameters through new technology for breeding, nutrition, and animal health presents a third reason for increased importance of accurate parasite detection. This increase in efficiency in animal production means that the need for parasite control also increases since parasitism is one of the greatest deterrents to efficient production. It often takes fewer parasites to cause a problem in a highly efficient animal than a poor performing animal. A good example of this is that a high-producing lactating cow exposed to just a few hundred infective *Ostertagia* larvae (which invade the gastric glands causing an increase in abomasal pH and decreasing digestion efficiency, producing a subsequent drop in dry matter intake) can experience plummeting milk production. Low-producing cows, on the other hand, can often carry relatively high levels of parasites before negative effects on production can be detected. One of the reasons for this is that poor producing cows often have management, nutritional, or health problems that mask the negative effects of parasitism.

More accurate diagnosis leads to healthier animals: A more recent reason that parasite diagnosis is gaining important is that over the past 25 years, internal parasites have been shown to affect a multitude of economic parameters in domestic livestock, but now new data regarding the effect of parasites on the immune system show an even stronger effect than previously thought. These data demonstrate that parasites can cause a suppression of the immune system negatively affecting an animal's ability to fight off other diseases. Not only do the animals suffer directly from the presence of parasitic infections but also these infections allow other disease problems to become more significant. Having the ability to accurately diagnose the presence of parasitic infections is, therefore, very important to the overall health of an animal.

Parasite diagnosis and control are also a very important part of animal health because nearly all animals encounter parasites sometime in their life. Although parasite exposure is highly variable, depending upon environmental contamination, many of these animals are exposed to high levels of parasitism at various periods throughout their lives. Often, the types of parasites and the level of parasitic infections that develop vary with the age of the animal and are influenced by the animal's immune system, the environmental and management conditions they are raised under, and the level of parasite contamination present in the animal's environment. Parasite exposure can also be influenced by many other factors, including housing or pasture conditions, contamination history, stocking rate or degree of animal concentration, individual animal behavior activities, and weather. The failure to detect the presence of parasitism, whenever it occurs in an animal's life, can have serious economic ramifications on production parameters or serious emotional importance for those animals raised as pets or with other special attachment.

Parasite resistance found in cattle, equine, and small ruminants throughout the world increases the need for better diagnosis: Overall, probably the most important reason for providing sensitive and accurate testing for parasites by veterinary clinics all across the country is that parasite resistance has now become a widespread problem in nearly all species of animals. Knowing whether or not treatment is successful can only be done through post-treatment monitoring. Parasite resistance to dewormers has been known to occur in equine and small ruminants (sheep and goats) for several decades, but during the past few years it has now become a widespread problem in cattle. Monitoring treatment to ensure success can be worth millions of dollars to producers and animal owners throughout the United States. Identifying treatment failures allows follow-up treatments before the resistant population can propagate and cause serious problems [19–21]. Fecal worm egg reduction tests conducted over the past 20 years show widespread resistance (efficacy less than 90%) for macrocyclic lactone pour-ons and injectible products while the efficacy of multi-formulations of fenbendazole have to maintain a high level of efficacy during the same period of time (see Figures 1.61 and 1.62). The combination or concomitant use of macrocyclic lactone pour-ons and injectables with fenbendazole, on the other hand, have demonstrated a high efficacy value for this combination use (see Figure 1.63).

Diagnoses for liver flukes: There are two different types of liver flukes of veterinary importance that can infect cattle in the United States. These flukes are *Fasciola hepatica*, the common liver (bile duct) fluke of cattle and *Fascioloides magna*, the giant deer liver fluke. Both flukes are completely different from each other in terms of their distribution, their infection process, diagnosis, and economic importance. *Fasciola hepatica* is endemic, mostly only in coastal areas of the country, but

Trial Summary for Fecal Egg Count Reduction Tests Reported on the Merck National Data Base Conducted with FDA Approved Macrocyclic Lactone Products (Updated May, 2021).

Products	No. of Trials	No. of Samples	Egg Counts/3 g*		Percent Efficacy (%)
			Pre-Rx	Post-Rx	
Injections					
Ivomec® Inj.	25	1352	70.1	37.1	47.0
Ivomec® Plus	17	823	102.6	55.7	45.7
Dectomax® Inj.	44	1791	64.1	15.4	76.0
Cydectin Inj.	12	614	36.9	5.3	85.7
Ivermectin Inj.	13	630	90.0	45.6	48.3
Ivermectin Plus	5	193	97.5	48.6	50.1
Inj. summary:	116	5403	76.8	34.6	54.9
Pour-ons					
Ivomec® PO	21	823	61.8	27.0	56.3
Ivermectin PO	81	3378	62.6	29.2	53.4
Dectomax® PO	23	941	67.9	23.7	65.1
Cydectin® PO	25	1044	60.9	14.5	76.1
Eprinex®	5	224	38.1	25.8	32.2
PO summary	155	6410	58.3	24.0	58.8
Overall summary:	271	11,813	68.4	29.8	56.4

* All samples taken at Rx and again 2 weeks post-RX.

FIGURE 1.61   Trial summary for fecal egg count reduction tests for macrocyclic lactone pour-on and injectable products.

Trial Summary for Fecal Egg Count Reduction Test Reported on the Merck National Data Base Conducted with Various Formulations of fenbendazole (Safe-Guard® and Panacur® – Merck Animal Health).

Product	No. of Trials	No. of Samples	Egg Counts/3 g*		Percent Efficacy (%)
			Pre-Rx	Post-Rx	
Panacur® Drench	32	1296	59.3	0.7	98.8
Safe-Guard® Drench	88	3694	62.1	0.8	98.7
Summary Drench	120	5110	60.7	0.8	98.7
Safe-Guard® feed	29	1459	51.6	0.1	99.1
Safe-Guard® 1.96%	19	803	38.6	0.7	98.1
Safe-Guard® mineral	16	620	30.7	1.1	96.2
Safe-Guard® paste					
Blocks, liquid feed	20	835	38.1	1.6	95.8
Overall summary:	175	7516	53.9	0.7	98.7

* All samples taken at Rx and again 2 wks post-Rx.

FIGURE 1.62   Fecal worm egg reduction test showing efficacy of multi-formulations of fenbendazole (Safe-Guard® or Panacur®).

Trial Summary for Fecal Egg Count Reduction Test Reported on the Merck National Data Base Conducted with Safe-Guard®/Panacur® in Combination with Various Endecticide Formulations (Updated May, 2021).

Combination Product	No. of Trials*	No. of Samples*	Egg Counts/3 g		Percent Efficacy (%)
			Pre-Rx	Post-Rx	
Safe-Guard/Panacur Drench plus:					
Ivomec® PO/Inj./Plus	21	805	79.4	0.4	99.4
Ivermectin PO/Inj.	34	1424	81.3	1.1	98.6
Dectomax® PO/Inj.	7	263	97.9	0.1	99.8
Cydectin® Inj.		1 41	134.2	0.7	99.4
Cydectin® Pour-on	11	447	64.0	0.2	99.7
Combination summary	74	2980	91.4	0.5	99.4

*Updated May, 2021.

FIGURE 1.63 Fecal worm egg reduction test showing efficacy for combination treatments*.

can be found in some limited river valleys away from the coast or on irrigated pastures. *Fascioloides magna* has a more widespread prevalence found throughout some 25 states (mostly in the midsection and upper Midwest region of the country), wherever the natural host, the white-tailed deer, are prolific. The deer fluke can be found in the upper Great Lakes region, lower Mississippi and Southern Atlantic seaboard, the Gulf Coast, the Rocky Mountain trench, and Northern Quebec and Labrador. Both flukes depend upon the distribution of an intermediate host, the lymnaeid snail, thereby limiting where enzootic areas are located. Even though fluke-infected animals are often moved throughout the country, these infections will not propagate unless the intermediate host snails are present.

The amount of economic loss caused by liver flukes in cattle is not well defined because infections are seldom uniform throughout a herd and the level of infection (number of flukes) in a particular animal cannot be quantified. Conducting fecal fluke egg counts is time consuming, and even if eggs are found, there is no way to know how many animals in a particular group are infected unless all animals are tested and the level of infection is impossible to know without necropsy. Even though damage by liver flukes cannot be accurately quantified, the fact that these flukes invade and live in a vital organ, their overall importance is seldom questioned by the veterinary practitioner. The questions for most producers are "How do I know whether flukes present in my herd, and, if so, which type of flukes do my cattle have, what are the economic consequences, how do I control these flukes and is treatment economically justified?"

Recent pharmaceutical advertisements indicate that the common fluke, *F. hepatica*, is spreading across the United States and has become a problem everywhere; however, there are no published documentation indicating that this is occurring [23]. Several USDA reports on liver condemnations indicate an increase in livers being condemned since 1973, a time when no approved products were available to flukes, but do not indicate whether this increase is normal due to weather fluctuations, better inspection techniques, or due to ineffective treatment. Technical experts (from a corporate sponsor) on a recent TV show told a producer from Minnesota and one from Virginia that treating cattle for flukes in their area was very important, however, they forgot to tell the callers that the liver flukes found in Minnesota and Virginia are almost exclusively deer flukes (*F. magna*) and that their product was not approved for use to control this parasite.

I. *Fasciola hepatica*, the common liver fluke of cattle is found mainly in Florida, Louisiana, the gulf coast of Texas, parts of California, Hawaii, the coastal Pacific Northwest, and some river valleys and irrigated pasture in the Northwest as far east as Montana (see Figure 1.64). Although this fluke can infect some wildlife species such as deer and small ruminants such

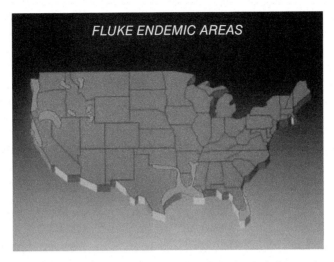

FIGURE 1.64   Map showing prevalence of the common liver fluke (*Fasciola hepatica*).

as sheep and goats, cattle are the main host and continued environmental contamination by cattle is required to perpetuate the infection.

A. **Life cycle:** Adult *F. hepatica* lives in the bile ducts of the liver and eggs are passed through the bile into the feces and back into the environment. When these eggs are deposited in warm moist environment, they hatch and develop into free-swimming organisms (miracidium) which invade a particular type of snail (*Lymnaea*) for further development. Once infected snails shed a tadpole-like organism (cercaria) which then migrates onto green plants where they form a protective cyst (metacercaria) and are con-sumed by grazing animals. Pastures showing ideal conditions for liver flukes survival on pastures requires moisture for a large part of the season (see Figure 1.65). The cysts will

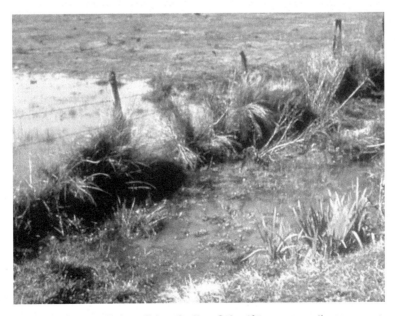

FIGURE 1.65   Pasture showing ideal conditions for liver flukes if *Lymnaea* snails are present.

die off after the water recedes and hot dry summer conditions arrive since these cysts are very susceptible to dry conditions. Snails survive cold winters or hot dry periods by burying themselves in the mud and waiting until favorable conditions return. Infected snails often release the cercaria in the spring when they emerge from the mud as temperatures begin to warm up and spring rains bring moisture which helps the infection process. Moving fluke-infected cattle to feedlots or areas of the country where lymnaeid snails are not present to complete the life cycle does not spread the infection. The yearly transmission cycle for *F. hepatic* on pastures is shown in Figure 1.66.

B. **Ecological requirements:** High rainfall areas, irrigation, or wet lands are required for fluke transmission and for the survivability of the intermediate snail host. Light loam or sandy soil is not conducive for snail survivability: therefore, the presence of liver flukes in Gulf States like Mississippi and Alabama is limited or nonexistent. Also, snails cannot survive in acid soils such as peat soil but prefer neutral, well-buffered heavy clay soils such as those found in Louisiana. Snails survive in shallow depressions in fields, springs, seeps, and slough that hold water over 180 days per year. Sustained heat and summer droughts end infection season.

C. **Prevalence:** Prevalence is relative low nationwide according to surveys conducted with feedlot cattle demonstrating a 5% condemnation rate throughout the United States [24, 25]. Surveys conducted with beef cattle operations demonstrated 19.2% (range 5.9–52.7%) prevalence in fluke endemic states as listed above but a much lower rate when prevalence is calculated with states where *F. hepatica* numbers are low or nonexistent [4]. The number of flukes per infected liver was not determined in this study. Recent advertisements indicate liver fluke prevalence is on the rise, spread by moving hay from infested to un-infested areas, but this claim is not substantiated and highly unlikely since metacercaria are killed during the drying process. Furthermore, if this statement is true, it would indicate that current approved products despite extensive use are not sufficiently effective to impact the prevalence of this parasite.

D. **Economics:** The economic threshold of liver fluke infections in terms of fluke burden and stage of infection from the common fluke has not been established. One study indicated economic loss occurred in cattle when a mean fluke count of 60.3 flukes per liver

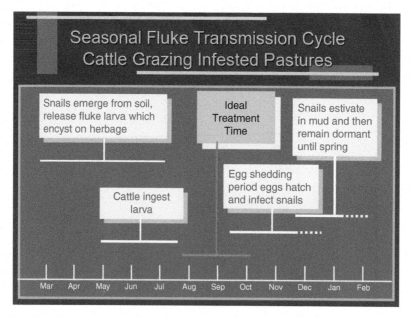

FIGURE 1.66   Fluke (*Fasciola hepatica*) yearly transmission cycle on pasture.

was found while clinical conditions developed when a mean fluke count of 171.2 flukes per liver was found [23]. The problem is that it is impossible to determine when fluke numbers are high enough to be a problem. In feedlots, the success from treatment for flukes in arrival cattle is confounded both by the age of the flukes upon arrival and recovery time of the liver following treatment even if treatment is successful. If the flukes are immature when treatment is given, these flukes will be missed by treatment and continue to develop and livers will be condemned at slaughter. Even if all flukes are killed, but the animals are sent to slaughter before livers have regenerated from previous fluke damage, the livers will be condemned despite treatment. In both cases, the economic loss due to liver condemnation is equal.

A study conducted at Louisiana State University with fluke-infected feedlot calves comparing albendazole (Valbazen®-Pfizer) and thiabendazole demonstrated better gains for albendazole [26]. The study was somewhat compromised because albendazole is a more efficient dewormer than thiabendazole as well as demonstrating some fluke efficacy. Two further studies conducted in 2001 and 2002 showed no benefit in treating flukes with ivermectin plus clorsulon @ 2 mg/kg (Ivomec® Plus – Merial) while using a full dose of clorsulon @ 7 mg/kg (Curatrem® – Merial), an economic benefit was realized [27, 28]. In the first study, young calves exposed to liver fluke-infested pastures gained significantly better when treated with doramectin injectable (Dectomax® – Pfizer) compared to a combination of ivermectin and clorsulon @ 2 mg/kg (Ivomec Plus-Merial). In the second (four-year) study, body condition score, weight gain, and pregnancy rates for heifers grazing fluke-infested pastures treated for gastrointestinal nematodes alone (injectable endecticide), flukes alone (clorsulon @ 7 mg/kg), both nematodes (injectable endecticide) and flukes (clorsulon @ 7 mg/kg) versus non-treated controls demonstrated significant improvement for those heifers treated with full-dose clorsulon (7 mg/kg) plus endecticide versus endecticide alone. Heifers treated for flukes alone did not have significantly higher pregnancy rate than untreated control heifers or heifers treated only for gastrointestinal nematodes.

E. **Diagnosis:** Finding *F. hepatica* eggs in fecal samples. Checking manure samples for *F. hepatica* eggs is just an extension of the Modified Wisconsin Sugar Flotation method. The residue in the bottom of centrifuge tube contains fluke eggs if any are present. To find any fluke eggs that are present, simply mix the residue with tap water and pour through the Fluke Finder and any fluke egg present will be on the final screen (see Figure 1.67).

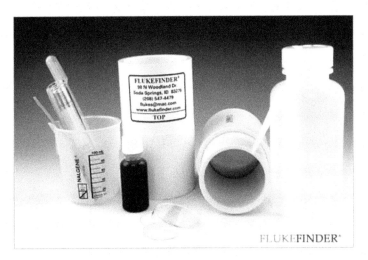

FIGURE 1.67   Commercial Fluke Finder with filtration device.
Source: FLUKEFINDER.

These eggs are identified (see Figures 1.68 and 1.69), counted, and reported as the number of fluke eggs present in a 3 g sample (see Chapter 2).

F. **Treatment:** For successful treatment of *F. hepatica* in endemic areas of the country, the flukes need to be sufficiently developed for the clorsulon (at 7 mg/kg) to work (>56 days old); therefore, strategic treatment for flukes should be given as soon as a majority of the invading flukes are sufficiently mature to be killed by the flukicide of choice, but before the flukes are mature enough to begin laying eggs back onto the pasture. With albendazole or ivermectin plus clorsulon (at 2 mg/kg), the flukes need to be mature (>90 days old) for treatment to be effective. Freedom of Information (FOI) studies indicated that in 100% of the studies reported, fluke eggs were found following treatment with albendazole. Since mature flukes are laying eggs back into the environment, treatment with these two products need to be given later in the year and most likely will not prevent pasture recontamination. Most transmission takes place in the spring when moisture

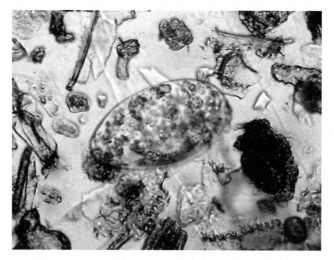

FIGURE 1.68   Fluke (*Fasciola hepatica*) egg found in fecal sample (40×).

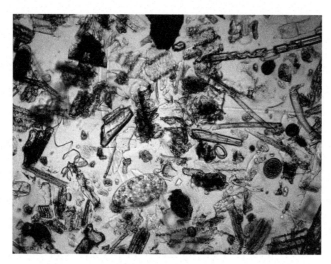

FIGURE 1.69   Fluke (*Fasciola hepatica*) egg found in fecal sample (10×).

levels are at the highest and before temperatures turn hot; so, in southern coastal states where flukes are present, depending upon spring moisture, flukes can mature by early to late July whereas in the Pacific Northwest, maturity usually takes place later. Most producers, however, apply fluke treatment in late fall or early winter after pasture recontamination has already taken place.

Fluke treatment for the common fluke, *F. hepatica*, is best applied where the infection occurs on pasture. Clorsulon (at 7 mg/kg) is currently the only effective treatment based on production trials. Ivermectin plus clorsulon (at 2 mg/kg) was shown to be no more effective than doramectin alone with fluke-infected animals [28]. Ideal treatment should be given to herds with greater than 25% prevalence levels and with greater than 40 flukes per animal. Treatment timing should occur just prior to maturation of the migrating fluke to adults.

Treatment for flukes in the feedlot is difficult because it is nearly impossible to know which cattle need treatment because flukes may not be mature. Also, cattle coming from fluke endemic parts of the country may not have sufficient level of infection to warrant treatment. Some of these cattle may have already received fluke treatment. Treating cattle upon arrival in the feedlot is usually too late to prevent damage to the livers and production loss in the animals since the flukes were consumed on the pasture and most likely the flukes have already completed the migration phase by the time the cattle arrive in the feedlot. Also, treating cattle for flukes on arrival in the feedlot does not prevent liver damage unless treatment is effective against all stages of the parasite [28, 29].

II. *Fascioloides magna*, the liver fluke of deer which can infect cattle and other domestic species such as sheep and goats. Deer are the natural host for this parasite. The flukes are flat, elongated worms found while slicing the liver usually surrounded by a fibrous capsule.

    A. **Prevalence:** *Fascioloides magna* occurs throughout the United States, but is mostly found in the Great Lakes area where deer populations are high and the necessary snail intermediate host is present to keep the infections going. In cattle, the encapsulation prevents eggs from escaping in the liver and therefore fecal checks for deer fluke eggs is not possible.

    B. **Economics:** There are no economic data demonstrating losses in cattle due to the deer fluke other than the cost of liver condemnation at slaughter. A field study reported from the Michigan State University Veterinary Extension under the Michigan Beef Improvement program demonstrates excellent slaughter results in heifer calves born and raised in Northern Michigan with nearly 100% of the livers infested with *F. magna* liver flukes [30]. It is assumed that liver damage in cattle has to be extensive (>90%) before clinical disease is observed. This parasite, however, is lethal in sheep and goats since the parasite is not encapsulated and continues migration through the liver until the organ is destroyed and the animal succumbs.

    C. **Treatment:** There is no approved treatment for *F. magna* in deer or cattle. High doses of albendazole and clorsulon showed some activity but albendazole levels (20–46 mg/kg) necessary for even marginal efficacy were dangerously close to lethal levels (>4.5 times recommended dose).

        Treatment for the deer fluke, *F. magna*, in cattle is currently not available and based on recent production studies probably unwarranted [29]. Limiting cattle's access to wet areas of a pasture by fencing off the creeks and areas where standing water may be present for a major portion of the summer may be the only way help reduce exposure to the deer fluke.

Dung beetles: Many of the anthelmintics (dewormers) on the market today may have a negative impact on dung beetles. The residue of a number of anthelmintic products passed in fecal material following treatment have been shown to have an impact on the natural development of parasite fauna in the fecal pats excreted by cattle. This impact may range from destroying fly larvae and the development of these flies to the inhibition of eggs and larval stages of the dung beetle. Most experts agree that the destruction of fly larvae is a good thing; however, the destruction of the eggs or development stages of the dung beetle may not be as universally acceptable for a number of reasons outlined below [31, 32].

The anthelmintic products that have been determined to have a detrimental effect on the dung beetle fauna are ivermectin, doramectin, and eprinomectin [33]. No differences were observed between the injection and pour-on formulations [31]. These avermectins showed larval mortality, mortality of immature adults, and reduced egg production for periods up to one month following treatment. In experiments performed under temperate and tropical conditions, the aging of the dung pat did not lead to significant lowering of the concentrations of ivermectin [32]. There are approximately six months of the year when treatment of cattle with avermectins would affect mortality of newly emerged dung beetles and three months of the year when avermectin would affect dung beetle oviposition or larval survival [34–36].

Fenbendazole, albendazole, and moxidectin have shown no effect on the dung beetle or its offspring [33, 37]. Even when fenbendazole was administered in a sustained release bolus, no detrimental effect on dung beetles was observed. At 42-days post-treatment, the solid matter of the control and fenbendazole-containing cow pats were reduced to crumbling, granular texture, while the cow pats from the ivermectin-treated animals were solid and compacted.

The dung beetle (see Figure 1.70) has been identified as environmental aid for the degradation of the fecal pat, which provides the re-fertilization of the pastures and aids in the natural destruction of infective parasitic larvae. Recent research has demonstrated that the dung beetle is

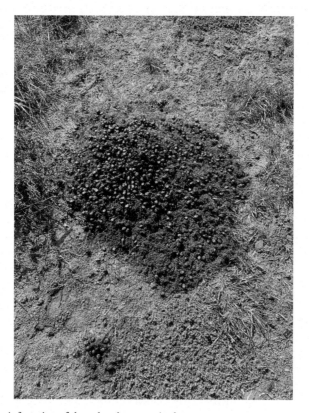

FIGURE 1.70 Heavy infestation of dung beetles on a single manure pat.

responsible for the natural destruction of infective larvae present in the fecal pat (see Figures 1.71 and 1.72), which develop from eggs passed from animals infected with gastrointestinal parasites. It is easy to spot pastures where ivermectin products have be administered to animals and intact fecal pats are visible. This is especially true of horse pastures found throughout the United States

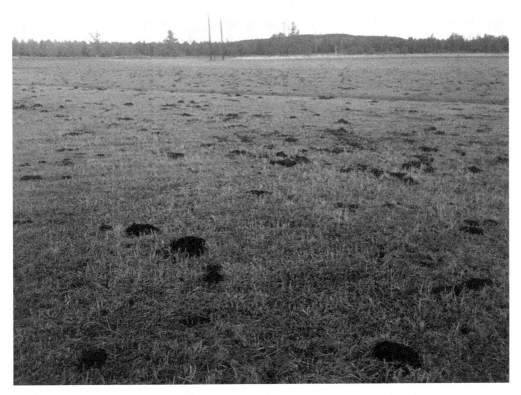

FIGURE 1.71   Intact manure pats seen in Oregon.

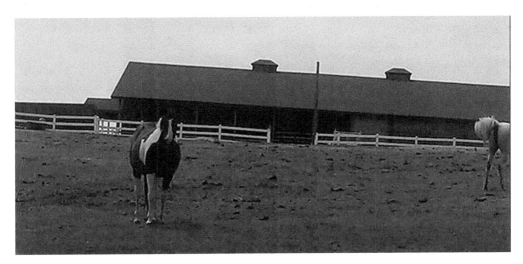

FIGURE 1.72   Intact manure pats on horse pasture in Wisconsin.

(see Figure 1.73). A number of studies have indicated that dung beetles naturally destroy from 60% to 80% of these larvae in any given fecal pat (see Figure 1.74). This may turn out to be an extremely important event that researchers have only just discovered since destruction of the dung beetle could lead to higher levels of parasite contamination on pastures grazed by avermectin-treated cattle [34, 37, 38].

Veterinary clinics are often involved in many situations where the early detection of potential parasite problems allows the clinics to alter or adjust their recommendations to prevent or otherwise curtail the development of a problem in the animals being treated. The degree of science that accurate parasite diagnosis by a veterinary clinic provides is hard to quantify but by simply having the knowledge and ability to detect certain parasites, these clinics can often prevent a high level of economic loss or unnecessary suffering to their clients' animals.

Books on clinical parasitology written for veterinarians describing the biology and treatment of parasites are numerous; however, a book specifically written for veterinarian technicians containing up-to-date information describing the newest and best techniques leading to the diagnosis of both clinical and subclinical parasitic infections is lacking. Such a book for veterinary

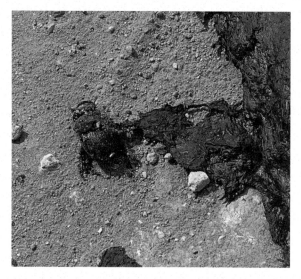

FIGURE 1.73   Fresh fecal pat in West Texas with active dung beetles.

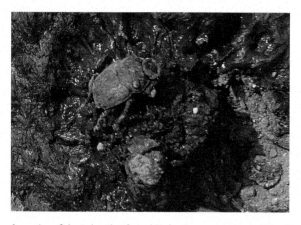

FIGURE 1.74   A second species of dung beetles found in fresh manure pat in West Texas.

technicians is especially important to help livestock producers strive for maximum efficiency for their animals and informed pet owners strive to protect their animals from as many harmful parasites as possible. Furthermore, many of these harmful parasitic infections require highly sensitive laboratory diagnosis in order to detect their existence. The goal of this book on parasitology, written for veterinary technicians, is to ensure veterinary clinics all across the country have the best, most sensitive, and specific laboratory tests to detect both clinical and subclinical economically important parasitism when and wherever they occur in both domestic animals and wildlife. We want to provide the best science available for veterinary clinics and veterinary diagnostic laboratories to help diagnose and treat parasitisms.

In summary, gastrointestinal parasites include a wide range of economically important organisms that infect nearly all domestic animals and wildlife sometime in their life. These parasites develop natural infections in animals depending upon environmental contamination causing anywhere from minor to major health problems which can even lead to death by the host animal if the infection becomes overwhelming. One of the keys to successful treatment is early detection; however, when the parasites exist in a subclinical state, detection can be a significant problem and economic losses or physical suffering can occur without the knowledge of its owner or the producer raising the infected animals. Veterinarians play a key role in diagnosing and prescribing treatment to control or prevent damage caused by these organisms. The first step in this process, however, is for veterinary technicians to know and have available the best and most sensitive technique in order to find and identify these organisms so proper treatment can be prescribed by the attending veterinarian.

REFERENCES

1. Drudge, J.L. and Lyons, E.T. (1986). *Internal Parasites of Equids with Emphasis on Treatment and Control.* Hoechst-Roussel Agri-Vet Company.

2. Bliss, D.H. and Kvasnicka, W.G. (1997). The fecal exam: a missing link in food animal practice. *Compendium Cont. Ed. Pract. Vet.* 4: 104–109.

3. Bliss, D.H. and Todd, A.C. (1977). Milk losses in dairy cows after exposure to infective trichostrongylid larvae. *Vet. Med. Small Anim. Clin.* 72 (10): 1612–1617.

4. Hoover, R.C., Lincoln, S.D., Newby, T.J., and Bliss, D.H. (1984). Controlling parasitic gastroenteritis in pastured cattle. *Vet. Med.* 79: 1082–1086.

5. Lawrence, J.D. and Ibarburu, M.A. (2007). Economic analysis of pharmaceutical technologies in modern beef production. *2007 Conference on Applied Commodity Analysis, Forecasting and Market Risk Management.* Iowa State University.

6. Bungarner, S.C., Brauer, M.A., Corwin, R.M. et al. (1986). Strategic deworming for spring-calving beef cow/calf herds. *Am. J. Vet. Res.* 189: 427–431.

7. Stromberg, B.E., Vatthauer, R.J., Schlotthauer, J.C. et al. (1997). Production responses following strategic parasite control in beef cow/calf herd. *Vet. Parasitol.* 68: 315–322.

8. Smith, R.A., Rogers, K.C., Hausae, S. et al. (2000). Pasture deworming and (or) subsequent feedlot performance with fenbendazole. I. Effects on grazing performance, feedlot performance and carcass traits in yearling steers. *Bov. Pract.* 34: 104–144.

9. Bliss, D.H. and Newby, T.J. (1988). Efficacy of the morantel sustained-released bolus in grazing cattle in North America. *J. Am. Vet. Med. Assoc.* 192: 177–181.

10. Bliss, D.H., Jones, R.M., and Condor, D.R. (1982). Epidemiology and control of gastro-intestinal parasitism in lactating, grazing adult cows using a morantel sustained release bolus. *Vet. Rec.* 10: 141–144.

11. Bliss, D.H. (1988). *The Cattle Producer's Handbook for Strategic Parasite Control.* Somerville, NJ: Hoechst-Roussel Agri-Vet Co.

12. Williams, J.C., Loyacano, A.F., Broussard, S.D. et al. (1995). Efficacy of a spring strategic fenbendazole treatment program to reduce numbers of *Ostertagia ostertagi* inhibited larvae in beef stocker cattle. *Vet. Parasitol.* 59: 17–137.

13. Bliss, D.H., Campbell, J., Corwin, R.M. et al. (1993). Strategic deworming of cattle (part 1-3), roundtable discussion. *Agri-Practice* 14 (5): 34–41, (6) 32–37, (7) 18–27.

14. Ballweber, L.R., Gasbarre, L., Stromberg, B., et al. (2008). Parasitic gastrointestinal nematode control practices in the US cow/calf operations. Insights from the (USDA) National Animal Health Monitoring System (NAHMS).

15. Capper, J.L. (2012). Is the grass always greener? Comparing resource use and carbon footprints on conventional natural, grass-fed beef production systems. *Animals* 2: 127–143.

16. Capper, J.L. (2013). The economic impact of withdrawing parasite control (fenbendazole) from U.S. beef production. *ADSA-ASAS Joint Annual Meeting*, Indianapolis, IN.

17. Gasbarre, L.C. (1997). Effects of gastrointestinal nematode infection on the ruminant immune system. *Vet. Parasitol.* 72 (3–4): 327–337.

18. Newport, A. (2017). Five ideas for parasite refugia. *Beef Vet.* 4: 14–16.

19. Bliss, D.H., Moore, R.D., and Kvasnicka, W.G. (2008). Parasite resistance in US cattle. *Am. Assoc. Bov. Pract. Conf. Proc.* 41: 109–114.

20. Gasbarre, L.C., Smith, L.L., Lichtenfels, J.R., and Pilitt, P.A. (2009). The identification of cattle nematode parasites resistant to multiple classes of anthelmintics in a commercial cattle population in the US. *Vet. Parasitol.* 166 (3–4): 281–285.

21. Sonstegard, T.S. and Gasbarre, L.C. (2001). Genomic tools to improve parasite resistance. *Vet. Parasitol.* 101: 387–403.

22. Li, R.W. and Gasbarre, L.C. (2008). A temporal shift in regulatory networks and pathways in the bovine small intestine during *Cooperia oncophora* infection. *Int. J. Parasitol.* 29: 813–824.

23. Griffiths, H.J. (1961). Fascioloidiasis of cattle, sheep and deer in Northern Minnesota. *J. Am Vet. Med. Assoc.* 140: 342–347.

24. Marley, S.E., Corwin, R.M., and Hutcheson, D.P. (1996). Effect of *Fasciola hepatica* on productivity of beef steers from pasture through feedlot. *Agri-Practice* 17 (1): 18–23.

25. Foreyt, W.J. and Todd, A.C. (1976). Liver flukes in cattle: prevalence, distribution and experimental treatment. *Vet. Med. Small Anim. Clin.* 71: 816–822.

26. Loyacano, A.F., Malone, J.B., Pontiff, J., and Nipper, W.A. (1980). A new weapon against liver flukes. *Louisiana Agric.* 23: 22–23.

27. Loyacano, A.F., Skogerboe, T.L., Williams, J.C. et al. (2001). Effects of parenteral administration of doramectin or a combination of ivermectin and clorsulon on control of gastrointestinal nematode and liver fluke infections and on growth performance in cattle. *J. Am. Vet. Med. Assoc.* 218 (9): 1465–1468.

28. Loyacano, A.F., Williams, J.C., Gurie, J., and DeRose, A.A. (2002). Effect of gastrointestinal nematode and liver fluke infections on weight gain and reproductive performance of beef heifers. *Vet. Parasitol.* 107 (3): 227–234.

29. Marley, S.E., Corwin, R.M., and Hutcheson, D.P. (1996). Effects of *Fasciola hepatica* on productivity of beef steers from pasture through feedlot. *Agri-Practice* 17 (1): 18–12.

30. Johnson, E. (1991). Effects of liver flukes on feedlot performance. *Agri-Practice* 12: 33–36.

31. Flincher, G.T. (1981). The potential value of dung beetles in pasture ecosystems. *J. Ga. Entomol. Soc.* 16: 301–316.

32. Knutson, A. (2000). Dung beetles – biological control agents of horn flies. *Texas Biological Control News* (Winter). Texas Agricultural Extension Service, The Texas A & M University System.

33. Floate, K.D., Cotwell, D.C., and Fox, A.S. (2002). Reductions of non-pest insects in dung of cattle treated with endecticides: a comparisons of four products. *Bull. Entomol. Res.* 92: 471–481.

34. Wardhaugh, K. and Ridsill-Smith, T. (1998). Antiparasitic drugs, the livestock industry and dung beetles – a cause for concern? *Aust. Vet. J.* 76 (4): 259–261.

35. Sommer, C. and Steffansen, B. (1993). Changes with time after treatment in the concentrations of ivermectin in fresh cow dung and in cow pats aged in the field. *Vet. Parasitol.* 48 (1–4): 67–73.

36. Ridsill-Smith, T.J. (1993). Effects of avermectin residues in cattle dung on dung beetle (Coleoptera: Scarabaeidae) reproduction and survival. *Vet. Parasitol.* 48 (1–4): 127–136.

37. Strong, L., Wall, R., Woolford, A., and Djeddour, D. (1998). The effect of fecally excreted ivermectin and fenbendazole on the insect colonization of cattle dung following oral administration of sustained-release boluses. *Vet. Parasitol.* 62 (2–3): 253–266.

38. Wardhaugh, K.C., Longstaff, B.C., and Morton, R. (2001). A comparison of the development and survival of the dung beetle, *Onthophagus tarus* (Schreb.) when fed on the feces of cattle treated with pour-on formulations of eprinomectin or moxidectin. *Vet. Parasitol.* 99 (2): 155–168.

CHAPTER 2

The Modified Wisconsin Sugar Flotation Method

The "Modified Wisconsin Sugar Flotation Method" is an extremely valuable and successful scientific tool for veterinary medicine in determining the presence or absence of gastrointestinal parasitism in all animal species.

A fecal exam is the best nonintrusive way to detect internal parasitisms and can be an extremely valuable scientific tool in veterinary practice for all species of animals. The most accurate way to know how many parasites, the species of parasites, the stage of parasite development, and the sex of the parasites is to conduct a necropsy (see Figures 2.1 and 2.2), but since this is impossible because a necropsy is a dead-end proposition, the next best answer is to perform the most accurate fecal exam possible. Since gastrointestinal parasites live within their host, to propogate their species, they must pass their eggs or larvae via the feces back into the environment to create a new generation with a new infective-stage larval parasite (see Figure 2.3). This is where the fecal exam becomes important. The fecal pat contains a lot of valuable information for the owner/producer but these larvae or eggs have to be recovered in order to predict reinfection levels (see Figures 2.4 and 2.5). Since many fecal exam techniques exist, the one selected should be the best and the most

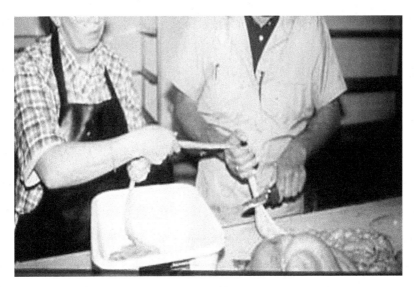

FIGURE 2.1   Animal necropsy is conducted to find and identify gastrointestinal parasites.

Large Animal Parasitology Procedures for Veterinary Technicians, First Edition. Donald H. Bliss.
© 2024 John Wiley & Sons, Inc. Published 2024 by John Wiley & Sons, Inc.

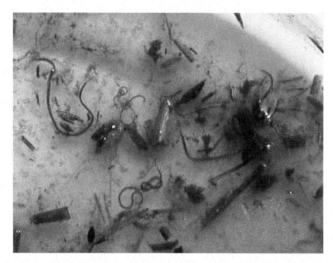

FIGURE 2.2 Worms found upon necropsy are identified to species, sex, age, and counted.

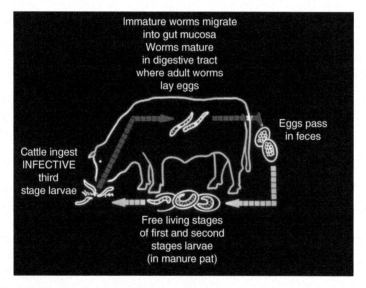

FIGURE 2.3 Typical *Trichostrongylus* parasite life cycle.

sensitive test available, otherwise, the exam may lead to erroneous, inaccurate, and possibly harmful conclusions. Telling a producer that their animals are "free of parasites" because the technique used was not sufficiently sensitive enough to detect the presence of an existing parasite or parasites, which is a serious mistake no veterinary practitioner wants to be responsible for. Suppose the parasite missed by the exam was deadly, such as whipworms (*Trichuris*) found in many animal species or threadworms (*Strongyloides*) often found to cause serious health problems in newborn calves or foals. While missing a pathogenic parasite can be a costly mistake for a pet owner, a similar situation also exists with livestock and wildlife, where costly production losses often occur daily when parasites go undetected.

For over 50 years, I have traveled all across North America conducting fecal worm egg counts at designated veterinary clinics and feed store for cattle, swine, equine, sheep, goats, and hoofed

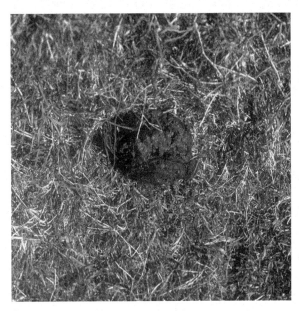

FIGURE 2.4   The fecal pat contains valuable information regarding parasite diagnosis.

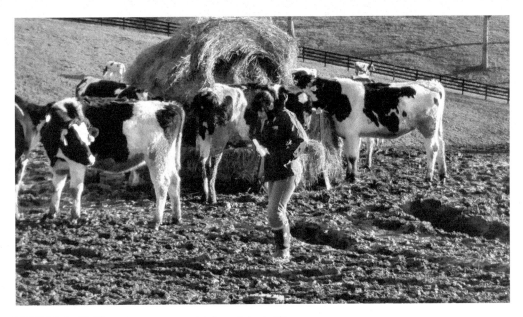

FIGURE 2.5   Picking up manure samples from dairy heifers.

wildlife inviting producers to bring fecal samples for parasite testing. Throughout these parasite evaluation clinics, I have personally have been told time and time again by producers that they thought their herd was parasite-free because samples they took to their veterinarian came back "free of parasites." Currently, many beef veterinarians use fecal examination techniques that are outdated or that were developed for small ruminants like sheep and goats (producing low fecal volume) and do not work with mature cows because of the large amount of feces produced daily. These techniques are also inaccurate with low worm egg-shedding parasites.

In the past, fecal examinations in food animal medicine were conducted only to determine the level of infection in a particular animal. These examinations, which followed outdated techniques, were unreliable. There are a number of commercial fecal exams sold to veterinary clinics involving no centrifugation recommendations but then also provide inaccurate results [1]. Using the wrong technique will lead to erroneous information, usually followed by an incorrect and flawed recommendation. This is especially true for cattle harboring subclinical levels of parasites. Even if the fecal examination is negative, the economic performance of the herd can be affected by undetected parasitisms if the fecal sample technique is inadequate. Most commercial techniques, fecal kits, and flotation solutions (see Figures 2.6 and 2.7) that are currently used were developed for use with sheep and goats for detecting the barber's pole worm (*Haemonchus contortus*) which is a high egg-shedding parasite in animals with low fecal output while missing low egg-shedding parasites like *Nematodirus*, nodular worm (*Oesophagostomum*), or whipworm (*Trichuris*). These techniques are also very inaccurate when used with cattle because cows have a very high output of fecal matter with normally low fecal worm egg output.

As a result, many food animal practitioners still regard the results obtained from fecal examination to be variable, controversial, and even inaccurate. Furthermore, many veterinary colleges still teach that fecal examinations are fundamentally of little importance to food animal practitioners. The reason the fecal is highly underutilized because there are many fecal exams being promoted that are inaccurate and provide erroneous information about the parasite status in all species. The goal of this publication is to demonstrate that by choosing the correct fecal exam which can be conducted easily and accurately, the clinic will benefit immensely from this new and powerful information. This fecal exam will provide the veterinary clinics with the science

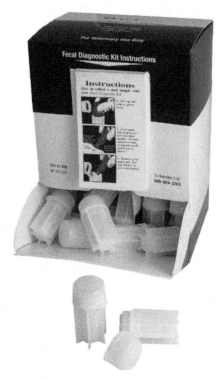

FIGURE 2.6   Fecalizer diagnostic kit sold to vet clinics.
Source: VetOne.

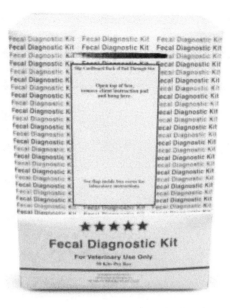

FIGURE 2.7   A generic fecal diagnostic kit for veterinarians.
Source: Petoly.

necessary to help make accurate deworming recommendations to all their clients for all species of animals. Conducting fecal exams is a professional value-added service for all clients.

Monitoring animals for parasites and instituting control strategies requires a basic knowledge of how the different types of parasitisms develop in the many different types of animal species a particular veterinary clinic may be exposed to. Dairy cows, for example, when kept in total confinement will have considerably less parasite exposure than animals which graze on permanent pastures. When the swine operations, in the mid-1990s, moved from family farms to large integrated totally confined systems, many of the common swine parasites disappeared. Swine lungworm (*Metastrongylus apri*), for example, requires the earthworm as an immediate host to survive and reproduce. Once hogs are moved indoors, this parasite, therefore, longer can be found. The only worm parasite in swine that has been shown to survive universally in confinement operations is primarily the large roundworm (*Ascaris suum*); occasionally threadworms (*Strongyloides ransomi*) and whipworm (*Trichuris suis*) will be found but usually only in old facilities. The nodular worm (*Oesophagostomum dentatum*) most commonly found in gestation sows and baby pigs are now only found in group gestation pens wherever bedding is routinely used. The swine kidney worm (*Stephanurus dentatus*), the lungworm (*M. apri*), and the thorny-headed worm (*Macracanthorhynchus hirudinaceus*) have all disappeared from swine held in confinement.

The same is true for pets such as dogs or cats living in a home with its owner since transmission seldom takes place inside the house. These animals have access to outside areas where parasite contamination and reinfection is possible. Sometimes, the only way pets become infected is through a play or exercise area such as a pen, yard, or kennel. The other possibility, of course, comes from when the owner takes their animals for a walk or to a pet park where other infected animals have contaminated the area when the wondering parasite-free animals get exposure.

When choosing fecal examination for the clinic, remember, the chosen fecal exam technique must be run properly and the samples examined must be collected, identified, and handled and (or) shipped correctly. Any deviation may make the entire process invalid. Samples that are not properly cooled, for example, will produce poor results because eggs can hatch and then will be missed. Also, for example, if the sugar solution is left open allowing evaporation to occur, which in turn, changes the specific gravity of the sugar solution, invalidating the results (see instructions for collecting, handling, and shipping samples later in this discussion).

The ideal fecal exam should have the following characteristics:

1. The test needs to be accurate with a high degree of sensitivity for use in animals producing large volume of manure such as horses, lactation dairy cows, adult beef cattle, and bison.

2. The test should produce consistent results with a high degree of repeatability.

3. The test should have of high degree of sensitivity such that negative results indicate the absence of adult parasites.

4. The test must also be sensitive enough to float all types of parasite eggs present even those with a high specific gravity like tapeworm (*Moniezia*) eggs or eggs from low shedding parasites such as whipworm (*Trichuris*) or the thread-necked worm (*Nematodirus* spp.).

5. The test should be easy to operate and inexpensive to run so that all producers can afford to have fecal worm counts conducted on their animals or groups of animals at routine intervals.

6. The test solution used should not distort the eggs or oocysts so they can easily and reliably be identified and enumerated.

The best overall fecal worm egg count test for all species that meet the above specifications is the Modified Wisconsin Sugar Flotation Technique [2]. The Modified Wisconsin Sugar Flotation Technique was first published in the Compendium entitled "The fecal Examination: A missing Link in Food Animal Practice." This test uses a 1.275 specific gravity sugar solution with a "horizontal swinging head" or free-swinging centrifuge technique. A comparison study conducted at the University of Wisconsin found that the Wisconsin Sugar Flotation Technique yields positive results for recovering worm eggs for 90% of a group of 270 dairy cows: the sodium nitrate method yielded positive for only 19% of these cows, while the McMaster's technique was positive for only 10% [1]. The Modified Wisconsin Sugar Flotation Method, therefore, has been shown to be excellent for use in all species providing the clinics with the single-most sensitive and accurate test for all clients. Other fecal exam techniques are discussed and specific tests for specific parasites will be explored later in this chapter.

The Modified Wisconsin Sugar Flotation Technique has been recommended by the World Association of Veterinary Parasitologists (WAAVP) [3] for conducting fecal worm egg count reduction tests to monitor anthelmintic resistance. Furthermore, the Modified Wisconsin Sugar Flotation Technique has also been extensively tested at Kansas State University (Dr. Dryden [4, 5]). The publication entitled "Comparison of common fecal techniques for the recovery of parasite eggs and oocysts" describes a number of critical issues that makes the Modified Wisconsin Sugar Flotation Technique better than all other tests examined.

The first key finding from Kansas State was that centrifugation consistently recovered more worm eggs than all other methods including direct smears or letting samples set for long periods of time. Second, the Sheather's sugar solution (specific gravity of 1.275) which is used as the flotation medium with the Modified Wisconsin Sugar Flotation Technique was equal to or better than magnesium sulfate, zinc sulfate, sodium nitrate, or saturated salt solution in both species of parasites recovered and in the total number of eggs found in the fecal material tested. A further benefit of the Sheather's solution used with the "Modified Wisconsin Sugar Flotation Method" is that the solution is neither hypotonic or hypertonic, so the eggs retain their shape and are not distorted due to the flotation media [6–8].

Several simple rules exist in fecal sample collection. Collecting samples rectally is the best way to get fresh samples, but working individual animals through a head gate or squeeze chute just to obtain individual fecal samples is time consuming, costly, and not very practical in most operations. The next best way of taking samples, therefore, are from animals observed in the act so the samples can immediately be collected off the ground. In pastured animals, especially open range country or large pastures, it is often possible to drive out to a group of resting animals and carefully get the animals up without spooking them, let them defecate, and then samples can readily be obtained off the ground.

Fecal collection is a simple process but it must be done correctly to ensure accurate results. Samples should be as fresh as possible. Ideally, samples should be collected immediately after expulsion. For pets and companion animals such as horses, take individual samples unless housed in large groups like rescue horses or racing dogs. For animals groups on pasture, it is best to get close without spooking the animals preferably when they are at rest, so one can get close to them by coming up slowly being careful not to spook the animals. As the animals get up, watch samples as they drop and identify whether it is a cow or calf sample for breeding animals or just random for all other uniform animal groups. Fecal sampling is basically a four-step process. Step one is to place an inverted sandwich bag over the hand (see Figure 2.8), Step 2 is to take a small golf ball sample from a freshly drop manure pat (see Figure 2.9), Step 3 is to reinvert the baggie (see Figure 2.10), and then the final step is to squeeze the air out of the baggie, seal and label the sample ready for the lab (see Figure 2.11).

Try to take samples equal to 5–10% representative samples but seldom more than 20 samples are needed for accurate results even for very large groups of animals. If a pasture, for example, has 50 cows and 50 calves present, a sample size of 4–5 cows and 4–5 calf samples would be an

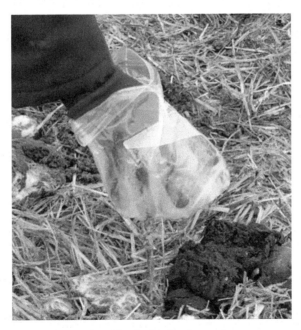

FIGURE 2.8   Step one – invert bag over hand for fecal collection.

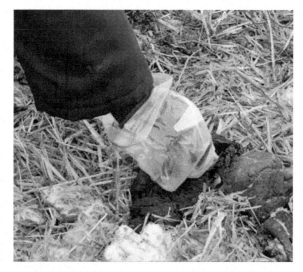

FIGURE 2.9   Step two – take golf ball-sized sample.

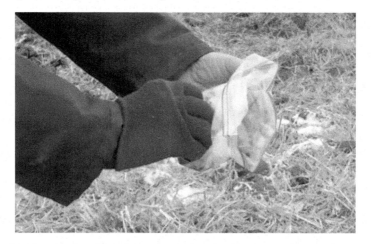

FIGURE 2.10   Step three – reinvert baggie.

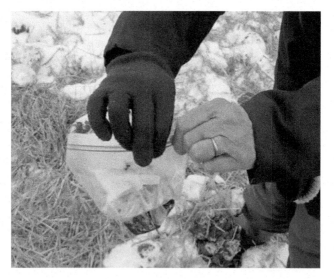

FIGURE 2.11   Step four – squeeze air out, seal baggies, and label.

accurate parasite assessment for that group. A golf ball-sized sample is the maximum amount of fecal matter needed for each sample with cattle, bison, swine, or horses. For all other groups like pets, poultry, small ruminants, and hoofed wildlife, a smaller sample size is good, but not less than three to five pellets or an approximate thimble-sized sample.

The sample should be fresh and then kept cool (refrigerated or kept on ice) until examined. When collecting samples from pastured animals, it is recommended to have an ice chest or cooler present in the vehicle so the samples can immediately be cooled until which time they can be run or placed in a refrigerator. The number one rule is that all samples should be collected fresh. Parasite eggs differ from different species, such that eggs of some species hatch faster than other species. Note: once the egg hatches in the manure, the worm egg can no longer be detected. Obviously, samples taken rectally will provide the most accurate results. In many cases, catching the animals to monitor fecals is not possible, so the next best technique is to quietly go among the animals to be tested and slowly get them up and move them so the defecate and fresh samples can easily be obtained.

Monitoring animals for fecal worm egg counts requires a plan. Identifying different species and their meaning to the host animals can be very important. Some parasites are very prolific and can lay thousands of eggs every day and can contaminate the environment of the host animals very rapidly and these parasites must be monitored regularly. An example is small strongyles in horses. It is not uncommon for a horse to be shedding 1000 eggs in 3 g samples which represents 15,000 eggs per pound of feces or 450,000 eggs per day if the animal excretes 30 pounds of fecal matter every day. Leaving this animal unprotected allows these parasites to contaminate the horses' environment very rapidly.

To conduct fecal exams to determine product efficacy, the American Association of Veterinary Parasitologists recommend a fecal exam to be taken on samples at the time or just prior to the time of treatment following a second treatment taken 2 weeks (14-days) following treatment. The process is called a Fecal Egg Count Reduction Test (FECRT). Samples should be taken from an individual animal or randomly from a representative number of animals in a group of animals all treated at the same time. For mass treatment in a herd or large group of animals, samples from at least 10% of the group or a total of 20 samples (with a large group <200 animals) is recommended [9].

In developing guidelines for parasite and monitoring schedule for a particular animal or group of animals, several key factors should be considered relating to the biology of most parasites. Parasites need warmth and moisture for worm eggs to hatch and the larval development to successfully reach an infective phase. So, although animals may carry parasites any time of the year, there are times of the year when parasite development is at its best and eggs shedding by the host should be at its lowest level in order to prevent a heavy reinfection pattern from developing. Another key time of the year in temperate parts of the United States is winter. Most often the reinfection of animals is at their lowest point during the winter; therefore, animals that are dewormed in late fall or early winter will stay worm-free until warm weather returns.

Samples are being sent in the mail or delivered to the lab as individual samples each placed in a small baggie, zipped locked bag, glove, or other small container marked as to animal identification or other identification such as animal group, pen, or location on the operation where sample was collected. Other information given is the farm or ranch name, location and address of the operation, and the date samples were collected. A return address, e-mail (carefully written or typed), or fax number is requested for returning lab results. All samples arriving at the lab are refrigerated upon arrival and remain refrigerated until process.

Collect fresh manure (golf ball-sized) from individual animals using an inverted resealable bag like a glove, reinvert, and then seal. Clearly identify each sample or group of samples if taken from more than one animal in a large number of animals is the same using a permanent marker. Samples should be cooled to refrigeration temperatures as soon after collection as possible. Samples can be refrigerated for several weeks if necessary. Heat causes worm eggs to develop and hatch, and freezing can destroy eggs. Take individual samples (do not composite sample).

Collect sufficient number of samples to profile herd (5–10% of each production class), i.e., take samples from adult cows, yearling cattle, replacement heifers, calves, and bulls. For dairies, take samples from different stages of lactation. For swine, take multiple samples from various age groups or pens. For horses, take individual sample. Label each sample with animal name or number, if samples are taken randomly; label age group of animals, pen, or pasture where samples were taken.

The Modified Wisconsin Sugar Flotation Fecal Exam is extremely accurate in detecting the presence or absence of parasitism in all animal species and can be used to predict the potential recontamination of the animals' environment whether it is a pasture, barnyard, pen, or yard. The fecal examination can also be useful in assessing an animal's or herd's response to treatment strategies. An excellent way to check and see if a dewormer is working properly for a particular location is to pull samples at the time of treatment and then again exactly two weeks later. Samples taken exactly two weeks after treatment give all dewormers plenty of time to remove the parasites (two weeks) but not enough time for a new patent infection to develop. To calculate percent reduction for any product in post-treatment samples, take the average number of eggs found in the pre-treatment sample and subtract the average number of eggs found in the post-treatment samples and then divide this result by the pre-treatment average to give an overall percent reduction. The results should demonstrate a 90% efficacy or better for the dewormer to be working properly. If the calculations fall below 90% efficacy, the dewormer used is showing parasite resistance. In conducting this test, if sample size is greater than 17, random samples can be examined to save time and labor. If the sample size is less than 17 head, collect from individual animals for the pre-treatment and post-treatment samples [9–11].

The first step is, of course, to have the best fecal exam possible while the second step is being able to interpret the exam results and subsequently be able to explain the results to the client. The Modified Wisconsin Sugar Flotation Technique when performed correctly provides three valuable answers for the client. The first is whether or not the samples being tested are free of worm eggs? Second, if positive, what type of parasite(s) is/are present? And third, what is the total daily worm egg output for the particular animal or animals being tested? While most people think the fecal worm egg count is indicator of how many worms are present in the animal being tested, but, of course, it does not tell how many worms are present, instead, it tells how many worm eggs are being shed in either a 1.0 g of 3.0 g samples depending upon species being tested.

The main question of how many worms are present in the animal being tested is the one mostly everyone misunderstands; there is a way, the following is an explanation of what the egg counts means. A fecal exam measures fecal worm egg output and determines environmental contamination [17]. It is a predictive value for future infections later in the year. Daily manure production by livestock was published by Statistics Canada on the "Geographical Profile of Manure Production in Canada" in 2006 [12]. Generally all types of cattle produced large amounts of manure: milk cows (136 lb/day); beef Bull (92 lb/day); beef cows (81 lb/day); steers (52 lb/day); heifers (52 lb/day); calves (26 kg/day); weaner pigs, sows, boars, and market hogs (2–9 lb/day); poultry (2 lb/day); horses (60–70 lb/day); lambs (2 lb/day); adult sheep (6 lb/day).

If a mature beef cow, for example, is shedding 10 eggs in a 3 g sample in early spring, we can multiply by 150 (454 g/lb) that means there are approximately 1500 eggs in one pound of manure shed by this cow. If this cow is producing 81 pounds of manure a day times 1500 equals 121,500 worm eggs being shed daily representing the daily contamination rate for just one animal on the pasture. This information is very valuable for the veterinarian because they can now match the count with the season to predict when is the best time to deworm for their client.

The math for a horse sample is the same as cattle, except it is not uncommon to find high counts in horses exceeding 500 strongyle eggs in a 3 g sample. A horse shedding 500 eggs in a 3 g sample, for example, translates into 75,000 eggs in one pound of manure, so on a daily basis this horse can excrete more than 4,500,000 eggs per day in 60 lb of manure excrete in one day on the pasture. One horse on one pasture can produce over 100-day period on one small pasture 4.5 million eggs per day, which translates into 400 million over a 100-day period on pasture. The only way to maintain a horse free from parasites is to prevent pasture buildup of larval contamination during the first two to three months of the season.

In the same calculations for small ruminants such as sheep, goats, alpaca, or hoofed wildlife, the math is different since the Modified Wisconsin Sugar Flotation Method uses only 1 g samples for these species. The reason for this is small ruminants produce smaller digested material such that these fine particles can make the sample hard to read; therefore, a smaller sample size is used for all small ruminants. Also, the fecal worm egg counts in small ruminants are much high than cattle due to low volume of fecal output and a reduced immune system against gastrointestinal parasites compared with cattle. This is especially true for goats since over the past thousands of years, they tend to be browsers; so, when they graze heavily contaminated pastures, it appears that their immunity against parasites are lower than, for example, cattle. Goat often develops very high worm egg counts. A fecal worm egg count for a goat with a worm egg count of 500 eggs/1 g samples when multiplied by 454 (grams per pound) shed 227,000 eggs per one pound of manure for a daily output of 5 lb of manure or 1,135,000 eggs per day for a single animal.

Fecal worm egg count, therefore, indicates first, whether or not worm eggs are present. If worm eggs present, the fecal worm egg counts determines what type of parasite(s) are present and, finally, the fecal exam provides an estimate of the daily fecal worm egg output of their animal(s) tested. This daily worm egg output provides an estimate of future contamination rates for the animal or groups of animals being tested. Of course, worm egg output alone does not tell the whole story. This answer is very complicated because there are a number of factors the veterinarian needs to consider first before answering the question. The first is what specie of animal is involved, because every animal species will have a different answer. The age of the animals is also important because a very young animal tends to suffer more from parasitisms than old more mature animals and have higher worm egg counts. And the third is what is the parasite specie or species involved in the worm egg count, since some species of parasite are higher egg shedders, than others. Another factor to consider is some parasites can cause damage in two ways, the first is direct, that is, how damaging is it to the host animal and the second is indirect, that is, how long does it live in the environment for reinfection (see individual chapters for specific recommendations).

1. **Winter-time:** The bovine veterinarian knows that wintertime provides the highest maintenance cost for cattle producers, so keeping brood cows worm-free during the winter reduces maintenance cost and keeps the cows in better body condition as calving begins. Second, if the cows are shedding worm eggs during the winter, they will immediately begin to contaminate the spring pastures as soon as the grass begins to green-up occurs. Winter-time is a great time to conduct fecals to make sure all animals are parasite-free during the winter months.

2. **Spring-time:** When conditions are right for grass growth, conditions are right for parasite development. Spring contamination determines the pasture contamination infection rate for the rest of the year [8]. Worm eggs that are deposited on the pasture in early spring have the propensity to live through the following spring. For spring-born calves, the new calves will readily become infected as soon as they are big enough to begin to graze the pasture. Another great time to conduct fecals to make sure all animals are parasite-free is during the first two to three months of the grazing season.

3. **Mid- to late-summer:** Deworming cows in the middle of the summer is most likely a waste of time, since the parasite contamination rate for the season is already developed and the contamination pattern of infection on the pasture has already been established, animals treated at this time will become reinfected immediately after treatment. The only time this is recommended if animals are clinically infected and, then in this case, the animals should be treated and removed from the pasture to a noninfected pasture or pen. During the summer months, the only time a fecal exam is useful is to check and see if the deworming program is working or if a client's animals are full of parasites and need help.

4. **Late-fall:** Fall deworming should be delayed until after a hard frost, since pasture contamination has already been established and treatment at this time is probably a waste of time and money for the operation since the animals in question will immediately begin reinfected as soon as they start to graze following treatment. If the treatment is delayed until a hard frost, the animal will stay parasite-free until the following spring as long as a highly effective (not parasite-resistance) dewormer is used. Another great time to check for parasites to access a client deworming program and get ready for a late-fall deworming (after a hard frost) and after the pastures are dormant for the winter. Late fall is also a great time to check if any animals going out on small grain pastures for the winter or corn stocks where reinfection will no longer occur.

Parasite evaluation clinics or designated fecal egg day or days set aside by the clinic for running fecals (see Figure 2.12). For the past 37 years, I have been conducting thousands of "Parasite Evaluation Clinics" all across the United States, Canada, and Mexico working with the

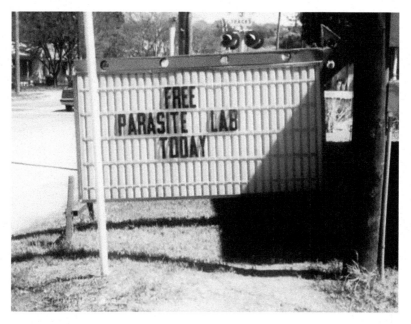

FIGURE 2.12   Free parasite testing – advertising clinic.

veterinary pharmaceutic industry, veterinary practices, feed dealer stores, and university ag extension offices (see Figures 2.13–2.21). The first clinic I conducted in Fredericksburg, Texas, working with the Hill Country Veterinary Clinic. Working with the clinic, we first set up a dinner meeting and invited producers from the area to attend a presentation on "strategic time deworming for beef cattle." At the end of the meeting, during a question and answering period, a producer announced

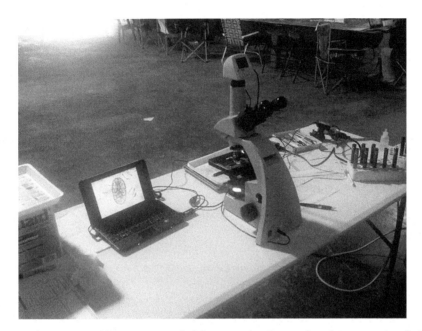

FIGURE 2.13   Microscope with camera, so technicians, veterinarians, and producers can view findings.

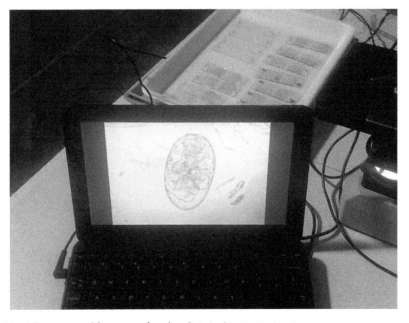

FIGURE 2.14   Microscope with camera showing *Ostertagia* egg on screen.

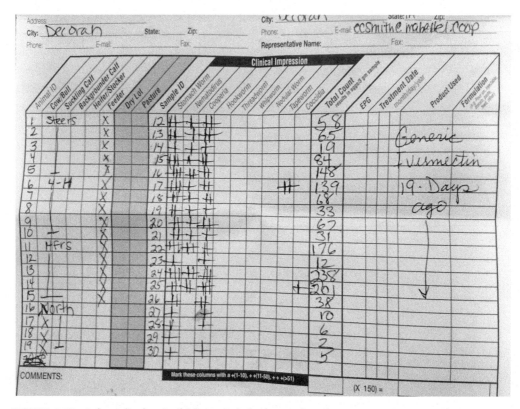

FIGURE 2.15 Lab results showing high counts in backgrounder calves.

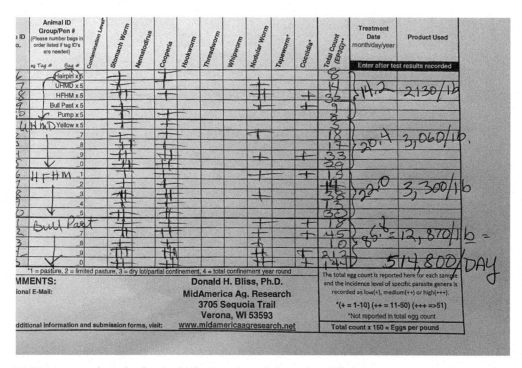

FIGURE 2.16 Lab results showing high counts in cattle located on different pastures.

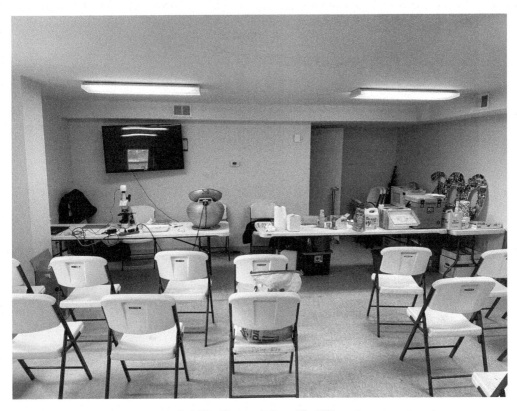

FIGURE 2.17   Parasite evaluation clinic (PEC) setup in Lowville, NY.

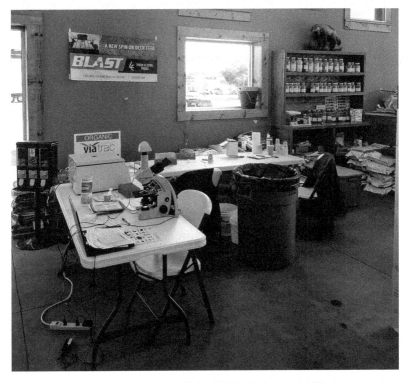

FIGURE 2.18   Parasite evaluation clinic setup with feed dealer in Southern Illinois.

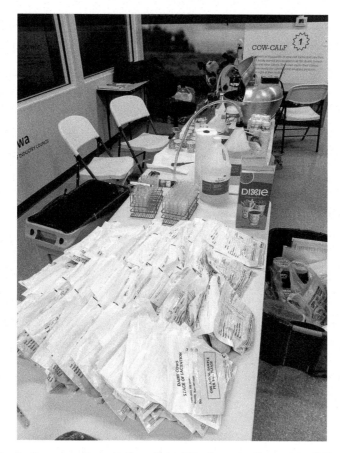

FIGURE 2.19 Conducting a parasite evaluation clinic at Northeastern Community College.

that he enjoyed our meeting but mentioned that we were talking to the wrong group of cattle producers because Texas A & M University School of Veterinary Medicine had recently published information that the beef cattle west of Interstate I35 were "parasite-free," especially those cattle from the Texas Hill Country around Fredericksburg. We then invited the producers attending the meeting to come back to the Hill Country Veterinary Clinic the following day with fresh fecal samples from their cattle herds and that we would run their samples free-of-charge and determine whether or not gastrointestinal parasites were present in their cattle (see Figure 2.22).

The following day we received a total of 195 samples that we evaluated for worm eggs conducting the "Modified Wisconsin Sugar Flotation Technique" and presented the producers with their results. One hundred percent of the samples were positive for parasite eggs with counts ranging from just a few eggs to over 500 worm eggs per samples following which the clinic sold over $25,000.00 worth of deworming products in the following 24-hour period.

I have now conducted thousands of "parasite evaluation clinics" over the past 38 years all across North America in every state except Alaska and all the southern providences of Canada including Prince Edward Island, Nova Scotia, New Brunswick, Quebec, Ontario, Manitoba, Saskatchewan, Alberta, and British Columbia. In Mexico, I have conducted parasite evaluation clinics in the states of Jalisco, Guanajuato, Hidalgo, Puebla, and Tabasco. Working with the Bank of Greece, I also helped conduct "parasite evaluation clinics" with working donkeys across a number of Greek islands and mountaintop villages in Mexico looking at the benefit of strategic

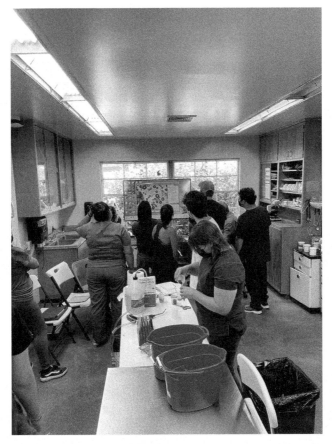

FIGURE 2.20   Vet Tech training (Cal Poly) on the "Modified Wisconsin Sugar Flotation Method."

deworming donkeys strategically on improved body condition scores and improved health of these working donkeys [13]. I also have spent a considerable amount of time setting up clinics working with Veterinary Tech schools and Veterinary Schools, training students on processing samples, reading samples, and interpreting results from samples conducted (see Figures 2.23–2.27).

The goal of these clinics has been to provide the producer a service and to raise awareness of parasitism as a production disease in cattle, buffalo, small ruminants, and equine. These clinics have also provided a service to veterinary clinics all across the country teaching their staff on how to use the "Modified Wisconsin Sugar Flotation Method" for conducting parasite exams and interpreting results for their producers.

As a further service, in 1985, I set up a veterinary parasitology laboratory to conduct mail-in fecals in Verona, Wisconsin, where producer all across the United States can mail in samples and test their animals for parasites at any time of the year. Over the past 38 years, I have personally read over a million fecal samples and our lab currently averages over 60,000 samples per year for all species (see Figures 2.28–2.30).

Many of the beef cattle sample results have been submitted to a national database which was established in 2000 and has been recently summarized for prevalence of parasite in each age group for non-treated cows, nursing calves, weaned calves, stockers, and feedlot cattle (see Chapter 3 for beef cattle).

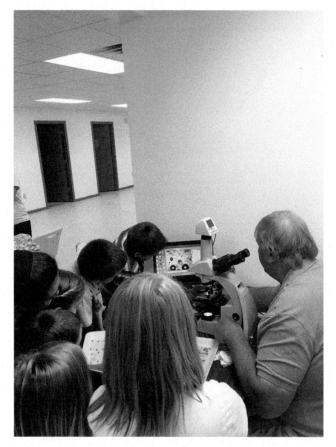

FIGURE 2.21   Young children looking at worm eggs on scope in Elma, Iowa.

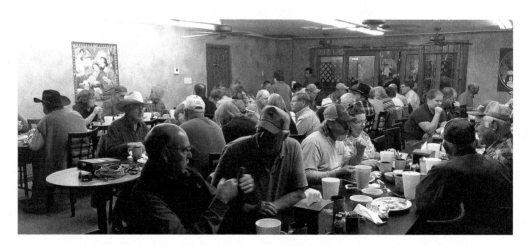

FIGURE 2.22   Dinner meeting for cattle producers in Victoria, Texas.

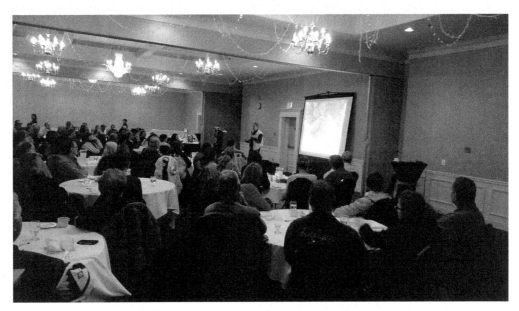

FIGURE 2.23   Cattle producer meeting discussing parasite control in South Texas.

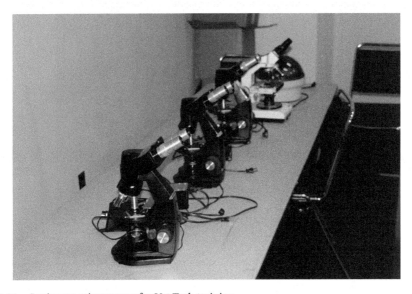

FIGURE 2.24   Setting up microscopes for Vet Tech training.

One of many deworming protocols developed for use in beef cows, is a unique protocol using strategically timed dewormings designed to reduce parasitism both in the animals themselves as well as in the animal's environment for an entire grazing season. Since beef cows are the main source of infection for calves, deworming the brood cow is necessary in order to reduce pasture contamination for their calves. The direct benefit to brood cows has been shown affecting many parameters (improved milk production, improved reproductive efficiency, better body condition scores, stronger immune system, lower over-wintering feed cost as well as improved weaning

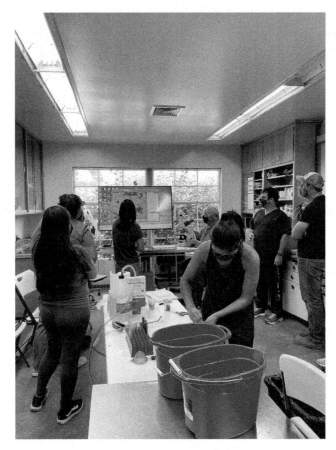

FIGURE 2.25 More Vet Tech training at Cal Poly San Louis Obispo, CA.

weights in their calves). This protocol has been tested under field conditions at a number of locations across the country.

The following specialized collection guidelines can be expanded to meet their clients' individual situation:

1. **Fecal exams for pets and companion animals:** Dogs and cats and other companion animals should be maintained as parasite-free as possible, especially those living in a home or in close contact with humans. Monitoring fecals can begin at a short interval equal to the shortest prepatent period for major parasites [16]. A sample taken 60–90 days following treatment will determine parasite pressure. If samples are positive 60 days following treatment, an aggressive treat and monitor program should be set up. If samples are negative 90 days following treatment, parasite pressure is probably low and a less aggressive deworming and monitoring scheme can be set up. Make sure the animals are negative for worm eggs during the winter months.

2. **Fecal exams for breeding, hunting, and sport dogs:** Animals held in kennels or outside dogs and cats should be dewormed regularly keeping in mind that some parasites such as *Ascaris* (roundworms) and whipworm eggs can live for years in the environment. Leaving these animals parasitized with these parasites can contaminate facilities for many years and make control very difficult. Keeping these animals' parasite-free will be more difficult; therefore, a routine deworming and monitoring schedule should be set up. If samples are routinely found to contain parasites, then the intensity of the program needs to be increased.

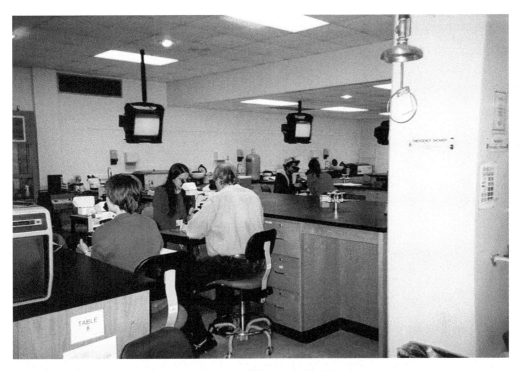

FIGURE 2.26   Microscope training at University of Wisconsin Vet School.

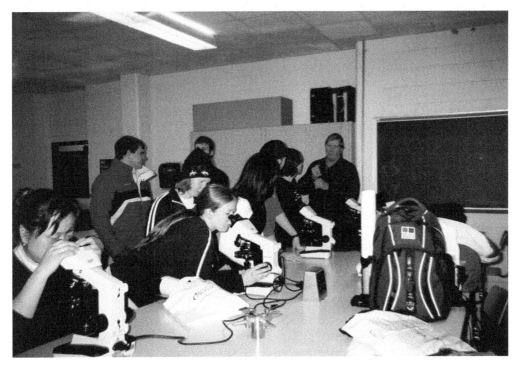

FIGURE 2.27   Microscope training at University of Minnesota Vet School.

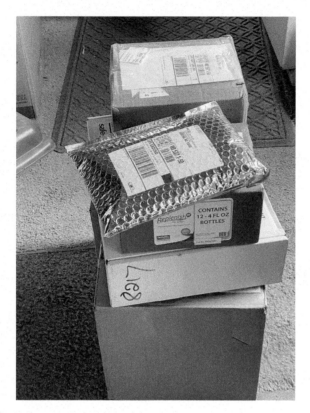

FIGURE 2.28   Fecal samples arriving by UPS to lab.

3. **Fecal exams for equine:** Horses are very difficult because they can transmit parasites in confinement was well as on pasture. Horses held in stalls or pens can develop high worm burdens because of several issues related to the horse. First of all, stall horse provide moisture for parasite development through urine and then when horse is bored, they will chew on contaminated boards, bedding, and feces; therefore, horses need to be maintained as parasite-free as possible for the entire year. Second, many horse parasites across the country have developed some resistance to several dewormers. Conducting a fecal worm egg reduction test is recommended for horses, where control seems to be difficult. Otherwise, individual horses should have a fecal exam several times a year, ideally, in mid-summer and again in mid-winter keeping in mind the winter fecal exam should be negative; otherwise, a deworming is warranted. A few worm eggs found in the summer exam is not bad unless these counts are greater than 100 eggs per sample. Most positive samples for horses warrant treatment.

4. **Fecal exams for confined cattle:** Confined cattle should be checked when moved into confinement such as feedlot cattle. Since parasite resistance is prevalent in cattle, FECRTs should be conducted, or the arrival deworming should be given with two unrelated products and then followed by a fecal exam (14 days later) to make sure the counts are negative.

5. **Fecal exams for swine:** Sows should be worm-free at arrowing, so a fecal check at farrowing is well worth the effort. Gower pigs moved into a grower facility should be worm-free if born from parasite-fee sows. The next best time to check grower/finisher pigs is six weeks into the grower facility. This will determine if the grower facility is contaminated.

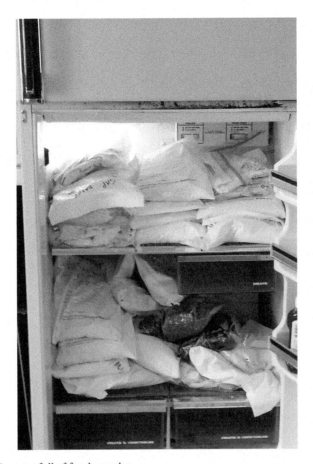

FIGURE 2.29   Refrigerator full of fecal samples.

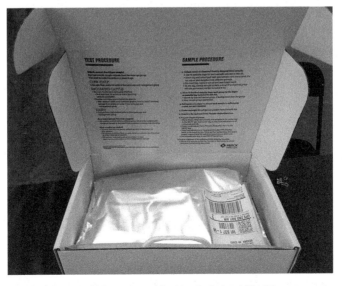

FIGURE 2.30   Mail-in Parasite Fecal kit sponsored by Merck Animal Health.

6. **Fecal exams for small ruminants:** All small ruminants should be parasite-free during the winter months. This means these animals will not immediately contaminate the spring pastures. Once spring grazing begins, all animals should be treated three times, three weeks apart to prevent summer buildup of pasture contamination. A mid-summer fecal check will indicate whether the spring treatment worked and parasite contamination is under control.

7. **Fecal exams for pasture cattle:** In pastured cattle, sheep, and goats, the program is more involved. Having cattle parasite-free during the months when the temperature is too cold or too hot and dry for pasture growth (and infective larvae growth). The winter months, therefore, is a great time to conduct a fecal exam. Cattle showing positive fecal results when samples are taken during the winter indicates that the fall deworming was most likely unsuccessful. For sheep and goats, positive winter fecals indicate resistance and that an alternate product should be used with a follow-up fecal to ensure efficacy.

All pasture animals should be worm-free as possible for first 60–90 days of grazing to prevent contamination of spring pasture. A fecal exam during this period will indicate egg shedding status. Most strategic deworming programs recommend a mid-spring deworming four to six weeks after grass green-up depending upon the age of the animals. A late summer or early fall sample is only meaningful if the worm egg counts are high. High summer fecal worm egg counts means that the spring deworming schedule needs to become more aggressive.

STANDARD OPERATING PROCEDURE FOR THE "MODIFIED WISCONSIN SUGAR FLOTATION TECHNIQUE"

Supplies needed for conducting the Modified Wisconsin Sugar Flotation Method:

1. Sugar solution (1 lb [454 g] of granulated sugar mixed with 12 oz [355 ml] of hot water). Commercially made sugar solution can be purchased in one gallon jugs from Jorgensen Laboratories, LLC (see Figure 2.31).

2. Dispensing bottle with attached 15 ml or larger dosing gun. A cattle drench gun works great. Leave the gun attached to sugar solution. Washing the gun is not necessary until changing sugar solution. Sugar crystals may form on nozzle sitting overnight but simply tap the end of the nozzle to clean the nozzle.

3. 3–5 oz paper cups (90 ml) (two cups per sample).

4. Tea strainer with handle.

5. Taper-bottom test tubes (15 ml).

6. Several test tube tracks.

7. Standard microscope slides.

8. 22 mm × 22 mm coverslips.

9. Tongue depressors (one per sample).

10. Small syringe (10 ml) to top of test tubes.

11. Centrifuge with a free-swing horizontal head with an ideal speed of 700 rpm depending upon the length of the swing arm.

12. Binocular Microscope with 40×, 100×, and 400× lens.

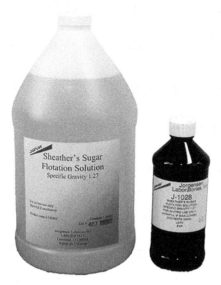

FIGURE 2.31   Commercial fecal flotation sugar solution made by Jorgensen Labs, LLC. (JorVet™) is available through normal veterinary distribution channels.
Source: Jorgensen Laboratories.

Laboratory procedure for processing fecal samples for worm egg counts:

Fecal solution mixture: The saturated sugar solution flotation medium is made by mixing 12 oz (355 ml) of hot water with every pound (454 g) of granulated white sugar used. The lab solution is made in a standard 2-gal wide-mouth plastic jug with well-marked lines indicating a 48-oz level. To make the sugar solution, forty-eight (48) oz of boiling water is measured into the jug. A 4.0 lb bag of sugar is added and shaken or stirred until solution is completely mixed and solution becomes clear. The final solution is allowed to cool to room temperature before being used. The cooled solution is poured through a small funnel into a 2-gal backpack attached to a 25 cc dosing gun. The backpack is hung on a hook (with an attached strap) over the lab bench where the samples are processed. The dosing gun is set to deliver 15 cc of the sugar solution each draw.

Standard operating procedure overview: The samples are hand massaged in the baggie to help mix sample before a corner is cut and a small sample is squeezed out on a wax paper and weighed on an electronic gram scale. The 3 g sample is then scrapped into a 3-oz paper cup containing 15 cc of saturated sugar solution with a wood tongue depressor stirring until the sample is completely mixed into the solution. The mixed solution is then poured through a standard tea strainer over a second 3-oz cup and pressed dry with the tongue depressor. The 3-oz cup containing the squeezed solution is poured directly into a 15 cc tapered test tube and placed in a free-swinging horizontal head centrifuge and centrifuged at 800 rpm for five minutes. After centrifugation, the test tube is placed in a test tube rack where additional sugar solution is added using a 15 cc syringe to form a slight meniscus on top of the tube where a standard 22 × 22 mm cover slip is added. The cover slip is left to stand on the top of the tube for a minimum of five minutes before placing on a numbered microscope slide for reading. If not read immediately, the rack with the tube and attached cover slip or the slide with cover slip is placed in the refrigerator until read. After processing, all samples are read within 72 hours.

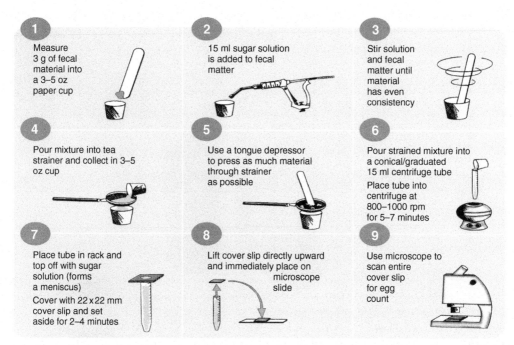

1
Measure 3 g of fecal material into a 3–5 oz paper cup

2
15 ml sugar solution is added to fecal matter

3
Stir solution and fecal matter until material has even consistency

4
Pour mixture into tea strainer and collect in 3–5 oz cup

5
Use a tongue depressor to press as much material through strainer as possible

6
Pour strained mixture into a conical/graduated 15 ml centrifuge tube

Place tube into centrifuge at 800–1000 rpm for 5–7 minutes

7
Place tube in rack and top off with sugar solution (forms a meniscus)

Cover with 22 x 22 mm cover slip and set aside for 2–4 minutes

8
Lift cover slip directly upward and immediately place on microscope slide

9
Use microscope to scan entire cover slip for egg count

FIGURE 2.32   Nine-step procedure for the Modified Wisconsin Sugar Flotation Method.

Modified Wisconsin Sugar Flotation Method – nine-step method (see Figure 2.32):

1. Measure 15–18 ml of sugar solution into 3–5 oz cup; the higher amount is for dry matter samples such as for equine samples and the lower amount is for watery samples such as samples from cattle soon after turnout on green pastures (see Figure 2.33).

2. Add 3 g of fecal material into a cup containing sugar solution for cattle, bison, swine, equine, and pets. Use 1-g samples for small ruminants, hoofed wildlife, fowl, or poultry and small animal species such as rabbits, snakes, and turtles (see Figure 2.34).

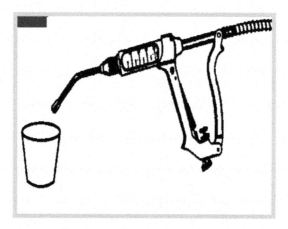

FIGURE 2.33   Add 15–18 oz solution to cup (easiest with a drench gun).

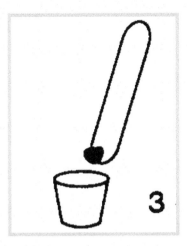

FIGURE 2.34   Add 1–3g manure to cup with solution.

3. Stir the solution and fecal matter with a tongue depressor until the material has an even liquid consistency. For animal feces consisting of pellets such as for sheep and goats, the pellet needs to be cut with the side of the tongue depressor and then crushed and stirred until an even liquid consistency has been reached (see Figure 2.35).

4. Pour the mixture into a tea strainer over a second 3–5 oz cup (see Figure 2.36).

5. Use a tongue depressor to press as much solution through the strainer as possible or at least until the material in the tea strainer appears dry. Pressing the finger low on the stick to press prevents breaking the stick and making sure the fecal matter is pressed dry.

6. Pour the solution from the cup into a 15-ml centrifuge tube with a tapered bottom (see Figures 2.37–2.38).

7. Place the test tube in the rack. Top the off with sugar solution until a meniscus bulges slightly over the top of the tube, sufficient to make contact with the cover slip. Do not overfill because worm egg can be lost in any solution that spills over down the test tube.

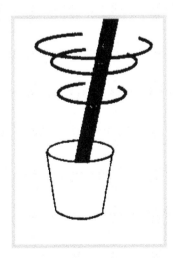

FIGURE 2.35   Stir manure into solution with tongue depressor.

FIGURE 2.36 Pour mixture through tea strainer into another cup, press until dry.

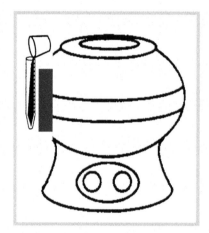

FIGURE 2.37 Pour strained solution into test tube and centrifuge at low rpm (700–800).

8. Cover the test tube with a cover slip and set aside for five minutes (see Figure 2.39).

9. Lift the coverslip straight up and place it on a microscope slide and scan the entire coverslip to identify and count the eggs present (see Figure 2.40).

The samples are read using 4× magnification. Each slip is read completely starting from upper left corner of the cover slip moving downward making five complete passes until the entire cover slip is read. All eggs are identified as to type and enumerated (see Figure 2.41). Each species egg will be identified later including level of coccidia oocyst shedding and level of tapeworm egg shedding (see Figures 2.42 and 2.43). See cattle worm egg chart listed below. Egg types are identified according to published identification keys of gastrointestinal nematode and flatworm (tapeworm) parasites. Whenever possible, the best response is usually achieved when the producer can see the worm eggs directly from the microscope and have the fecal worm egg counts interpreted as to their full meaning (see Figure 2.44).

Artifacts and funny objects are often found in samples, but although they are mostly annoying, only a few like mite eggs can cause confusion for the average reader. The most important

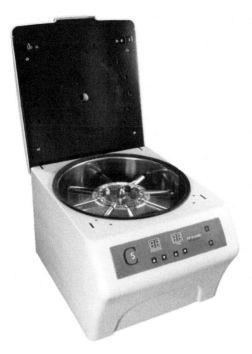

FIGURE 2.38   Example of a centrifuge with horizontal free-swinging head.

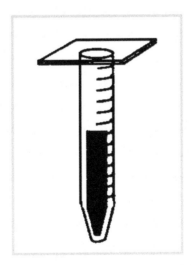

FIGURE 2.39   Put tubes in rack and add solution to form meniscus and place cover slip on test tube after centrifuging.

artifact to identify is the oribatid mite egg commonly found throughout North America (see Figures 2.45–2.49). The following artifacts are commonly seen: Common objects and artifact found in fecal samples are listed in Figures 2.45–2.62. Further worm egg identification (see Figures 2.63 and 2.64 for cattle and equine) will be covered in separate chapters. Examples are given below: (see individual chapters for specific worm egg identification.) Positive or negative (0) results are recorded on a fecal worm egg count reporting form for each specie tested (Figures 2.65–2.71).

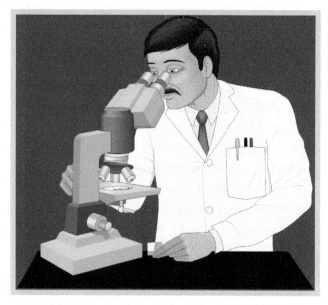

FIGURE 2.40   Read entire cover slip, identify eggs, and count total number eggs found on entire cover slip.

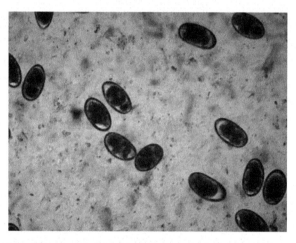

FIGURE 2.41   Screen shot of eggs from microscope camera.

INTERPRETATION OF FECAL WORM EGG COUNTS IN SHEEP, GOATS, AND CAMELIDS USING THE MODIFIED WISCONSIN SUGAR FLOTATION TECHNIQUE

Understanding the meaning of worm egg counts will provide veterinarians the necessary insight needed to help clients build a deworming strategy for a particular operation or operations. Factors that affect fecal worm egg shedding are numerous, so a number of these factors need to be considered every time an analysis is made and a fair assessment of the worm egg counts generated. The age of the animal, the season of the year, the amount of exposure to pasture and the stocking rate of the animals on pasture all affect worm egg counts. The amount of rainfall or moisture on the pasture and the number of degree days with temperatures sufficient to promote parasite development on pasture are also very important to future infections. These factors directly affect egg count interpretation as infection levels build on the pasture and ingestion of these larvae increases and

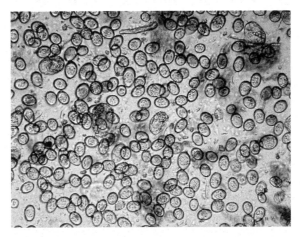

FIGURE 2.42 Heavy coccidia oocysts present plus a few threadworm eggs found in some dairy calves (10×).

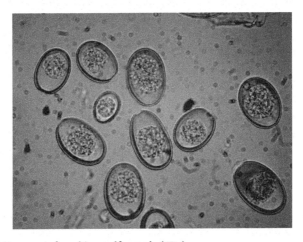

FIGURE 2.43 Coccidia oocysts found in a calf sample (40×).

worm burdens rise in the animals themselves. Furthermore, the health of the animals, the stage of gestation, stage of lactation, and the numbers and type of parasites present at each examination must be considered. Post-lambing worm egg counts, for example, are almost always higher than pre-lambing counts.

The five most common types of internal nematode parasites in sheep and goats that are routinely diagnosed present in fecal exams are: Stomach worms (primarily the barber's pole worm – *Haemonchus* sp.), intestinal worms (*Cooperia* sp.), threadworms (*Strongyloides* sp.), whipworms (*Trichuris* sp.), and nodular worms (*Oesophagostomum* sp.). All eggs are counted and included in the worm egg count total, except for tapeworms and coccidia. Tapeworms and coccidia are commonly found but are listed on the worm egg count forms simply as positive at a low level (+) 1–10 eggs, medium level (++) 11–50 eggs, or high level (+++) 50 eggs or greater. One egg/g equals 454 eggs/lb of manure, i.e., a count of 500 equals 227,000 eggs/lb of feces, so 5.0 lb of feces per day would yield 1,100,000 eggs per day on the pasture per animal.

I have detailed the quick assessment for each species group in their respective chapters; however, I have outlined sheep, goats, and camelids below as an example to review here.

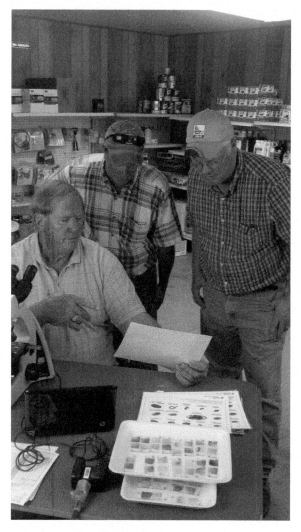

FIGURE 2.44 Talking to producers about their results.

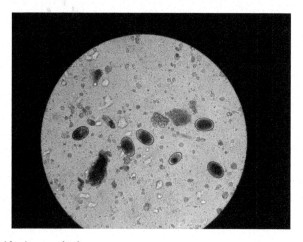

FIGURE 2.45 Oribatid mite eggs (4×).

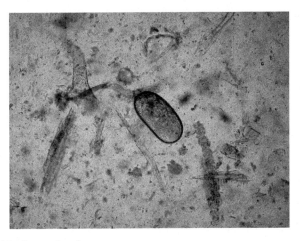

FIGURE 2.46   Oribatid mite egg (10×).

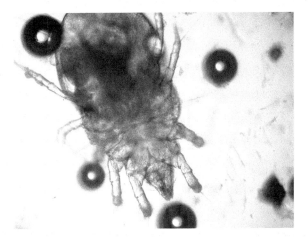

FIGURE 2.47   Oribatid mite (40×).

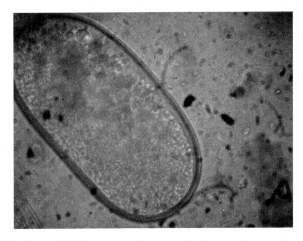

FIGURE 2.48   Oribatid mite egg (40×).

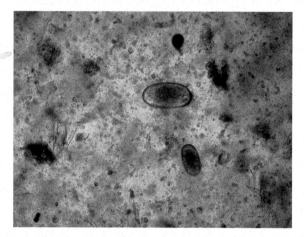

FIGURE 2.49   Oribatid mite egg with *Ostertagia* eggs (10×).

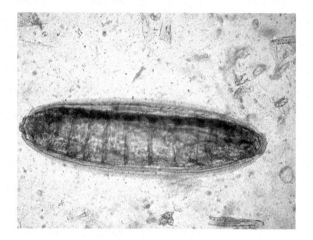

FIGURE 2.50   Fly pupal (10×).

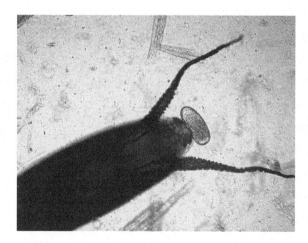

FIGURE 2.51   Fly larvae with parasite egg (40×).

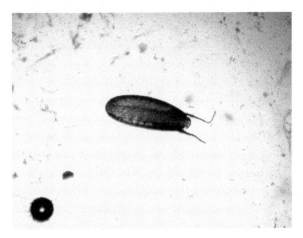

FIGURE 2.52   Fly larvae (10×).

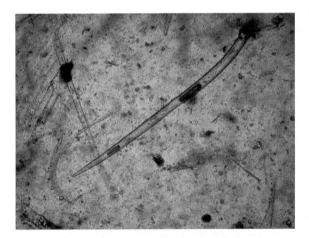

FIGURE 2.53   Hair follicle.

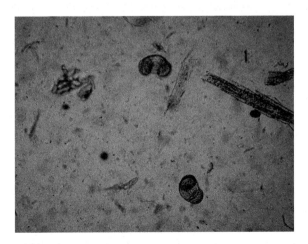

FIGURE 2.54   Pollen grain (10×).

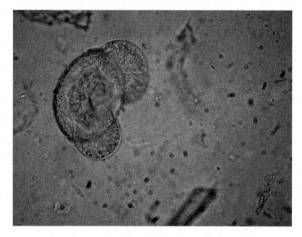

FIGURE 2.55   Pollen grain (40×).

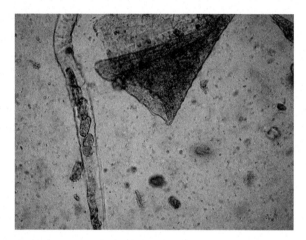

FIGURE 2.56   Gravid female threadworm (*Strongyloides*).

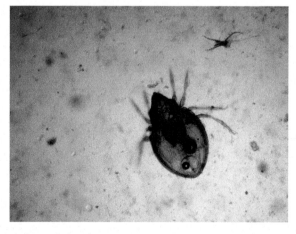

FIGURE 2.57   Tick in stool sample (10×).

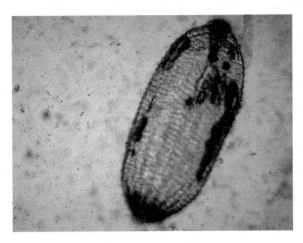

FIGURE 2.58　Corn-like artifact.

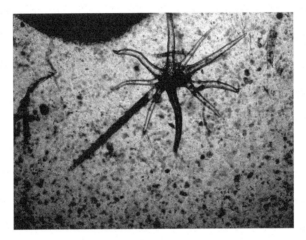

FIGURE 2.59　Allergy artifact (10×).

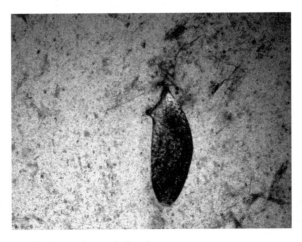

FIGURE 2.60　Random artifact in stool sample (10×).

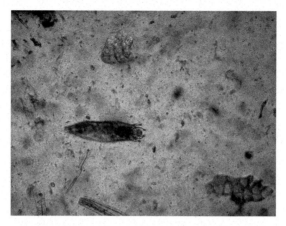

FIGURE 2.61   Feline mite (10×).

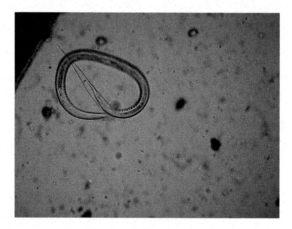

FIGURE 2.62   Infective larvae found in fecal sample.

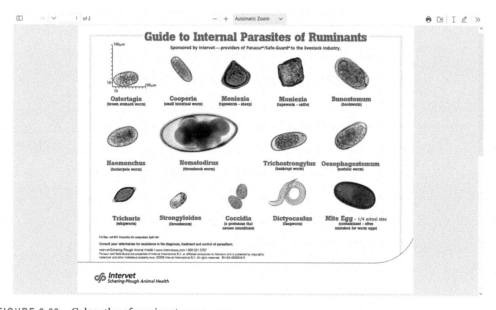

FIGURE 2.63   Color atlas of ruminant worm eggs.

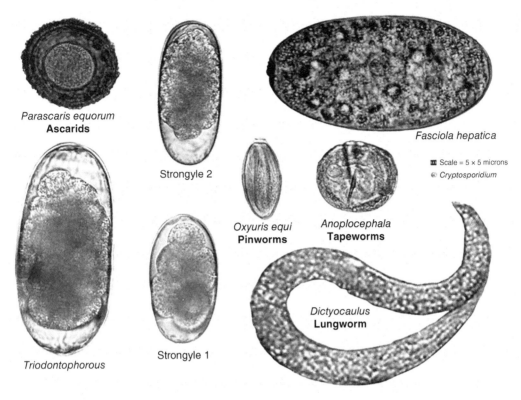

FIGURE 2.64   Worm egg chart for equine.

QUICK ASSESSMENT FOR SHEEP, GOATS, AND CAMELIDS BASED ON FECAL WORM EGG COUNTS

	Eggs/g Count	Estimated Parasite Level
Nematode egg counts	1–10 eggs	Low
Recorded on sheets	11–50 eggs	Moderate
	50+ eggs	High*
	300+ eggs	Very high*

*At this level, it appears that parasites begin to stop developing and undergo inhibition in tissues.

Positive worm egg counts for sheep and goats (other than very high counts) for the most part only indicate the presence or absence of parasites within a particular animal. It is impossible to determine how many parasites are present at any given time primarily because Haemonchus undergoes a phenomenon called inhibition or period of arrested development. This parasitic stage remains in the tissues for long periods of time and follow an annual development and inhibition cycle. The primary inhibition period begins about 45–60 days into a grazing period as the parasite contamination level on pastures buildup. These inhibited larvae can stage in the tissues through the beginning of the following grazing season.

The overall infection process begins when an infected animal grazes a pasture, it sheds worm eggs on a daily basis that pass in the manure. These eggs hatch and the larval offspring develop into infective larvae which recontaminates the pasture, thus exposing all animal grazing this pasture to new infections. If the pasture is already contaminated with infective larvae, the animals pick up

Dairy and Beef Cattle Parasite Evaluation Form

PEC ☐   Mail In ☐   Page____ of____

Collection Date: _____   Consultant: _____

Name of Farm: _____   Sponsor: _____

Producer's Name: _____   Sponsor Contact: _____

Producer's Address: _____   Sponsor Address: _____

City _____ Phone _____   City _____ Phone _____

State _____ Zip _____ Fax _____   State _____ Zip _____ Fax _____

E-Mail: _____   Representative: _____

Sample ID	Animal ID	Contamination Level*	Stomach Worm	Nematodirus	Cooperia	Hookworm	Threadworm	Whipworm	Nodular Worm	Tapeworm	Coccidia	Total Count (EP3G)**	Treatment Date month/day/year	Product Used
													Enter after test results recorded	

*1 = pasture, 2 = limited pasture, 3 = dry lot/partial confinement, 4 = total confinement year round   **(+ = 1-10) (++ = 11-50) (+++ =>51)

COMMENTS:

Eggs/Pound Manure [ ]

Total count x 150 = Eggs per pound

FIGURE 2.65   Parasite evaluation form for cattle and bison.

new infections at the same time they shed eggs back on the pasture contributing future contamination levels. This process continues until the grazing season ends. Depending upon temperature and moisture, these parasite eggs hatch, develop into infective larvae, and move away from the manure pats onto the vegetation where the reinfection process begins.

The biggest and least understood issue with sheep and goats is that once Haemonchus infections reach a high level, the physiology of the gut changes. The parasites respond by stopping their development undergoing an arrested development period waiting for the physiology of the gut to return to normal. This why the simple guide (listed above) to predict parasite levels within an animal based on worm egg counts can be misleading.

The time of the year when the assessment is made can also have an impact on worm eggs as follows:

1. **Winter:** As winter progresses, animals are no longer ingesting infective larvae off pasture, existing worm burdens begin to mature and die off as they age, conditions in the gut then start to return to normal which, in turn, triggers inhibited parasites to become active. If counts come back following treatment, this means inhibited are present or if worm egg counts are

Small Ruminants & Wildlife Parasite Evaluation Form

PEC ☐   Mail In ☐   Page____ of____

Collection Date:	Consultant:
Name of Farm:	Sponsor:
Producer's Name:	Sponsor Contact:
Producer's Address:	Sponsor Address:
City Phone	City Phone
State Zip Fax	State Zip Fax
E-Mail:	Representative:

Lab ID	Animal ID (If testing specific animals please number sample bags in consecutive order)	Stomach Worm (Haemonchus)	Nematodirus	Cooperia	Hookworm	Threadworm	Whipworm	Nodular Worm	Tapeworm*	Coccidia*	Total Count (EPG)	Treatment Date month/day/year	Product Used
												Enter after test results recorded	

COMMENTS:

*(+ = 1-10) (++ = 11-50) (+++ =>51)
*Not reported in total egg count

FIGURE 2.66   Parasite evaluation form for small ruminants.

high during the winter these counts indicate that heavy worm challenge existed from the previous season.

2. **Spring:** When inhibited larvae are being released form the gastric glands, egg shedding can reach a high level which indicates the presence of high worm burdens carried over from the previous season. High egg shedding levels at this time is dangerous because egg shedding in the spring determine contamination levels for the rest of the year.

3. **Summer:** Once animals are on pasture and grazing begins, worm counts will begin to rise within three weeks. Once egg counts exceed 100 eggs/g (45,400/lb of manure), worm burdens have reached a point when incoming larvae undergo arrested development and become inhibited larvae in the gastric glands of the abomasum.

4. **Fall:** The quick assessment chart (listed above) is most accurate in the fall at the end of the grazing season. Low counts indicate successful control of worm burdens while high counts indicate economic loss may be occurring and trouble controlling these infections due to inhibited worm burdens may be occurring.

Alpaca/Llama Parasite Evaluation Form

PEC ☐　　Mail In ☐　　　　　　　　　　　　　　　　　　Page____ of____

Collection Date:		Consultant:
Name of Farm:		Sponsor:
Producer's Name:		Sponsor Contact:
Producer's Address:		Sponsor Address:
City _____ Phone _____		City _____ Phone _____
State _____ Zip _____ Fax _____		State _____ Zip _____ Fax _____
E-Mail:		Representative:

Lab ID	Animal ID (If testing specific animals please number sample bags in consecutive order)	Stomach Worm (Haemonchus)	Nematodirus	Cooperia	Hookworm	Threadworm	Whipworm	Tapeworm*	E. mac*	Coccidia*	Total Count (EPG)	Treatment Date month/day/year	Product Used
												Enter after test results recorded	

COMMENTS:

*(+ = 1-10) (++ = 11-50) (+++ =>51)
*Not reported in total egg count

FIGURE 2.67　Parasite evaluation form for camelids.

Other techniques for fecal examination are also available to veterinarians. Three methods (or modifications) are commonly used for fecal examination: direct smear, dilution, and flotation. The direct smear has little value to the food animal practitioner because the amount of feces that can be microscopically examined is small, especially in relation to the total amount of feces produced daily by an adult cow. The chance of consistently finding eggs, oocysts, or trophozoites by this method is minimal. The dilution technique suffers from the same disadvantage as the smear technique and is of little value unless the animal is passing a large number of worm eggs. The dilution techniques such as the quantitative McMasters Method are commonly used; but because of its ability to detect subclinical infections, it is of little use in veterinary practice, especially in adult cattle. Commercial fecal flotation kits are available for the veterinary use but they all are simple flotation kits (Fecalyzer, Ovassay, and Ovatector) and all very inaccurate especially when it comes to running cattle feces (see Fecalyzer Technique listed below). These kits are also all expensive and require disposal of plastics.

Direct smear: A small amount of feces is mixed with a few drops of water and physiologic salt solution on a glass slide, a cover slip is placed on top and then examined. This is a quick way to examine feces for worm eggs but very inaccurate. A positive count may save time and money but a negative count means a better technique is necessary and thus the direct smear can be considered a waste of time. The best use of this technique is to detect motile parasite stages such as protozoan trophozoites and helminth larvae passed in the feces. Larvae of the threadworm

Swine Parasite Evaluation Form

PEC ☐   Mail In ☐   Page_____of_____

Collection Date:		Consultant:
Corporate Name:		Sponsor:
Name of Farm:		Sponsor Contact:
Producer's Address:		Sponsor Address:
City: Phone:		City: Phone:
State: Zip: Fax:		State: Zip: Fax:
E-Mail:		Representative:

Lab ID No.	Animal ID/ Pen #	Management*	Large Roundworm	Whipworm	Nodular Worm	Threadworm	Coccidia	Total Count** (EP3G)	Treatment Date month/day/year	Product Used
									Enter after test results recorded	

COMMENTS:

*Management:
1 = Nursery, 2 = Grower, 3 = Finisher,
4 = Lactating Sow, 5 = Gestation Sow,
6 = Gilt, 7 = Boar

**(+ = 1-10) (++ = 11-50) (+++ =>51)

FIGURE 2.68   Parasite evaluation form for swine.

(*Strongyloides stercoralis*) often associated with diarrhea in young puppies can be found in a direct smear. Also, Giardia trophozoite stages can also be seen on direct smears. A drop of dilute Lugol's iodine solution (10.5%) to immobilize larvae/trophozoite movement for microscopic examination is often necessary.

Fecalyzer technique: This method employs a small plastic well within a covered container to which is added a small amount of fecal material. A plastic cylinder is tightly fitted over the well and half filled with a flotation solution. The fecal material is thoroughly broken up by use of an applicator stick. Then, a small plastic sieve strainer is pushed down into the cylinder. The flotation medium is added until the cylinder is completely full and a convex meniscus has formed at the surface. A coverslip is placed over the meniscus and the system is allowed to stand for 20 minutes. The coverslip is then carefully transferred to a slide by means of thumb forceps. Counting and identification of parasite ova is conducted.

Concentration of feces by flotation: Fecal flotation methods all differ in solutions used and procedures. The most common solutions used for flotation are Sheather's sucrose (1.275 specific gravity), zinc sulfate (1.18 specific gravity), and sodium nitrate (1.20 specific gravity). The Sheather's solution is made by adding 1.0 lb (454 g) of sugar in to 355 ml of hot water (12 oz of hot water). The zinc sulfate solution can be made using 350 g of granular zinc sulfate dissolved in 1000 ml of water. The sodium nitrate solution can be made with 378 g of granular sodium nitrate dissolved in 1000 ml of water.

Poultry Parasite Evaluation Form

PEC ☐   Mail In ☐   Page___of____

Collection Date	Tested:	Consultant	Dr. Don Bliss	Representative
Corporate Name		Sponsor	
Name of Farm		Sponsor Contact	
Producer's Address		Sponsor Address	
City	Phone	City	Phone
State	Zip	Fax	State	Zip	Fax
E-Mail:		E-Mail:

Lab ID No.	Animal ID/ Pen # (Please number sample bags in order listed on form) eg. *Name or group* Bag #	Management*	Ascaridia	Heterakis	Capillaria	Syngamus	Coccidia*	Other	Total Count** (EPG)	Treatment Date month/day/year	Product Used
										Enter after test results recorded	

COMMENTS:
Additional E-Mail:

Donald H. Bliss, Ph.D.
MidAmerica Ag. Research
3705 Sequoia Trail
Verona, WI 53593

For additional information and submission forms, visit: www.midamericaagresearch.net

The total egg count is reported here for each sample and the incidence level of specific parasite genera is recorded as low(+), medium(++) or high(+++).

*(+ = 1-10) (++ = 11-50) (+++ =>51)
*Not reported in total egg count

FIGURE 2.69   Parasite evaluation form for poultry.

Use example: A small amount (1–2g) of feces is mixed with 15 ml of saturated sodium nitrate and strained into a paper cup; a 22 mm square coverslip was floated on top the liquid surface. After 20 minutes, the coverslip is placed on a glass slide and examined (see the Modified Wisconsin Sugar Flotation Technique for proper technique). There are a few parasites that are missed or become distorted because of the high specific gravity of the Sheather's sucrose solution. For those exceptions, zinc sulfate (sp. Gravity 1.18) is often used to identify potential infections with parasitic protozoan species like *Giardia lamblia* and the recovery of delicate larval stages of lungworm parasites like *Oslerus* and *Filaroides* in dogs and *Aelurostrongylus* in cats. Studies have shown that zinc sulfate as a flotation medium for detecting *Giardia* infections is nearly twice more reliable than Sheather's sucrose.

Concentration by centrifugation: A small amount (1–2g) of fecal material is thoroughly mixed with 15 ml of saturated sugar solution. This material is strained through gauze, poured into a test tube, and centrifuged at 1500 rpm for five minutes. Several drops from the surface of the centrifuged material is transferred to a glass slide, a cover slip is added on top and examined (see the Modified Wisconsin Sugar Flotation Technique for proper technique and centrifugal speed).

Wisconsin double centrifugal sugar flotation method: A small amount of feces (5g) is mixed with 15 ml of water in paper cup, strained through tea strainer, and pour-on into a centrifuge tube and centrifuged at 1500 rpm for 10 minutes. The tube is decanted; the sediment is mixed with 15 ml of sugar solution, mixed vigorously, a sugar solution meniscus is added, and a coverslip

Equine Parasite Evaluation Form

PEC ☐   Mail In ☐   Page____ of____

Collection Date		Consultant	
Name of Farm		Sponsor	
Producer's Name		Sponsor Contact	
Producer's Address		Sponsor Address	
City	County	City	Phone
State Zip	Phone	State Zip	Fax
E-Mail	Fax	Representative	

Lab ID No.	Animal ID	Age/Gender *	Contamination Level**	Strongyles	Roundworm	Threadworm	Tapeworm	Pinworm	Coccidia	Total Count (EPG)	Treatment Date month/day/year	Product Used
											Enter after test results recorded	

* 1 = Mare, 2 = Stallion, 3 = Gelding, 4 = Yearling, 5 = Weanling, 6 = Foal, 7 = Other

**1 = pasture, 2 = limited pasture, 3 = dry lot/partial confinement, 4 = total confinement year round

COMMENTS: Conducted by:

(+1 = 1-10) (++ = 11-50) (+++ =>51)

Eggs/Pound Manure ☐

Total count x 150 = Eggs per pound
(based on a 3 gram sample)

FIGURE 2.70   Parasite evaluation form for equine.

is placed on the tube and recentrifuged at 1500 rpm for 10 minutes. The coverslip is placed on a glass slide and examined for eggs and oocysts (see the Modified Wisconsin Sugar Flotation Technique for proper evaluation).

The McMaster method of egg counting: A small amount (2 g) of fecal material is weighed and mixed in a small volume of water (2–5 ml). Saturated saline solution is added to make a volume of 60 ml. Lead pellets are added; the bottle is capped and thoroughly agitated for one minute to ensure breakup and mixing of fecal material. By means of a syringe, a small representative volume is quickly transferred to a McMaster glass counting chamber. After three to five minutes of settling, the chamber is examined and the eggs identified and counted.

A multiplication factor of 100 gives the number of eggs/g of fecal material. A count or value of 1000 eggs or more indicate goats need treating. Goats reportedly can die with egg counts of only 2000 eggs/g (see the Modified Wisconsin Sugar Flotation Technique for proper evaluation). One of the main problems with this technique is that the sensitivity is very low in animals that produce high volume of manure [14, 15]. In the case of Dr. Levin's publication, he conducted a survey on the prevalence of parasitism in Illinois cattle, which was published in the 1960s. The publication has misled many veterinarians and producers over the years not to deworm their cattle until they had fecal worm egg counts over 300 epg.

Dog and Cat Parasite Evaluation Form

PEC ☐   Mail In ☐

Page____ of____

Collection Date _____

Name of Farm _____

Producer's Name _____

Producer's Address _____

City _____ County_____

State _____ Zip _____ Phone _____

E-Mail _____ Fax _____

Consultant _____

Sponsor _____

Sponsor Contact _____

Sponsor Address _____

City _____ Phone _____

State _____ Zip _____ Fax _____

Representative _____ Fax _____

Sample ID	Animal ID	Animal Type*	Roundworm		Tapeworm		Hookworm				Whipworm	Threadworm	Other	Total Count (EPG)	Treatment Date month/day/year	Product Used
			Toxocara	Toxascaris	Dipylidium	Taenia									Enter after test results recorded	

*1 = Male Dog 2 = Female Dog, 3 = Male Cat, 4 = Female Cat

COMMENTS:

Conducted by:

(+1 = 1-10) (++ = 11-50) (+++ =>51)

Eggs/Pound Manure [ ]

Total count x 454 = Eggs per pound
(based on a 1 gram sample)

FIGURE 2.71   Parasite evaluation form for dogs and cats.

Fecal concentration method: A small amount of feces is mixed in 9–10 ml of 10% buffered formalin with a tongue depressor or applicator sticks in a paper cup or flat bottomed tube. Let set for 30 minutes for fixation then add 3 ml of ethyl acetate (or ethyl ether) and 3 ml of surfactant (Triton-X-100 Rohm and Hass). The mixture is shaken vigorously for 30 seconds then filtered through dampened gauze held in a funnel, into a 15-ml centrifuge tube. The filtrate is centrifuged at 2000–2500 rpm for 10 minutes. The supernatant is decanted. The sediment is examined for coccidia oocysts, helminth eggs and larvae, and protozoan cysts.

Liver fluke diagnostic system: A commercial available product called Flukefinder® Test is available (see Figure 2.72). The Flukefinder isolates liver fluke eggs by differential filtration followed by differential sedimentation (see Figures 2.73 and 2.74). The test can be modified and improved both in efficiency and accuracy by combining this test with the "Modified Wisconsin Sugar Flotation Technique." This is done simply by running the sample being checked for flukes for worm egg counts first and then taking the sediment at the bottom of each tube selected for the fluke test and washing that sediment through the fluke finder counting all flukes found as fluke eggs in a 3 g sample. Flukefinder diagnostic system also works excellent for *Giardia,* trophozoites, and cysts, which are concentrated to a minimal volume and can be streaked onto a glass slide for identification and enumeration.

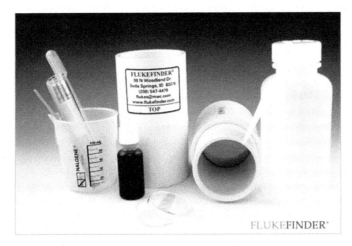

FIGURE 2.72   Commercial FlukeFinder™.
Source: FLUKEFINDER.

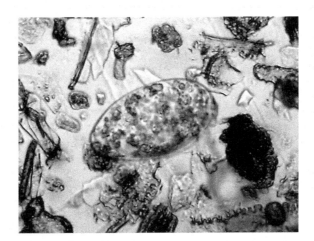

FIGURE 2.73   Fluke (*Fasciola hepatica*) egg (40×).

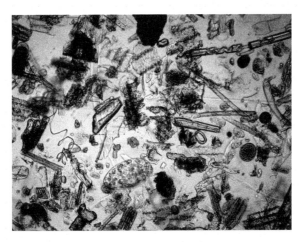

FIGURE 2.74   Fluke (*Fasciola hepatica*) egg (10×).

Mite eggs and other artifacts found in fecal samples: Many common artifacts are found in fecal samples and all most all are easily distinguished from worm eggs except those eggs passed by pasture or grain mites (Oribatid mites). The eggs from Oribatid mites found in fecal samples from all livestock and poultry come in many different egg sizes and stage of development and are easily distinguished using a couple key items to note, namely larger in size (5–20 times large) and intense granulation within the egg showing no distinguishing worm egg cells. Often a mite head and front legs are visible in the egg. Although harmless to people and animals, these mites often play a role in the transmission of tapeworm eggs. As the tapeworm grows, pieces of it break off and are transmitted out of the animal's digestive system along with the tapeworm eggs. Mites living in the soil ingest tapeworm eggs, and the cycle starts all over again. Grain mite or pasture mite eggs are very common found in fecal material from most species animals tested. See Figures 2.45–2.49 for mite eggs and other common artifacts routinely found in fecal samples of all species.

REFERENCES

1. Todd, A.C., Myers, G.H., Bliss, D.H., and Cox, D.D. (1972). Milk production in Wisconsin dairy cattle after anthelmintic treatment. *VM SAC* 66: 1555–1564.

2. Bliss, D.H. and Kvasnicka, W.G. (1997). The fecal examination: a missing link in food animal practice. *The Compendium* 4: 104–109.

3. Woods, I.B., Amaral, N.K., Bairden, K. et al. (1995). World Association for the Advancement of Veterinary Parasitology (W>A>A>V>P>) second edition of guidelines for evaluation of anthelmintics in ruminants (bovine, ovine, caprine). *Vet. Parasitol.* 58: 181–213.

4. Dryden, M.W., Payne, P.A., Ridley, R., and Smith, V. (2005). Comparison of common fecal flotation techniques for the recovery of parasite eggs and oocysts. *Vet. Ther.* 6: 15–28.

5. Dryden, M.W., Payne, P.A., and Smith, V. (2006). Accurate diagnosis of Giardia spp. and proper fecal examination procedures. *Vet. Ther.* 7: 4–14.

6. Sheather, A.L. (1924). The detection of worm eggs and protozoa in the feces of animals. *Vet. Rec.* 4: 552–557.

7. Ewang, T.G. and Slocombe, J.O.D. (1981). Efficiency of the Cornell-Wisconsin centrifugal flotation technique for recovering trichostrongylid eggs from bovine feces. *Can. J. Comp. Med.* 45: 243–248.

8. Whitlock, H.V. (1948). Some modifications of the McMaster helminth egg-counting technique and apparatus. *J. Council Sci. Indust. Res. Aust.* 31: 177–180.

9. Stromberg, B., Newcomb, H., Bliss, D. et al. (2007). Proposed Standardized testing for anthelmintic resistance determination. *Proceedings of the 52nd American Association of Veterinary Parasitologists,* Washington, DC (14–17 July 2007).

10. Coles, A.C., Bauer, B., Borgsteede, F.H.M. et al. (1992). World Association for the Advancement of Veterinary Parasitology (W.A.A.V.P.) Methods for the detection of anthelmintic resistance in nematodes of veterinary importance. *Vet. Parasitol.* 44 (1–2): 35–44.

11. Coles, G.C., Jackson, F., Pomroy, W.E. et al. (2006). The detection of anthelmintic resistance in nematodes of veterinary importance. *Vet. Parasitol.* 136: 167–185.

12. Statistics Canada (2006). Geographical Profile of Manure Production in Canada, 2001, Catalogue no. 21-601-M (accessed 19 October 2008).

13. Bliss, D.H., Georgoulakis, I., Grosomandis, S. et al. (1985). The strategic use of anthelmintics in working donkeys raised under Mediterranean climatic conditions. *Vet. Rec.* 1110: 141–144.

14. Faler, K. (1984). Improved detection of intestinal parasites. *Modern Vet. Pract.* 65: 273–276.

15. Levine, N.D. and Aves, I.J. (1956). The incidence of gastrointestinal nematodes in Illinois cattle. *J. Am. Vet. Med. Assoc.* 129: 331–332.

16. Blackburn, B.L., Schenker, R., Gagne, F., and Drake, J. (2008). Prevalence of intestinal parasites in companion animals in Ontario and Quebec, Canada, during the winter months. *Vet. Ther.* 9: 169–175.

17. Dewhirst, L.W. and Hansen, M.F. (1961). Methods to differentiate and estimate worm burdens in cattle. *Vet. Med.* 56: 84–89.

Parasites in Beef Cattle

Deworming beef cattle has evolved over the past 40 years to become a standard recommended practice on most progressive cow/calf and stocker operations throughout the United States. The emphasis on the economic benefits of deworming has brought about this change [44]. Beef producers recognize the value of deworming as a safe and effective tool to greatly improve the efficiency and quality of their animals. Cattle producers know that they need pasture for their cattle (see Figure 3.1), but they also know that where there is grass, there are parasites. The overall goal of strategic timed deworming is to reduce parasite exposure to their cattle. Preventing parasite development on the pasture is better than waiting until the animals are loaded with parasites before treatment is given (see Figures 3.2 and 3.3). One of the first signs of parasitism in cattle is rough hair coat and a pasty rear end due to diarrhea (see Figure 3.4). If the parasitism becomes severe enough, animals will become emaciated and begin to show "bottle jaw" (see Figures 3.5 and 3.6). Finally, some animals will succumb to parasitism if burdens get high enough (see Figure 3.7).

Each year, more and more producers are deworming their cattle at strategic times of the year to prevent economic losses caused by parasitism rather than waiting until after the cattle are harboring high levels of parasites and parasitic damage to the animals has already occurred. Conducting a fecal worm egg count (using a proper test) will tell the producer if parasites are

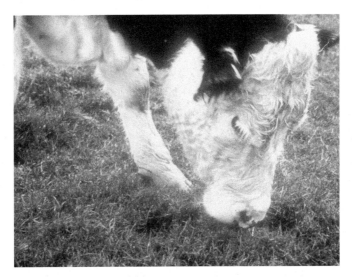

FIGURE 3.1 Cows grazing spring pastures ingest infective larvae that survived the winter, develop into adult parasites and begin contaminating these pastures.

Large Animal Parasitology Procedures for Veterinary Technicians, First Edition. Donald H. Bliss.
© 2024 John Wiley & Sons, Inc. Published 2024 by John Wiley & Sons, Inc.

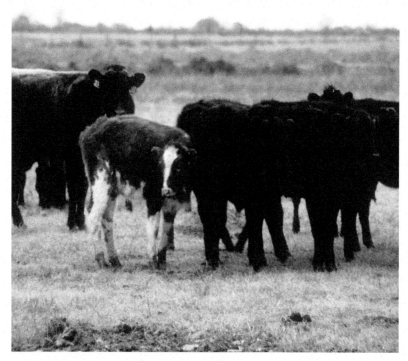

FIGURE 3.2   Yearling cattle showing signs of parasitism demonstrating that prevention is always better than treatment.

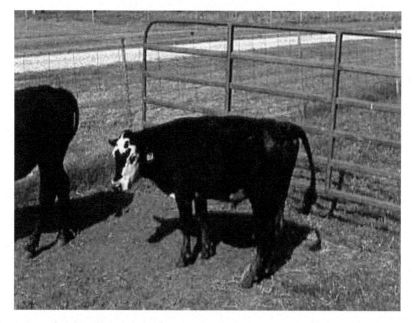

FIGURE 3.3   Steer showing clinical signs of parasitism.

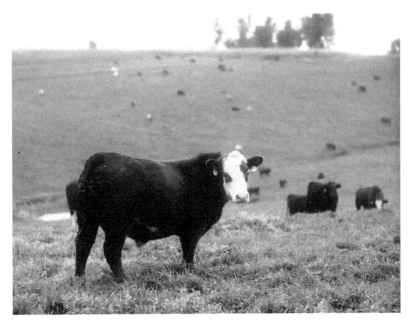

FIGURE 3.4   Grazing steers showing loose and pasty stool.

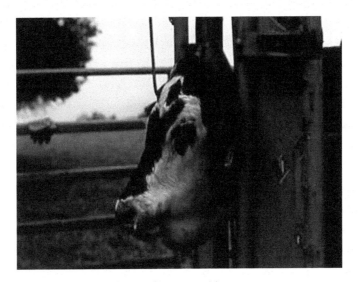

FIGURE 3.5   Steer showing "bottle jaw" due to heavy parasitism.

becoming a problem (see Figure 3.8). Over the past 40 years, I have conducted fecal worm egg counts on thousands of animals all across North America, and parasitism is everywhere cattle are present including big range country in the northern plains and high desert in the Southwest (see Figures 3.9 and 3.10).

Most producers are concerned about deworming at the optimal time to achieve maximum benefit. These producers appreciate having highly efficacious formulations that are safe and easy to apply and trust that the advertised efficacies of the dewormers they use are accurate.

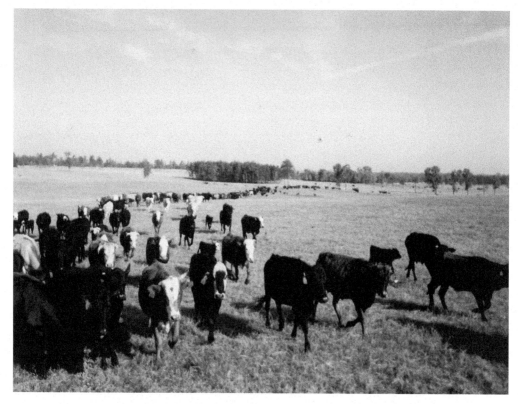

FIGURE 3.6 Clinical parasitism in Georgia cows.

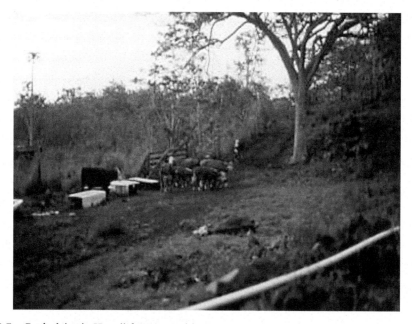

FIGURE 3.7 Cattle dying in Hawaii due to parasitism.

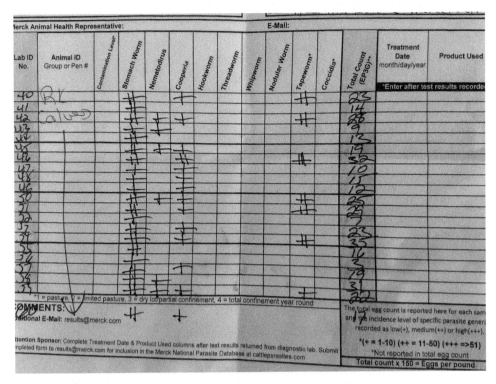

FIGURE 3.8   Lab results from Nebraska calves showing high fecal worm egg counts.

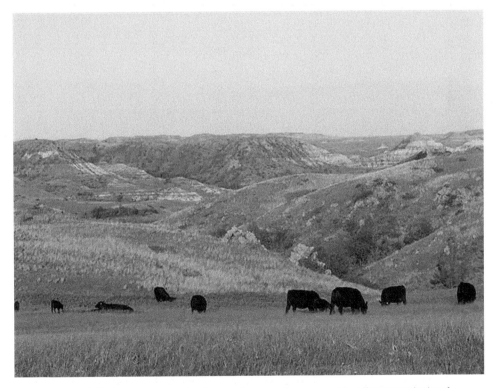

FIGURE 3.9   North Dakota cattle on extensive grazing operations respond well to strategic timed dewormings.

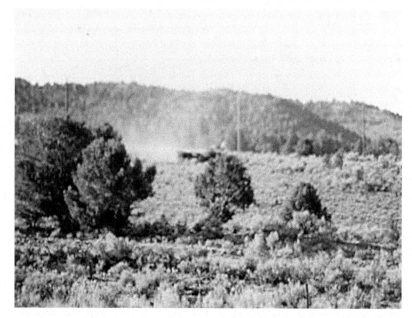

FIGURE 3.10   Parasite in cattle grazing dry range country survive drought periods significantly better when parasite burdens are low.

Many of the progressive producers have discovered that an aggressive strategic deworming program conducted on an annual basis will keep parasite burdens low throughout the year allowing their animals look better and perform better. Strategically dewormed animals have been shown to produce more milk, have increased feed efficiency, increased dry matter intake, increased reproductive efficiency, produce higher carcass quality, obtain higher body condition scores, and have a stronger immune system to fight off other diseases. Gastrointestinal parasites both directly and indirectly affect the animals in a number of ways. Animals are harmed by adult parasites living within the animals themselves but also through daily ingestion of infective larvae that begin attacking the animal's immune system as soon as the infection process begins.

The key to parasite control involves preventing parasite buildup in the animals and their environment through strategic timed deworming programs rather than waiting until the animals are harboring high levels of parasites to treat. It is possible to feed pass the parasite affects if the cost of feed is no problem. One the other hand, cattle grazing during dry period or drought conditions are more susceptible to the effects of parasites (even if worm burdens are low) because when nutrition is low, the negative effect from parasites are magnified. Often times, waiting until the animals appear parasitized before deworming, means that parasite damage has already occurred before the deworming is instituted. It is also important to note that worm-free cattle on worm-free ground stay worm-free. Otherwise, worm-free cattle turned on to a rye grass pasture or corn stalks stay worm-free (see Figure 3.11). Cattle treated going into a feedlot will stay worm-free through going to market. Bison and Cattle housed on dirt dry lots or concrete lots will stay free if dewormed properly upon arrival (see Figure 3.12).

Dr. Judith Capper, a livestock sustainability consultant, conducted a study (see Figure 3.13) on all peer-reviewed published data using a parasite control compound (fenbendazole) seasonally with the stated objective to quantify the effects of withdrawing this parasite control compound

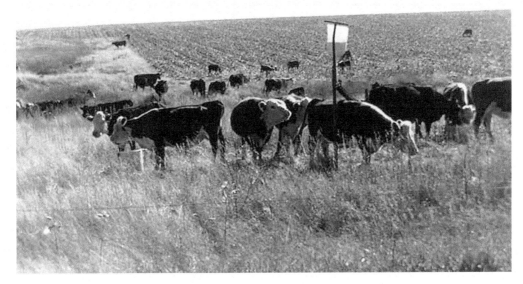

FIGURE 3.11   Cattle grazing on corn stalks.

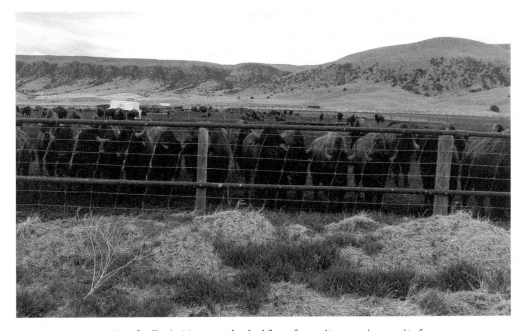

FIGURE 3.12   Bison in a feedlot in Montana checked free of parasites remain parasite-free.

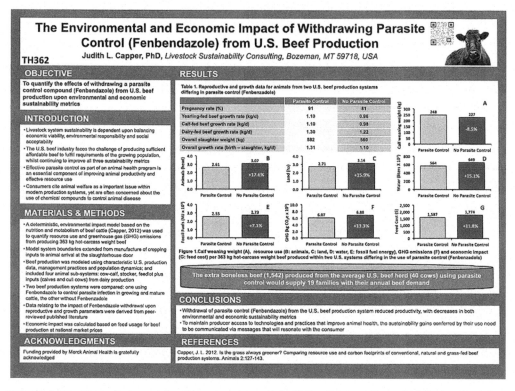

FIGURE 3.13 The environmental and economic impact of withdrawing parasite control (fenbendazole) from US beef production.

(fenbendazole) from US beef production studying its effect upon environmental and economic sustainability metrics [11, 12]. Dr. Capper found as follows:

1. 10.0% Better Pregnancy Rate

2. 8.5% Better Weaning Weights (+46.2 lb)

3. 11.8% Lower Feed Costs (−187 lb/head)

4. 17.6% Fewer Animals Needed

5. 15.4% Better Land and Water Utilization

6. 7.1% Less Fossil Fuel Used

7. 13.3% Less Green House Gas Emissions

The extra boneless beef produced from deworming the average US cow herd (40 cows) using fenbendazole (seasonally) would supply 19 families with their annual beef demand (1542 lb). Dr. Capper concluded that effective parasite control is an essential part of animal health for improving animal production and effective resource use.

Based on the research that has been conducted on the benefits of strategic timed deworming, considerable efforts have been made to teach veterinarians, nutritionists, pharmaceutical representatives, feed company representatives, and producers about these benefits [4, 5, 8, 9, 28, 32, 34, 40, 42]. A number of companies have created FDA-approved formulations that facilitate the ease of deworming for the producer. These formulations include many non-handling forms such as medicated blocks, medicated free-choice minerals, medicated range cube or cake supplements, medicated complete feeds and top-dressed feed formulations as well as topically applied pour-ons [3, 14, 26, 40].

STRATEGIC DEWORMING ENTAILS MORE THAN SIMPLY APPLYING A DEWORMER

The goal of strategically timed deworming application is to prevent economic loss and reduce environmental parasite contamination by eliminating worm egg shedding for a period of time at least equal to the life cycle of the parasites removed [1, 5, 23–25, 28, 33, 35, 40, 41, 48]. The timing of the deworming is very important in relation to the season of the year, type of grazing programs practiced, and the overall management goals of the operation. The success or failure of these strategically timed programs depend upon a number of factors, of which, one of the most important being the ability of the dewormer to effectively stop parasite eggs being shed back on the pastures, especially during the early part of the grazing season. If the dewormer fails and cattle continue to shed worm eggs back on the pasture following treatment, the benefit for pasture cleanup is greatly reduced or, in many cases, eliminated. The number one goal of strategic deworming cattle is to reduce the buildup of pasture larval contamination, so cattle are not eating a month full of larvae every time they take a mouthful of grass.

THE ECONOMICS OF AN AGGRESSIVE DEWORMING PROGRAM

Performance data of yearling cattle dewormed strategically on pasture and then re-dewormed upon arrival in a feed-yard were compared with non-treated cattle over the same period (see Figure 3.14). These data demonstrated that parasites adversely affected all parameters measured including weight gain, feed conversion, carcass quality, and herd health data. The strategically dewormed steers received a total of four treatments throughout the study using Safe-Guard® for an approximate cost of $1.25–$1.50 per head depending upon weight at the time of treatment or between $5.00 and $6.00 an animal for the entire trial period. At the start of the study and again upon arrival in the feedlot, the treated cattle were dewormed orally with Safe-Guard suspension.

Feedlot Finishing Gain (239 days) data showing long term effects of parasite treatment on pasture.				
Pasture	Control		FBZ	
Feedlot	Control	FBZ	Control	FBZ
No. pens	20	20	20	20
No steers	155	160	159	160
Total gain	584	652	663	686
Daily gain	3.63	4.15	3.86	4.03
Advantage		68 lb	78 lb	103 lb

Oklahoma/Colorado Strategic Deworming Trial

FIGURE 3.14   Feedlot health data showing that pasture treatment affects feedlot performance.

Since the cattle were already being worked for other management reasons, no extra labor cost were required to administer these treatments. While the cattle were on pasture, Safe-Guard was administered twice via a medicated free-choice mineral so again no significant labor cost was involved in any of the deworming treatments (Table 3.1).

The benefits of maintaining cattle relatively parasite-free throughout the trial began with an average advantage of 48.0 pounds per head at the end of a 118-day grazing period. Subsequently during the feeding period, the benefits were magnified with an average additional gain of 50.0 pounds resulting in a total weight of 98.0 pounds for the treated group versus the controls during the entire trial period. During the feeding period, the treated group averaged 0.33 pounds less feed for every pound of gain. None of the treated cattle died during the feeding period compared to four animals that died in the control group (see Figure 3.15). The number of animals pulled

Table 3.1 A "grazing through feedlot deworming performance trial [32]" demonstrated that Safe-Guard® given strategically had a significant production advantage compared with non-dewormed cattle as follows.

	Treatment Group		
Parameters	Non-dewormed Cattle	Dewormed Cattle*	Deworming Advantage
Weight gain on pasture	110.0 lb	158.0 lb	+48.0 lb
Avg. daily gain on pasture	0.93 lb/day	1.34 lb/day	+0.41 lb/day
Weight gained in feedyard	486.0 lb	536.0 lb	+50.0 lb
Avg. daily gain in feedyard	3.85 lb/day	4.46 lb/day	+0.61 lb/day
Feed-to-gain conversion	5.75 lb/lb gain	5.42 lb/lb gain	+0.33 lb/lb gain
Total weight gained	596.0 lb	694.0 lb	+98.0 lb
Percent choice	29.0%	55.2%	+26.2%
No. of animals that died	4	0	100% improvement
No. of animals pulled for Rx	22	4	Greater than 100% improvement

* Treated cattle were dewormed strategically on pasture (treatments at 0, 4, and 8 wks) and again upon arrival into the feedyard with fenbendazole (Safe-Guard®/Panacur®).

Feedlot health data showing that pasture treatment affects feedlot performance.

Pasture	Control		FBZ	
Feedlot	Control	FBZ	Control	FBZ
No. dead	4	0	1	0
No treated	22	13	6	4
Percent of total	4%	29%	13%	9%
No treatments	34	13	6	4
Percent of total	60%	23%	10%	7%

Oklahoma/Colorado Strategic Deworming Trial

FIGURE 3.15 5 Feedlot finishing data (239 days) data showing long-term effects of parasite treatment on pasture.

during the feeding period for unrelated health problems was five times greater in the control than in the treated group (22 versus 4). Additionally, 26.5% more of the treated cattle graded choice than the control cattle. Overall the return on a $6.00 per animal deworming investment netted a return greater than 10-fold just in the weight gain advantage alone. These data demonstrate that an aggressive deworming program applied strategically using a highly effective product such as Safe-Guard can greatly improve the efficiency and profitability of an operation [40].

Deworming, applied strategically, is a valuable tool to prevent production loss and allow animals to reach their maximum genetic potential. A parasite-infected animal can also be fed past the parasitism if the cost of production is not a factor. The more efficient the animal is in terms of genetic potential and management; however, the higher the costs are to feed past the parasitism. Depending on production levels and physiological needs, at some point it becomes nearly impossible to feed past the problem. In a highly efficient animal, all it takes is a few parasites to cause an economic problem. An example of this is feedlot cattle gaining over 4.0 lb/head/day are more susceptible to parasite problems and the effects of parasitism than cattle gaining 2.0 lb/head/day. Achieving weaning weight in calves greater than 700 lb requires a better deworming program that weaning calves at 500 lb. Also, cattle grazing extensive range conditions can be nutritional stressed due to a lack of available forage, and therefore, benefit greatly from deworming even though these cattle most often harbor fewer parasites than cattle raised on lush or adequate pasture situations.

The physiological effect of gastrointestinal parasites is anti-nutrition. The process whereby a 1000 lb Angus steer can be harmed by a few tiny parasites is complicated. Physical damage caused by parasites in the abomasum changes the physiology of the digestive system (see Figure 3.16). One parasite specie, *Ostertagia*, for example, completes it life cycle by spending time as a developing larva in the gastric gland. This larva can live within the gland for months at a time. While this larva is in the gland, it undergoes a molting process, growing and expanding within the gland. The inflamed gastric glands with inhibited larvae can be easily seen on postmortem (see Figure 3.17). The parasite mechanically destroys the gland temporarily shutting down acid production and causing blood leakage back into the gut tract. When a number of parasitic larvae are present in the gastric glands, acid production is reduced, the abomasal pH rises, digestion efficiency is reduced, appetite decreases, and dry matter intake drops off. It only takes several hundred to several thousand parasites to cause economic loss. Internal parasites, in simple terms,

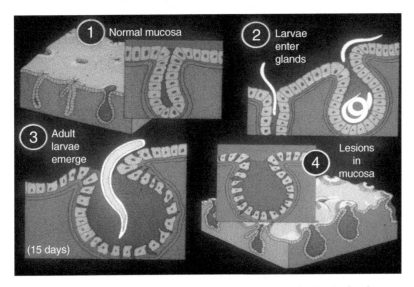

FIGURE 3.16   Parasite larvae destroy gastric glands and reduce acid production in the abomasum.

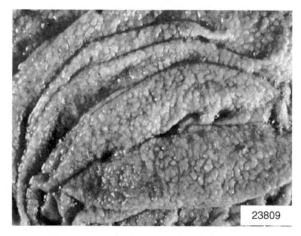

23809

FIGURE 3.17   Inhibited *Ostertagia* larvae on the surface of the abomasum.

are anti-nutrition. Producers spend millions of dollars to improve their animals' nutritional status; however, little is gained if the gastrointestinal tract is riddled with internal parasites. As the grazing animal becomes more and more parasitized, the pH in the abomasum begins to rise and digestion starts to slow down. An aerial view of a pasture with dewormed and non-dewormed cattle grazing separate paddocks, it is clearly shown that the dewormed cattle grazed the short pasture while the poorly grazed pastures were occupied by the wormy cattle (see Figure 3.18).

As the spring to summer progresses for non-treated cattle, the pastures become heavily contaminated, and when the worm burdens build within the animals, problems start to occur within the gastrointestinal tract. Of course, as the worm burdens build to a high level in the grazing animals, clinical signs of parasitism starts to show, and the physiological conditions of the gut

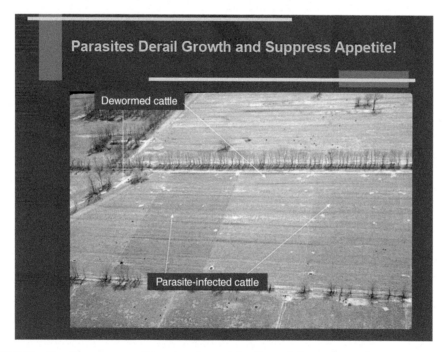

FIGURE 3.18   Parasites cause appetite suppression and derail growth in grazing cattle.

start to change which in turn seem to trigger the larvae to stop development and to inhibit or become inhibited. In parts of the country where grazing starts in March, inhibition starts to occur approximately three months later, thus later in May or June, whereas in the parts of the country where grazing begins later in April, May, or June, inhibition does not start to occur until later in the summer or early fall (see Figure 3.19). Keeping parasite levels low on the pasture is the single best method of preventing inhibition from occurring. **Internal parasites can also adversely affect the immune system**. Recent data indicate that gastrointestinal parasites have a strong effect on the animal's immune system [19, 26, 40]. One benefit of deworming, that is often overlooked, is its impact on the effectiveness of vaccinations (see Figure 3.20). Cows that are infected by parasites

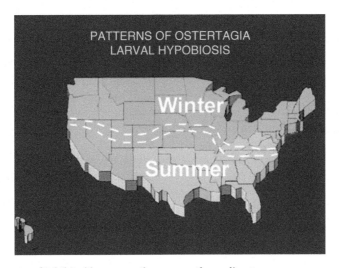

FIGURE 3.19   Patterns of inhibited larvae, northern vs southern climate.

ELSEVIER

Available online at www.sciencedirect.com

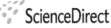
ScienceDirect

Veterinary Parasitology 148 (2007) 14–20

veterinary
parasitology

www.elsevier.com/locate/vetpar

Infection with parasitic nematodes confounds vaccination efficacy

Joseph F. Urban Jr.[a,*], Nina R. Steenhard[b], Gloria I. Solano-Aguilar[a], Harry D. Dawson[a], Onyinye I. Iweala[c], Cathryn R. Nagler[c], Gregory S. Noland[d], Nirbhay Kumar[d], Robert M. Anthony[e], Terez Shea-Donohue[f], Joel Weinstock[g], William C. Gause[h]

[a] Diet, Genomics, and Immunology Laboratory, Beltsville Human Nutrition Research Center, Agricultural Research Service,
United States Department of Agriculture, Beltsville, MD 20705, United States
[b] Danish Centre for Experimental Parasitology, Department of Veterinary Pathobiology, Copenhagen University,
DK-1870 Frederiksberg C, Denmark
[c] Center for Immunology and Inflammatory Diseases, Division of Rheumatology, Allergy, and Immunology,
Massachusetts General Hospital, Charlestown, MA 02129, United States
[d] Department of Molecular Microbiology and Immunology, The Johns Hopkins University Bloomberg School of Public Health,
Baltimore, MD 21205, United States

FIGURE 3.20   Publication describing parasite effect on vaccine efficacy.

have compromised immune systems caused by the negative nutritional impact gastrointestinal parasites have on the immune system. In addition to this indirect impact, some parasites have a direct impact on the immune system through mechanical damage they cause to the animal itself.

Immune suppression occurs when parasites actively hinder one or more of the host's defense mechanisms. For example, *Ostertagia* secrete substances that suppress the host's immune system. Because the *Ostertagia* larvae damage the glands of the abomasum during development, they disrupt metabolism and are thought to affect development of immunity simply by reducing the necessary substances such as protein and trace minerals. It has been shown that some parasites can cause cows to create immune cells that shut down the production of antibodies and macrophages, key components in a functioning immune system. Such measures ensure that the parasite will survive and be able to reproduce in the cow. These immune-suppressive tactics that protect the parasite leave the cow susceptible to other invaders such as bacteria and viruses. As noted previously, immune suppression interferes with the host's ability to respond to a vaccination, our most effective tool for preventing infectious diseases [40].

Strategic deworming is based on seasonal parasitic contamination patterns: Gastrointestinal parasites have two basic functions in life; the first function is to completely live off the animals they invade while the second function is to reproduce into the environment by producing eggs that pass out of the animals with the feces. The reproductive goal is to contaminate the environment of their host animals, thus maintaining their life cycle keeping their species alive. Fortunately, in most parts of the country, parasitic larvae have a seasonal survival and infection pattern. When a parasite egg is shed on the pasture in the feces, this egg begins development, embryonating into a first-stage larva (L_1), then molting into a second-stage larva (L_2), and finally molts again into a third and infective stage larva (L_3). During the first two larval stages in the fecal pat, the larva is fairly immobile staying in the fecal pat feeding off the bacteria and other debris found in the feces.

Egg development is greatly dependent upon temperature and moisture. Eggs that are passed in the middle of winter will not develop until warm weather returns in the spring. Eggs that are passed in the middle of drought or other unfavorable conditions may develop into infective larvae in the feces but without moisture cannot move away from the pat where they can be consumed by a host animal. Eggs that are shed during the summer grazing season, however, can develop into infective larvae in just a few days if temperatures are warm and moisture is plentiful (see Figure 3.21). Also, the eggs shed on the pastures earlier in the year, but that have been dormant

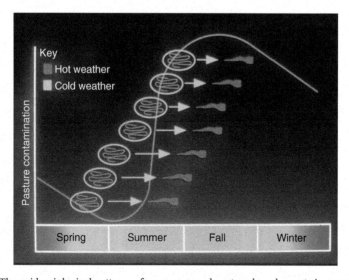

FIGURE 3.21 The epidemiological patterns of worm egg and pasture larval counts in a normal year.

in the environment will develop at this time as well. Because of this, pasture contamination can build rapidly especially during rainy conditions or where moisture is sufficient to allow the larvae to move away from the fecal pats onto the vegetation. As the seasonal pattern of infective larvae available to the cattle increases, the cattle grazing these pastures stop growing, and in some cases, actually lose weight some of which they had gained previously (see Figure 3.22).

During the final molt into an infective L_3 larva, this developing infective L_3 larva maintains an external sheath covering that provides extra protection from environmental conditions allowing L_3 larvae to survive severe winter or summer drought conditions (see Figure 3.23). This sheath also

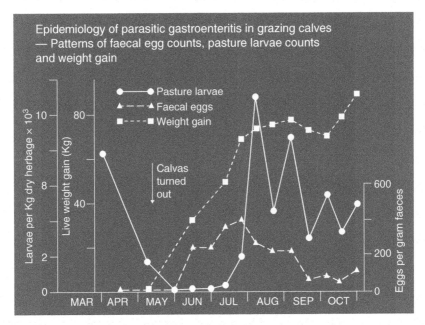

FIGURE 3.22   Seasonal parasite contamination adversely affecting weight gain during the last part of the grazing season.

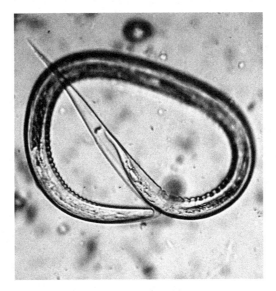

FIGURE 3.23   Infective larvae with protective outer sheath which prevents feeding, so larva must live off stored food supply.

prevents the L$_3$ larvae from feeding because the mouth parts are covered with the sheath forcing the L$_3$ larvae to live off internal stored food supply. Occasionally, infective larvae will show up in a fecal float (see Figure 3.24). Because of this feeding limitation, L$_3$ larvae have a limited life span especially after winter survival. In the spring when temperatures begin to warm and grass begins to grow, the infective L$_3$ larvae which have survived the winter become active moving with moisture trails away from the fecal pat onto the vegetation in order to be consumed by grazing cattle When temperatures are sufficiently warm (>65–70 °F), the larvae will move continuously using up internal body food supplies while trying to find a host animal. It appears that somewhere between two and three months (60–90 days) into the grazing season, the larvae surviving the winter will expire and die if no host is found.

Strategic deworming works during this period of time by preventing worm egg contamination and repopulation of the pastures during the first three months of the grazing season while the pasture are "naturally becoming de-contaminated." The specific goals of strategic deworming are to prevent parasite contamination in the environment by reducing the ability of the gastrointestinal parasites to reproduce during the first three months of the grazing season (see Figures 3.25–3.27).

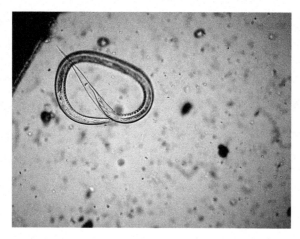

FIGURE 3.24   Infective larvae found on a fecal exam.

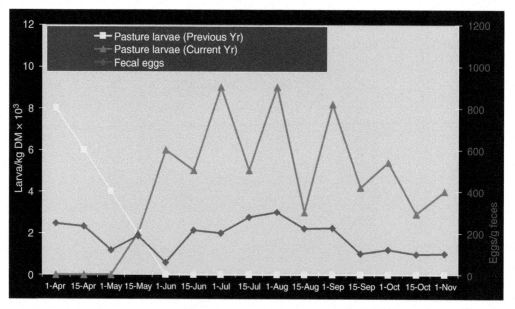

FIGURE 3.25   Epidemiological patterns of seasonal worm egg and pasture larval counts.

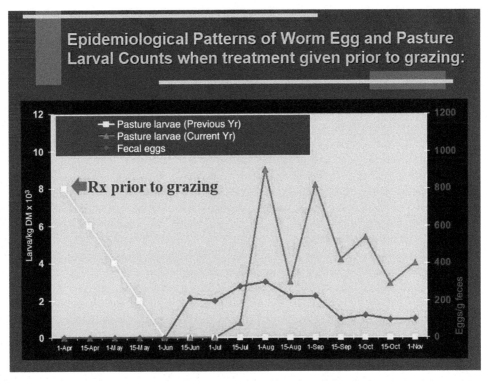

FIGURE 3.26   Deworming prior to grazing – effect on pasture contamination.

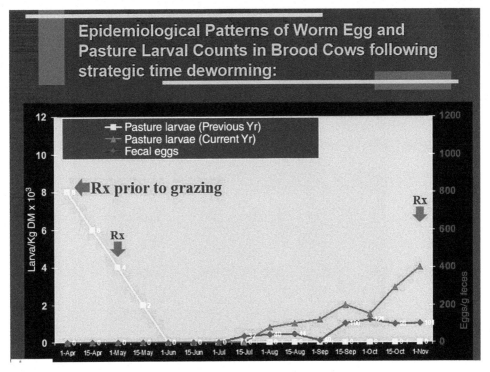

FIGURE 3.27   Epidemiological patterns of worm egg and pasture larval counts following both a winter and mid-spring deworming.

Strategic deworming is simply the use of dewormers to interrupt the life cycle of the parasites by allowing the cattle to consume infective larvae while grazing but timing treatment to kill these parasites before they have time to develop into an adult parasite producing eggs. The cattle work like vacuum cleaners picking up larvae while grazing but these larvae are killed by strategic treatment before they have a chance to recontaminate the environment. If no parasite eggs are shed on the pastures for the first three months, the second three months of grazing will be relatively parasite-free. Strategic deworming, therefore, provides approximately six months of "parasite-safe" pastures (see Figure 3.28).

Strategic deworming recommendations for cow/calf operations: This first goal of strategic deworming is to make sure the cattle are parasite-free during the winter and at the beginning of the grazing season. If cattle are harboring adult worm population in late winter or early spring, these parasites will begin contaminating the pastures immediately as temperatures warm up. In most parts of the United States, parasite challenge is minimal during the winter months (see Figure 3.29). Cattle dewormed at the beginning of winter in late November or early December will most often remain relatively parasite-free until the following spring (see Figure 3.30). The dewormer used must have a high degree of efficacy; otherwise, a second treatment given in early spring is required to remove all adult parasites before grazing begins.

Strategic deworming occurs after spring grazing begins. This spring deworming(s) needs to be given after the cattle have had a chance to graze but before the invading larvae have developed into adult parasites. Grazing cattle begin consuming the larvae as soon as they begin grazing. Within six weeks after ingestion, larvae will have time to reach maturation to an adult and begin laying worm eggs. This is the ideal time when the cattle should be dewormed strategically to prevent worm egg contamination back on the pastures In adult cows, it takes approximately six weeks from the time of larval ingestion until an egg-laying adult worm is present whereas with younger animals this time period is shorter. A treatment given six weeks after spring grazing in brood cows will remove all parasites ingested during the first six weeks of grazing. Even if cattle ingest larvae immediately following treatment, it will be another six weeks before adult parasites are present. This strategic spring treatment in adult cows prevents worm egg shedding for the first 12 weeks or 3 months of the grazing season. Therefore, adult cows given a deworming in late November or early December and then again six weeks after spring grazing begins, prevents parasite contamination of the environment for at least six months. These strategically treated animals would remain parasite-free throughout the winter and for at least 3 months (12 weeks) into the grazing season, the spring parasite contamination cycle is broken. Research using "split pasture" design indicates

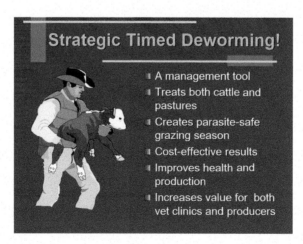

FIGURE 3.28 Strategic timed deworming provides beef producers increased value to their herd.

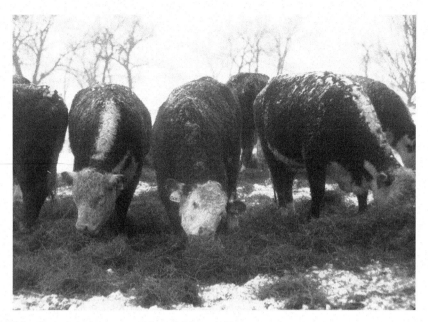

FIGURE 3.29   Overwintering cows can have high maintenance costs.

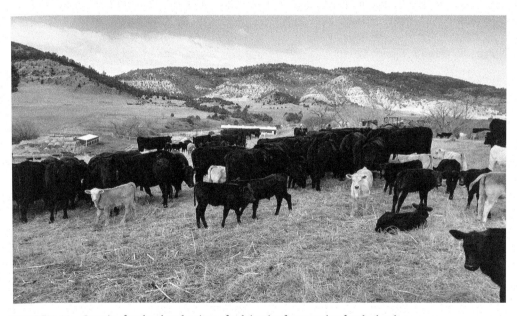

FIGURE 3.30   Parasite-free herd at the time of calving is of great value for the herd.

that yearly parasite contamination levels can be reduced by 80% or greater for the entire season (see Figures 3.31 and 3.32) [1, 4, 22-24, 40, 47, 48].

In southern United States and parts of the country where grazing begins prior to 1st April, two spring dewormings given six weeks apart is often recommended. Example: if spring grazing starts the first week in March, the first strategic deworming would occur around the 15th of April with a second deworming during the last week in May or the first week in June (see Figure 3.33). This is necessary whenever the length of the season is greater than 150–180 days (see Figure 3.34).

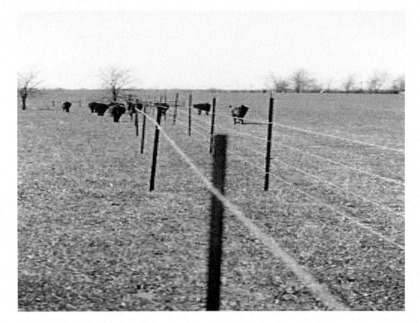

FIGURE 3.31   Split pasture design with double strand protection.

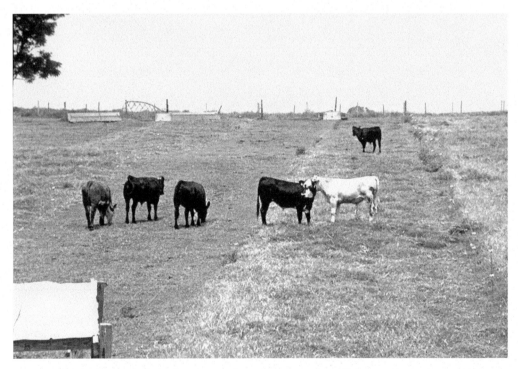

FIGURE 3.32   Split pasture design is necessary in studying treatment effects on pasture.

Strategic deworming recommendations for grazing yearling heifers and stocker operations: The deworming strategy is designed to be more aggressive for younger cattle than it is for older cattle. The larval development time within adult cattle is longer than it is in yearling

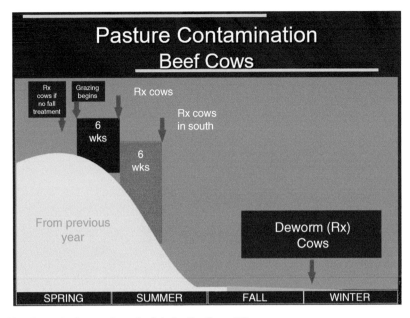

FIGURE 3.33   Strategic deworming schedule for Southern US.

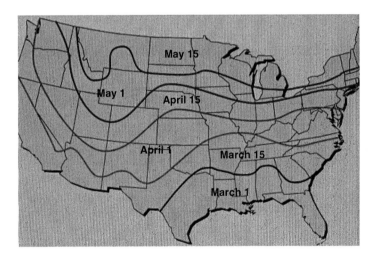

FIGURE 3.34   Treatment zones based on expected start for grass growth.

cattle and young calves due to an increased level of immunity against larval infestation by the older animals. The time it takes from larval ingestion until a mature adult parasite is present in young animals can be as rapid as three weeks in young calves up to four weeks in yearling cattle or bred heifers. To achieve parasite-free status during the first 12 weeks of the grazing season, the strategic deworming recommendations for young calves or yearling cattle is for these animals to be free of parasites at the beginning of the grazing season and then to receive two additional deworming, the first given 4 weeks after grazing begins and the second given 4 weeks later (see Figure 3.35). This program is called a "0–4–8 week" program. Since it will be another 4 weeks after the last deworming before worm eggs are shed, this program protects the young animals from shedding worm eggs back on the pasture for 12 weeks much like the strategic program for adult cows.

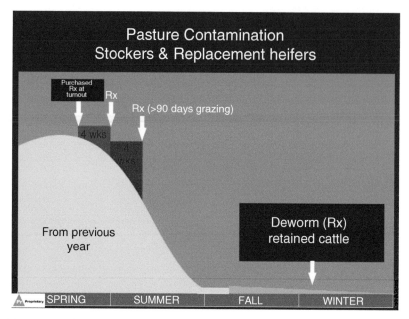

FIGURE 3.35   Strategic deworming for stockers and replacement heifers.

The timing of when dewormer use can have the greatest benefit and the number of deworming necessary to achieve this benefit varies from location to location in the country but the principals involved remain the same. The main reason the timing varies from location to location is due to the seasonal weather patterns. The intensity of a deworming program is also often dictated by the efficiency of the operation or goals of the operation where a purebred operation may use a more aggressive deworming strategy than a commercial operation. Some producers use different formulations of dewormers at different times of the year depending on whether the animals are on pasture or are being fed a supplement. Some producers alternate their deworming products depending upon the season. Over all, deworming given at the right time with the right product can add to the efficiency and economics of a deworming strategy.

Pour-on failures and avermectin/milbemycin (endectocide) resistance: Endectocides are compounds that demonstrate the ability to kill internal and external parasites in cattle [2, 10, 20, 21, 35, 48]. Although these endectocide compounds have showed efficacy against internal parasites, the failure of the endectocide pour-ons to eliminate worm egg shedding was identified soon after the endectocide pour-ons were first introduced on the US market [7, 13, 19]. This continual shedding predisposed the surviving parasites and their progeny to the development of parasite resistance to the avermectin and milbemycin family of compounds which are used in the pour-on formulations (see Figure 3.36). Since parasite survival and continual egg shedding is occurring while these chemical compounds are still active in the animals and their feces, both the worms themselves and their eggs are being shed on the pasture after exposure to the chemical compounds or residue of the compounds in the feces. This reduced efficacy and continual product exposure by the parasites over time creates the potential for parasite resistance to develop to these compounds [2, 7, 13, 19, 29, 30, 32, 36].

The reason for the reduced efficacy with endectocide pour-ons has been identified as the lack of consistent and adequate level of absorption by the endectocide pour-ons into the bloodstream when compared to injectable formulations of the same products [7, 17, 29]. Blood level determinations following treatment with doramectin in an injectable formulation demonstrated 90%

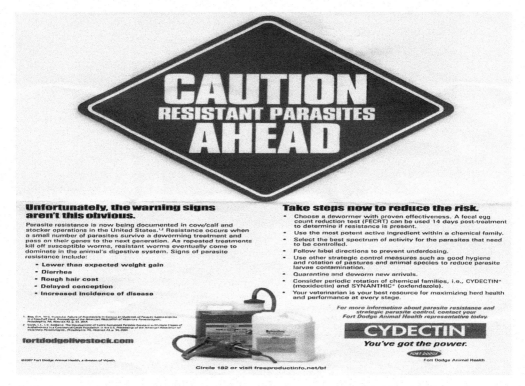

FIGURE 3.36   Caution: resistant parasites ahead.

absorbed while the pour-on formulation was only 15% absorbed as described by Pfizer, Inc. [16], as follows:

- 200 mg/kg injectable will deliver maximum concentrate in plasma 32 ng/ml.
- 500 mg/kg pour-on will deliver maximum concentrate in plasma 12 ng/ml.

This reduced blood level (12 versus 32 ng/ml) indicates that many animals may not be receiving a therapeutic dose following treatment with endectocide pour-on formulations and the parasites and their offspring are predisposed to parasite resistance. Also, the adult parasites and newly developing adults that survive pour-on treatment continue to produce eggs that are shed back into the environment of the animals, therefore, rendering these pour-on products unsuitable for use in a strategic deworming program.

The problem with the reduced blood levels exhibited by the pour-ons is compounded by the "persistent efficacy" exhibited by most of the endectocide pour-on products [16]. Based on FDA approvals, these products exhibit persistent residues in the animals ranging from 14 to 42 days following treatment depending upon the product and species of parasite involved. The persistent residues indicate prolonged exposure of the surviving parasites and parasite offspring to endectocide, thereby greatly increasing the chance for the development of parasite resistance to these compounds. Endectocide pour-ons that have poor efficacy against internal parasites may promote resistance. Recent data, in fact, indicate that parasite resistance is now a real threat in operations where the pour-ons have been used for several years or more [7, 13, 31, 39]. Endectocide pour-ons have become popular among cattlemen because of ease of application and reduced cattle stress compared to injectable formulations of the same product. However, recent field trials have indicated, in some cases, that these pour-ons lack sufficient efficacy to be considered an efficient dewormer. Three fears result from this lack of efficacy:

1. Production losses occurring due to failure of pour-ons to remove internal worm burden.

2. Continued egg shedding in pastures with continued parasite contamination in the environment.

3. Parasites and parasite eggs left following treatment most likely develop resistance to compound used (Table 3.2).

University trial measuring duration of protection with endectocide pour-ons demonstrated low level of efficacy with two popular endectocide pour-ons: The persistent efficacy indicated on the label claims protection from reinfection during the persistent period. Once the animal is reinfected, the parasite undergoes a prepatent period during which time it develops into an adult stage. Another four to six weeks are required before worm eggs should appear in feces. In the above study, none of the pour-on chemistry exceeded 85% reduction in fecal worm counts. The WAAVP (World Association for the Advancement of Veterinary Parasitology) has set a standard that if the efficacy of a product does not reduce worm egg counts greater than 90% following treatment, this product is designated as a "parasite-resistant product [49]."

Summary of pour-on failures to adequately control gastrointestinal parasites:

- The control of gastrointestinal and the efficacy of dewormers have become economically more important as the genetic potential of cattle improves.

- Incomplete parasite control by the endectocide pour-ons means cattle will continue shedding parasite eggs on pasture, leading to increased parasite burdens further into the grazing period, the potential for the development of parasite resistance, and failure of strategic deworming programs to be effective.

- Producers can ensure their animals are parasite-free by having fecal samples run for parasite eggs following treatment.

Fecal worm egg counts and the fecal egg reduction test (FECRT) are valuable tools to determine the parasite status within a herd. The Wisconsin Modified Fecal Flotation Method [6] is recommended (see Figures 3.37–3.39). The most important part in determining parasite contamination level is the fecal examination technique used. There is a lot of valuable information in the fecal pat (see Figure 3.40). Using the wrong fecal technique will lead to erroneous

Table 3.2   A trial conducted at Louisiana State University [37] by Dr. Williams indicates extended efficacy does not occur and parasite resistance is probable for ivermectin pour-on or doramectin pour-on formulations using the "Fecal Egg Count Reduction Test."

Treatment* Group	Days Post Treatment (Worm Eggs/3 g Samples)									
	0	7	14	21	28	35	42	49	56	70
Controls	193.7	96.8	93.0	100.7	73.1	53.0	77.0	111.3	98.3	55.5
Ivermectin	128.2	26.1	53.7	24.6	19.0	24.6	12.1	27.8	32.2	24.8
% Efficacy		73%	43%	76%	74%	54%	85%	75%	68%	56%
Doramectin	217.8	36.7	42.5	41.5	37.2	27.3	18.1	33.6	21.1	20.0
% Efficacy		62%	55%	59%	50%	49%	77%	70%	79%	64%

* Ivermectin pour-on (Ivomec® pour-on – Boehringer) and doramectin pour-on (Dectomax® – Pfizer).
Source: von Samson-Himmelstjerna and Blackhall [37]/with permission of Elsevier.

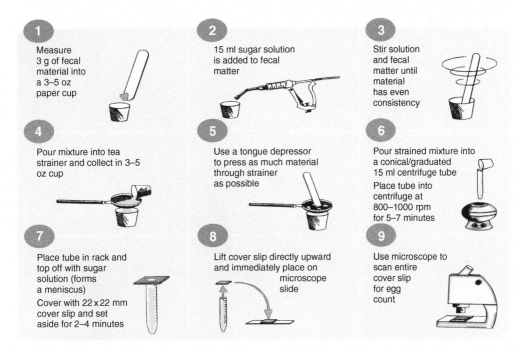

FIGURE 3.37   Modified Wisconsin Sugar Flotation Method.

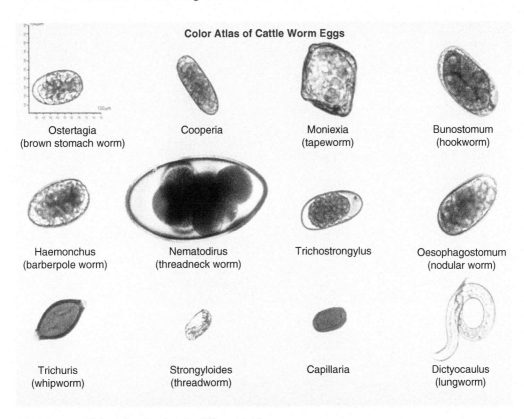

FIGURE 3.38   Color atlas showing the different cattle worm eggs.

Dairy and Beef Cattle Parasite Evaluation Form

PEC ☐   Mail In ☐   Page_____ of_____

Collection Date:		Consultant:	Dr. Don Bliss
Name of Farm:		Sponsor:	
Producer's Name:		Sponsor Contact:	
Producer's Address:		Sponsor Address:	
City	Phone	City	Phone
State	Zip	Fax	State	Zip	Fax
E-Mail:		Representative:	

Sample ID	Animal ID	Contamination Level*	Stomach Worm	Nematodirus	Cooperia	Hookworm	Threadworm	Whipworm	Nodular Worm	Tapeworm	Coccidia	Total Count (EPG)**	Treatment Date month/day/year	Product Used
													Enter after test results recorded	

*1 = pasture, 2 = limited pasture, 3 = dry lot/partial confinement, 4 = total confinement year round

**(+ = 1-10) (++ = 11-50) (+++ =>51)

COMMENTS:

Donald H. Bliss, Ph.D.
MidAmerica Ag. Research
3705 Sequoia Trail
Verona, WI 53593

Eggs/Pound Manure ☐

Sponsor's E-mail:

For additional information and submission forms, visit: www.midamericaagresearch.net

Total count x 150 = Eggs per pound

FIGURE 3.39   Dairy and beef cattle parasite evaluation form.

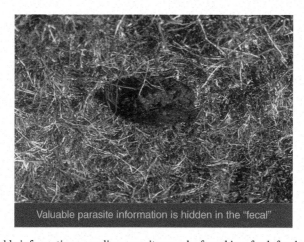

Valuable parasite information is hidden in the "fecal"

FIGURE 3.40   Valuable information regarding parasites can be found in a fresh fecal pat.

information, an incorrect diagnosis, and a flawed recommendation. This is especially true for cattle harboring a subclinical level of parasites. Most commercial fecal exams kits sold to veterinary clinics such as the "Fecalyzer" or "McMasters" are unsuitable for determining worm egg counts in cattle. These techniques were developed for sheep or small animal parasite diagnosis where a low fecal output and high worm egg counts are common. Adult beef cows produce 30–50 pounds of manure a day so the technique used must be very sensitive. A sugar flotation test such as the Modified Wisconsin Centrifugal Flotation Method is the only method sensitive enough to provide satisfactory results in brood cows. The necessary concentration of sugar to float worm eggs out of the fecal material is 1.0 lb white table sugar/12 oz of hot water (454 g of sugar in 355 ml of water).

Advantages of the "Modified Wisconsin Sugar Flotation Method":

1. Requires no specialized equipment and can be conducted in a small area, even under field conditions.

2. Can be used to examine a large number of samples in a short period of time. One person can set up 100 samples in a couple of hours.

3. This technique is sensitive enough to detect low egg counts in lactating dairy cows producing 80–100 lb of manure a day.

4. This technique is sensitive enough to detect eggs from non-prolific worm species such as whipworms (*Trichuris*) and threadneck worms (*Nematodirus*).

5. This technique breaks up tapeworm proglottids allowing tapeworm (*Moniezia*, *Anoplocephala*, and *Taenia*) eggs for easy detection.

6. This technique is sensitive enough to float coccidia, cryptosporidium, and giardia cysts and for species identification of coccidia oocysts.

7. This technique is sensitive enough to show the difference in egg shedding associated with various dewormers and is the recommended technique for the FECRT (fecal egg count reduction test).

8. Does not distort worm eggs thus allowing general parasite genus identification through egg morphology.

9. Can be used to float lungworm (*Dictyocaulus*) and threadworm (*Strongyloides*) larvae from fresh rectal fecal samples.

10. Samples do not have to be read immediately. Prepared samples can be stored in a refrigerator for several days before reading if necessary.

INTERPRETATION OF FECAL WORM EGG COUNTS IN CATTLE USING "THE MODIFIED WISCONSIN SUGAR FLOTATION TECHNIQUE"

Understanding the meaning of worm egg counts will provide veterinarians and producers the necessary insight needed to help build a seasonal deworming strategy for a particular dairy, beef, or feedlot operation. Factors that affect fecal worm egg shedding are numerous, so a number of these factors need to be considered every time an analysis is made and a fair assessment of the worm egg counts generated. The age of the animal, the season of the year, the amount of exposure to pasture, the condition of the pasture, and the stocking rate of the animals on a particular pasture, all affect worm egg counts. The amount of rainfall or moisture and the number of degree days with temperatures sufficient to promote parasite develop for a particular operation are also very important to egg count interpretation. Other factors to be considered are the health of the animals, the stage of gestation, stage of lactation, and the numbers and type of parasites present at each examination.

The problem with a simple guide (listed below) is that due to an innate immune response, non-treated adult brood cows often have their highest counts in the spring when worm burdens are the lowest and the lowest counts in the fall when the worm burdens are at their highest level. For calves and yearling cattle, the opposite is true such that worm egg counts increase as the season progresses. In calves and yearling cattle, however, the type of parasite present may be more important than the overall count. Most importantly, worm egg counts determine future contamination of the pasture. 1 egg/3 g equals 150 eggs/lb of manure. A worm egg count of 10 means 1500 egg/lb of manure or 75,000 eggs (in 50 lb of manure) excreted daily per cow back into their environment.

A. **Simple worm egg count guide:** Simple guide assessing whether the overall average worm egg counts are low, moderate, or high are as follows:

Category	Low	Moderate	High
Cows	5 or less	6–20	Greater than 20
Yearlings	1 or 10	11–30	Greater than 30
Calves	1–20	21–50	Greater than 50

B. **Worm egg count guide for parasites in calves and yearling cattle:** Parasites in calves or yearling cattle often differ from adult animals depending upon how the youngstock are raised. A number of the parasites commonly found in young cattle are sufficiently pathogenic such that the animals develop a strong immunity against the parasites later in life and, therefore, some parasites common in young cattle are rarely found once the animals mature. This state of immunity has been given the term known as "age immunity." Nematodirus (threadneck worm) is probably the most well-known cattle parasite that is routinely found in yearling cattle but almost never found in mature adult cows. Nematodirus is very pathogenic in young animals and, therefore, the infected cattle appear to develop a very strong immunity against reinfection later in life. Several other parasites commonly found in very young calves (even nursing calves on pasture) are: whipworms (*Trichuris*) and threadworms (*Strongyloides*). Therefore, based on the immune status and presence of barnyard infections in younger cattle, the interpretation of worm egg count in young cattle will be different than adult cattle and are as follows:

Assessing differential fecal worm egg counts in calves and yearling cattle as to whether they are low, moderate, or high based on parasite or parasite category:

Categories	Parasite name	Low	Moderate	High
Stomach worms	(Hot complex)*	10 or less	10–50	>50
Nematodirus	Threadneck	1–3	4–10	>10
Trichuris	Whipworm	1–3	4–10	>10
Bunostomum	Hookworm	1–5	6–10	>10
Strongyloides	Threadworm	5 or less	5–25	>25
Oesophagostomum	Nodular worm	5 or less	5–25	>25
*Moniezia***	Tapeworm	1–10 (+)	11–50 (++)	>50 (+++)

* *Haemonchus*, *Ostertagia*, and *Trichostrongylus*.

** Tapeworm eggs are released from proglottids, so specific counts are not conducted.

C. **Worm egg count guide for dairy cattle:** Interpretations and Treatment Recommendations with Dairy Cattle Based on Fecal Exams are as follows:

1. All lactating dairy cows with positive worm egg counts during the first trimester of lactation should be dewormed. The ideal goal for lactating dairy cows is to be worm-free during the first 100 days following calving when nutritional demands required by production are the greatest.

2. Dry cows with positive worm egg counts should be dewormed at the time of or just prior to freshening. Deworming can be given during the final stages of transition as long as reinfection does not occur prior to calving.

3. Dairy cows held in total confinement or given access to dirt yards or dry lots with positive worm egg counts should be dewormed once a year either in late fall or prior to freshening, otherwise no deworming is necessary in confined dairy cows.

4. Calves and yearling animals held in confinement, on the other hand, can harbor significant "barnyard infections." Barnyard infections are usually made up of whipworms, threadworms, tapeworms, Nematodirus, and hookworms. These animals may require frequent treatment (sometimes monthly) to prevent production loss.

5. Worm egg counts found in late lactation seem to have little economic impact on these animals. Deworming cows in late lactation should only be done when deworming the entire herd going into winter housing conditions to make sure all cows are worm-free during winter.

D. **Worm egg count guide for brood cows and calves:**

1. Worm egg counts are not as important in grazing beef cattle as it is in dairy cattle for determining whether to deworm or not since these animals are all on pasture and exposed to parasitism seasonally. Where fecal worm egg counts often prove advantageous for the veterinarian is with producers who doubt whether parasitism is present in their herds. A positive fecal demonstrates the presence of parasites and the need for strategic timed deworming is recommended. Cows should always be negative during the winter months when maintenance costs are the highest.

2. Fecal worm egg counts in beef cattle should be conducted to make sure the dewormers used are working. Strategic deworming guidelines for deworming beef cattle indicate key deworming times are in late fall after the end of the summer grazing season and again once or twice six weeks apart (depending upon location) in mid-spring soon after the beginning of spring grazing to reduce parasite challenge on pasture. Branding time is a great time to treat young calves for parasites acquired on the calving pasture before the grazing season gets underway (see Figure 3.41). There is a common parasite found in bedding around the calving pasture called the threadworm (*Strongyloides*) and causes nonspecific "white scours." Infection can be severe especially during a wet calving season (see Figure 3.42). Calves can become infected through the skin as soon as they hit the ground during the birthing process. Adult *Strongyloides* breed and lay eggs outside the host animals, the eggs are embroynated when passed. These eggs develop into larvae on pasture and infect the calves immediately upon contact. The *Strongyloides* will eventually self-cure but in the meantime considerable damage is caused to the calves. It is not uncommon for beef producers across the Midwest to lose calves to these scours.

3. Fecal worm egg counts taken in the winter or a minimum of two weeks following the fall deworming will determine whether the dewormer used is working.

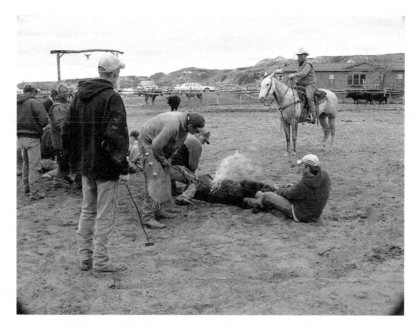

FIGURE 3.41   Branding calves in North Dakota.

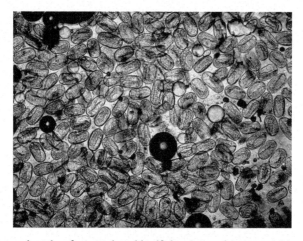

FIGURE 3.42   Fecal samples taken from 10-day-old calf showing a white scour with a very heavy thread-worm (Strongyloides) infection.

E. **Worm egg count guide for confined feedlot beef cattle:**
1. Cattle with positive fecal worm egg counts should be dewormed upon arrival as long as the positive counts average more than 5 eggs/3 g and over 70% of the cattle tested showing positive counts. Deworming 800 lb steers with an average worm egg count of 8 eggs/3 g demonstrated an extra 25 lb gain for the feeding period.
2. For best results, a minimum of 20 samples should be analyzed for this interpretation especially where cattle from different sources are mixed together as stockers on pasture or in a background yard or feedlot.
3. Cattle showing positive worm egg counts after arrival into a feedyard should be dewormed or re-dewormed when average counts are greater than 10 eggs/3 g due to endecticide resistance or product failure. Either a change in dewormer or concomitant use of two different classes of dewormer is usually necessary to solve this problem.

FECAL EGG COUNT REDUCTION TEST (FECRT)

The World Association for the Advancement of Veterinary Parasitology (WAAVP) Guidelines for Anthelmintic Testing recommends the FECRT for parasite resistance testing [38]. This procedure simply involves taking a random fecal sampling of 5–10% of the herd at the time of deworming application followed by a second sampling taken 10–15 days later from a similar number of animals. If the worm egg counts taken after treatment are not reduced by 90% or greater, parasite resistance is suspected and an unrelated dewormer should be used.

PRODUCT PROFILE OF FENBENDAZOLE (SAFE-GUARD®/PANACUR® – MERCK ANIMAL HEALTH)

Fenbendazole was approved for equine in the United States in 1979, for cattle in 1984, for swine in 1986, and for lactating dairy cows in 1996. Fenbendazole has been used in hundreds of thousands of animals over the past 25 years with a flawless safety record. For cattle, fenbendazole is approved as an oral suspension, oral paste, in a free-choice mineral to be fed over a three to six period, in a medicated block to be fed over three days, as a top-dress crumble, pellet, or meal or can be mixed in the ration in a one-day feeding. Research data on the efficacy of fenbendazole given in a single dose versus a single dose spread multiple days was excellent either way [12, 34, 43]. These data indicate that fenbendazole accumulates in the parasite and when sufficient product is ingested over time, the parasite is destroyed. Fenbendazole's high degree of efficacy in swine with an approved label recommendation to be fed over three to 12 days is proof of this particular valuable characteristic especially with non-handling formulations of fenbendazole. Every time cattle are worked, injury to the animals or crew working the cattle can happen, so a dewormer that can be administered in a medicated free-choice mineral, cubes, or other non-handling feedgrade formulation is a valuable tool (see Figures 3.43–3.45). Deworming animals in a chute or in a cattle-working alley is time-consuming, can be harmful to the animals, and hard on the people working the cattle (see Figures 3.46 and 3.47). Being able to deworm animals without touching them reduces both stress and working cost since labor costs need to be added to the drug costs when working cattle

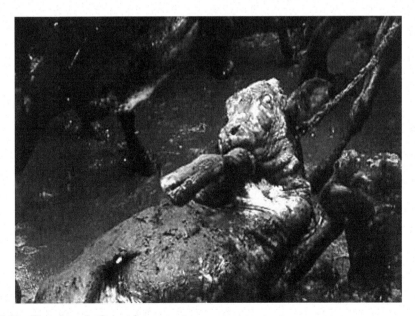

FIGURE 3.43   Steer down in the mud.

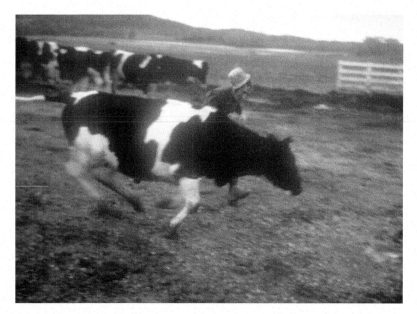

FIGURE 3.44   Man chasing a dairy heifer.

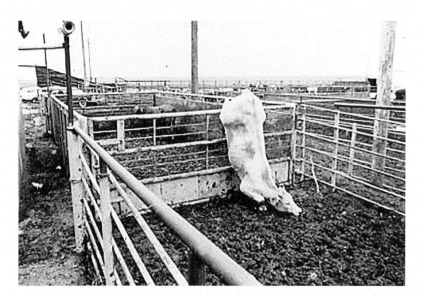

FIGURE 3.45   Steer stuck on scale.

for treatment. With non-handling formulations of fenbendazole (Safe-Guard/Panacur – Merck Animal Health), cattle deworm themselves by simply consuming fenbendazole-medicated supplements (see Figures 3.48–3.50). Safe-Guard medicated mineral is an excellent way to deworm brood cows with since no animal handling is required (see Figure 3.51). Safe-Guard has no smell or taste so the cows don't know they are receiving treatment. Some cattle will come to the mineral feeders every day while other cows will come up and hangout for a bit around the feeders and then you don't see them again for a couple days. The way safe-Guard works is that it is cumulative in the parasite so when the parasite comes in contact with the product it can ingest or absorbs the product but can't excrete the product so when the cattle finally gets back to the feeder it then receives its

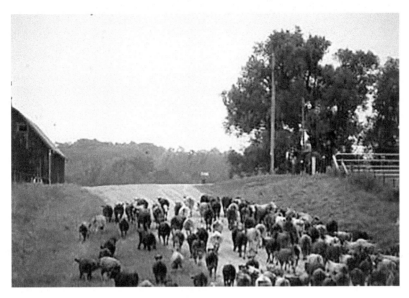

FIGURE 3.46 Working cattle in Wisconsin using dogs to help.

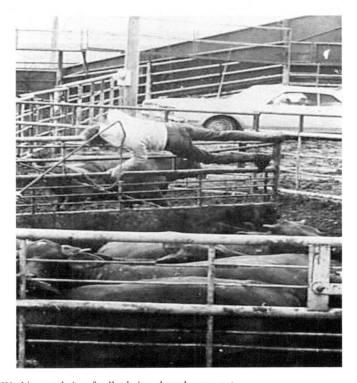

FIGURE 3.47 Working cattle in a feedlot being chased over a gate.

adequate dose to provide excellent efficacy [14]. The mineral is designed to be eaten over a four to six day period but if it takes slightly longer it is no problem (there is a 13-day meat withdrawal when Safe-Guard is administer in the mineral).

Fenbendazole (Safe-Guard – Merck Animal Health) has a 100× margin of safety and can be used at any stage of gestation or lactation safely. Fenbendazole is also safe for the environment

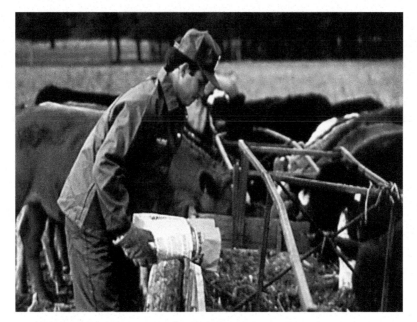

FIGURE 3.48   Topdressing cattle feed with Safe-Guard pellets.

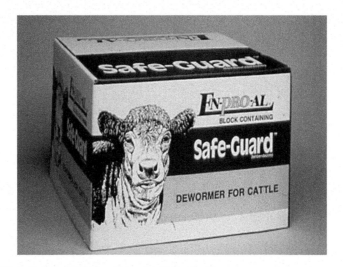

FIGURE 3.49   25 lb Safe-Guard® block will treat 8200 lb of cattle.

with no detrimental effects on fecal fauna such as dung beetles. The reason for fenbendazole's high degree of safety is due to its mode of action and ability to kill parasites by destroying their ability to metabolize food stuff while nearly all other dewormers kill by destroying the nervous system of the parasite. By destroying the ability of the parasite to utilize food stuff, it kills the parasites rapidly removing them within the first 24 hours after product exposure.

Recent data following fecal worm egg counts following treatment with different formulations demonstrated equally high efficacy levels between the different formulations. No differences were observed in the efficacy levels achieved between different formulations of fenbendazole based on fecal egg counts (Table 3.3) [23].

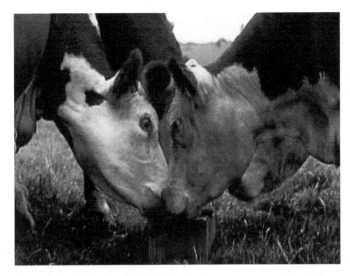

FIGURE 3.50   Cows licking Safe-Guard® medicated block.

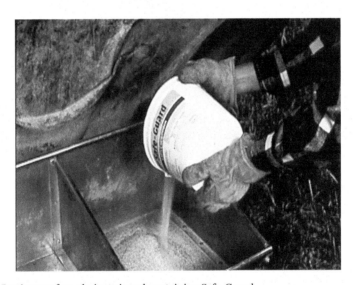

FIGURE 3.51   Putting out free-choice mineral containing Safe-Guard.

Table 3.3   Fecal worm egg counts taken one to two weeks following treatment with fenbendazole (FBZ) using different formulations.

Formulation Containing FBZ	Oral Suspension	Blocks	Medicated Mineral	Medicated Feed
Number of operations	26	4	9	31
Number of samples	173	30	57	200
Number positive	4	5	7	7
Number negative	169	25	56	193
Range	0–6	0–33	0–9	0–6
Percent negative	98%	83%	88%	97%
Average post Rx				
Worm egg counts	0.1	3.2	0.4	0.06

TREATMENT TIMING

1. **Fall deworming regime (includes Grub and Lice Control):** At the end of the grazing season when pastures are dormant (preferably after a hard frost), pour cows with an endecticide pour-on and drench with Safe-Guard liquid drench or fed cows Safe-Guard pellets at the rate of 1.0 lb per 1000 lb of body weight (Safe-Guard 0.5%) or 4 oz per 1000 lb body weight (Safe-Guard 1.96%). If feeding area is limited, spread the dose over several days to make sure all animals consume the pellets or mix Safe-Guard 1.96% flake meal in a weeks-worth of free-choice mineral. Other non-handling forms of Safe-Guard can be used such as medicate cubes (or cake) and medicated liquid feed.

2. **Mid-spring-early summer strategic timed dewormings:** Using Safe-Guard 1.96% flake meal, mix correct dose (4 oz per 1000 lb of cattle treated) in four to six days of free-choice mineral mix. Begin treatment five to six weeks after turn out or five to six weeks after first spring grass growth. Repeat treatment four to six weeks later if located south of the Mason–Dixon Line. Other Safe-Guard formulations will also work including Safe-Guard medicated liquid feed or Safe-Guard medicated cubes or cake mix. The bigger calves will consume the medicated mineral formulation, so add additional product to include (250 lb or larger) calf weights in calculation. It is also recommended to deworm calves with Safe-Guard anytime they are handled such as at branding.

3. **Fall deworming:** Repeat fall program listed above.

GASTROINTESTINAL AND LUNGWORM PARASITES FOUND IN BEEF CATTLE

Parasitism in dairy cattle can be broken into five main categories: *Stomach worms, Intestinal worms, Liver Flukes, Lungworms*, and *Protozoa*.

STOMACH (ABOMASAL) WORMS

The barber's pole worm (*Haemonchus placei, Haemonchus contortus*) is a blood-sucking parasite. This is a very economically damaging parasite in cattle but is especially damaging in sheep and goats becoming one of the most important causes of death in these animals. Larval stages have been found in the rumen and abomasal tissues and are extremely hard to kill. Eggs are easily identified in a fecal exam (see Figures 3.52–3.55).

The Brown Stomach Worm (*Ostertagia ostertagi*) is probably the most studied and most prevalent parasite of cattle. Larval stages invade and destroy the gastric glands. Large numbers of parasites can significantly reduce digestion efficiency. Larval stages can undergo inhibition and remain in the glands for months before emerging into lumen of the abomasum to develop into an adult worm. Eggs are easily identified in a fecal exam (see Figures 3.56–3.58).

***Trichostrongylus axei, Trichostrongylus colubriformis* (bankrupt worm)** Sucks gastric fluids from mucosa, causes necrosis of the mucosa, and, therefore, can be very damaging in large numbers. Has a kidney bean-shaped egg but most parasitology (see Figures 3.59–3.61). Technicians do not distinguish this egg separately from Ostertagia and Haemonchus but rather group them together under the heading of "stomach worms."

INTESTINAL NEMATODE PARASITES

Cooper's worm (*Cooperia punctate, Cooperia pectinata, Cooperia oncophora, Cooperia spatulata, Cooperia bison*) disrupts digestive functions of the small intestine. Probably the second most prevalent parasite of cattle. Eggs easily found in a fecal exam and are distinct because of

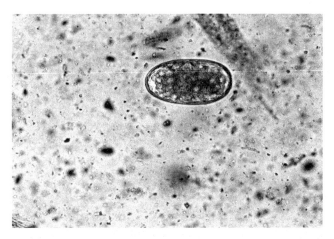

FIGURE 3.52   *Haemonchus* egg (10×).

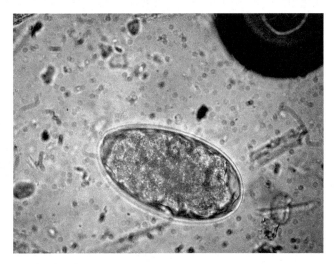

FIGURE 3.53   *Haemonchus* (40×).

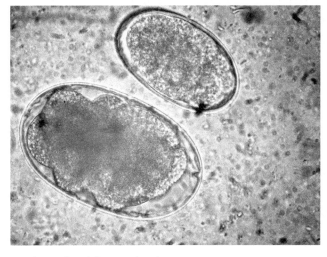

FIGURE 3.54   *Haemonchus* and Nodular eggs (40×).

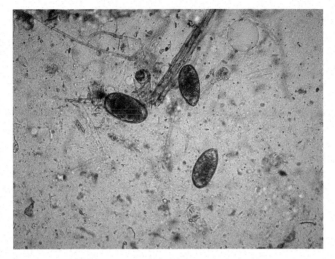

FIGURE 3.55 *Haemonchus* egg plus two smaller *Ostertagia* eggs (10×).

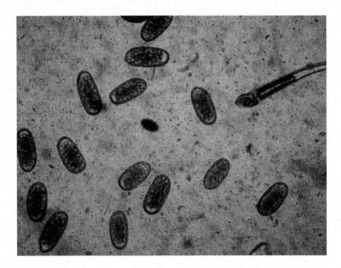

FIGURE 3.56 *Ostertagia* egg (10×).

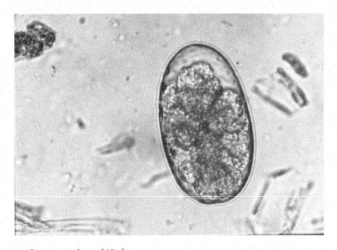

FIGURE 3.57 *Ostertagia ostertagi* egg (40×).

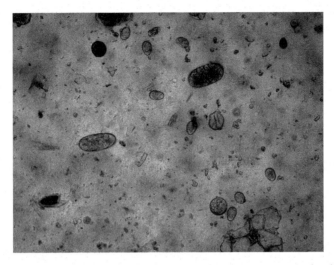

FIGURE 3.58   *Ostertagia* (smaller egg) and *Haemonchus* eggs with coccidia oocysts (10×).

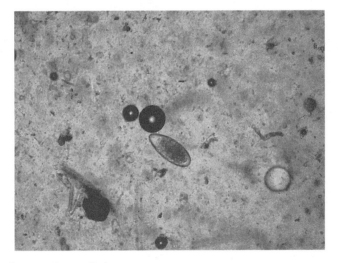

FIGURE 3.59   *Trichostrongylus* egg (4×).

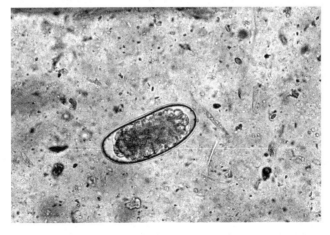

FIGURE 3.60   *Trichostrongylus* egg (40×).

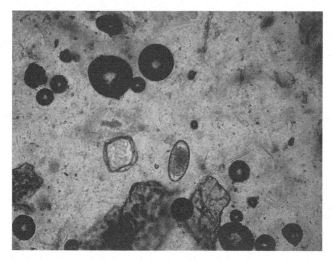

FIGURE 3.61   *Trichostrongylus* plus tapeworm eggs (10×).

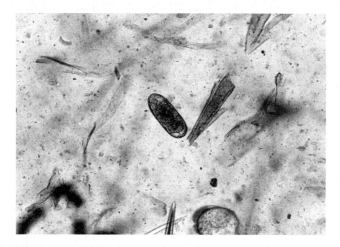

FIGURE 3.62   *Cooperia* spp. egg (10×).

elongated parallel sides (see Figures 3.62 and 3.63). Cooperia eggs are easily distinguished from Nematodirus eggs (see Figure 3.64). Cooperia is an underrated parasite in terms of damage caused by this worm. The prepatent period (time from ingestion until egg laying mature adult worm is short (17–21 days).

Threadneck worm (*Nematodirus helvetianus*) is most commonly found in young animals and is seldom found in adult cattle. Larvae survive well in cold weather and can live for several years on pasture. One unique feature with this parasite that helps survival of the egg and larvae is that the first two molts (L_1 and L_2) remain protected in the egg (see Figure 3.65). The Nematodirus egg is very large being roughly twice the size of other bovine gastrointestinal nematode eggs and is easily identified in fecal exam but almost never found in mature cows and only occasionally in first calf heifers (see Figures 3.66–3.71).

Nematodirus is a common cause of diarrhea, loss of body condition, and, oftentimes, even the cause of death in young calves and yearling cattle (see Figures 3.72 and 3.73). Because it is

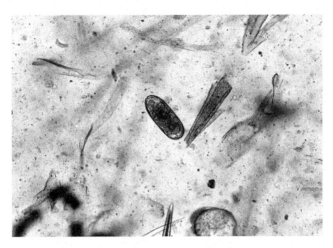

FIGURE 3.63   *Cooperia* spp. egg (40×).

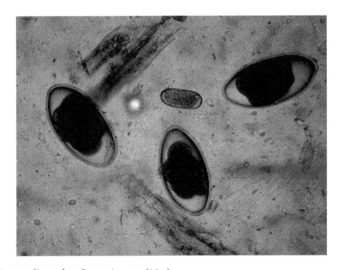

FIGURE 3.64   *Nematodirus* plus *Cooperia* eggs (10×).

very pathogenic in young animals, older animals seem acquired a strong immunity against this parasite. Nematodirus eggs are almost never seen in the feces of brood cows and older animals. At necropsy, adult worms are visually seen on the surface of the small intestine (see Figure 3.74) and easily identified with the naked eye (see Figures 3.75 and 3.76). When subjected to the electronic microscope, the adults worms apparently wind through the villa of the small intestine denuding the surface and disturbing nutrient adsorption (see Figure 3.77).

   Threadworm (*Strongyloides papillosus*) can gain entrance through the skin, orally passed to babies through the milk and through ingested infective larvae. These larvae pass through the lung and then back to the intestine. Threadworms can cause dermatitis, pneumonia, weight loss, and a "white or gray" scours (see Figure 3.78). Adult worms can cause hemorrhage in the small intestine. Most prevalent in young calves born in wet or muddy calving area or unclean pens. The eggs are small with blunt ends and thin shells and contain fully developed embryos when passed in the feces (see Figures 3.79–3.81).

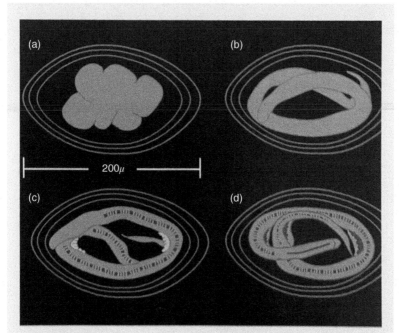

Preparasitic development to the infective stage occurs within the egg. Hatching occurs when this stage is reached, and when environmental conditions are right.

FIGURE 3.65   *Nematodirus* eggs develop slowly to reach an infective stage within the egg.

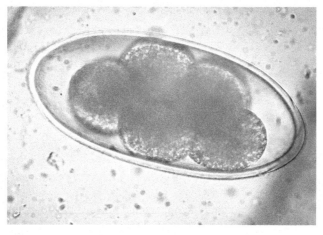

FIGURE 3.66   *Nematodirus helvetianus* egg (40×).

Whipworm (*Trichuris discolor*) is another very damaging parasite in young cattle. Oftentimes symptoms are confused with coccidiosis because of the bloody diarrhea associated with this parasite. Several hundred worms can kill a young calf. The egg is very characteristic and looks like a football with polar caps on each end (see Figures 3.82–3.84). The female worm is not prolific and eggs are often missed in the fecal exam unless carefully conducted.

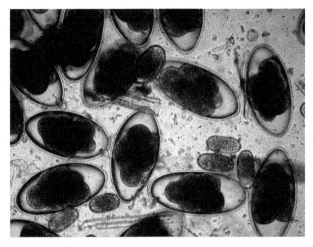

FIGURE 3.67   Heavy *Nematodirus* with Cooperia, *Haemonchus*, and *Ostertagia* eggs (10×).

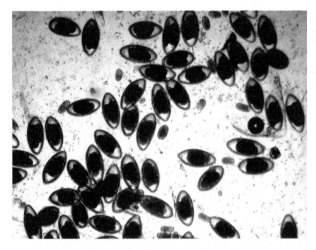

FIGURE 3.68   Heavy *Nematodirus* plus *Ostertagia*, *Haemonchus*, and *Cooperia* (4×).

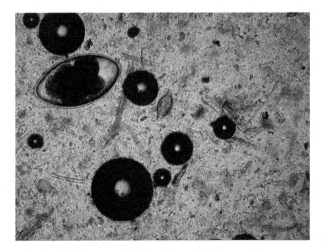

FIGURE 3.69   Nematodirus and Whipworm (*Trichuris*) eggs (10×).

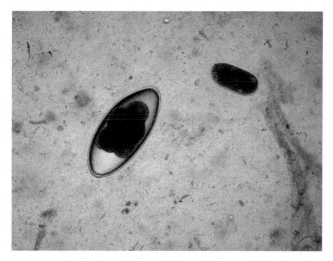

FIGURE 3.70   Nematodirus and Hookworm (*Bunostomum*) eggs.

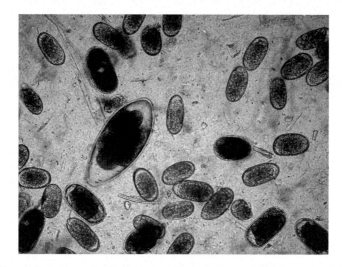

FIGURE 3.71   *Nematodirus, Cooperia, Bunostomum, Haemonchus,* and *Ostertagia* eggs.

Capillaria (*Capillaria bovis*). Often found in the feces for all ruminants but only in small numbers. The egg differs from *Trichuris* (whipworm) egg because the polar plugs on the eggs of football-shaped egg do not project as do the whipworm egg (see Figures 3.85 and 3.86). *Capillaria* has never been reported to cause problems in cattle.

Hookworm (*Bunostomum phlebotomum*) adults suck blood feeding on a plug of mucosa in the intestine. The larvae penetrate the skin and migrate through the lungs causing dermatitis and pneumonia. Calves on manure packs in the winter often become infected with hookworms. Eggs are easily identified in a fecal exam. Often these large eggs are in the 8–16-cell stage when passed (see Figures 3.87–3.90).

Large Roundworm in cattle (*Neoascaris [Toxocara] vitulorum*) is a parasitic Ascaris found mostly in tropical and subtropical climates. Infections have been recorded throughout North America. A fecal worm egg count survey in Wisconsin in 1973 found 49 herds positive for round-worm eggs out of 1003 farms surveyed. Calves can become infected by ingesting embroynated eggs

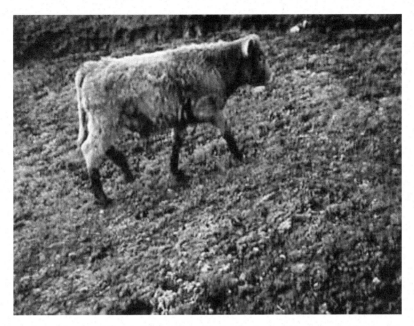

FIGURE 3.72   Clinical *Nematodirus* infections found in beef calves with counts over 50 eggs per 3 g sample.

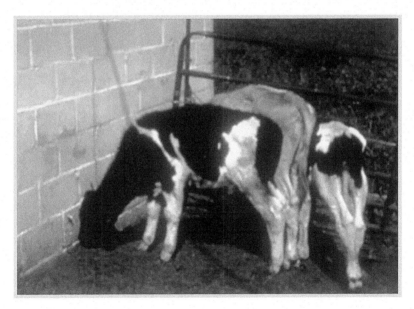

FIGURE 3.73   Clinical parasitism in dairy calves caused by pure infection with *Nematodirus*.

found in the environment or passed to the calf via the milk or prenally. Neoascaris eggs passed in the feces can survive for long periods of time in the environment (see Figures 3.91–3.93). After a Neoascaris outbreak in Florida, dirt was sent to our lab and we were able to recover embryonated Neoascaris eggs from around water troughs [15]. Patent roundworm infections can be seen in young calves up until four months of age, at which point, adult worms are most often spontaneously eliminated.

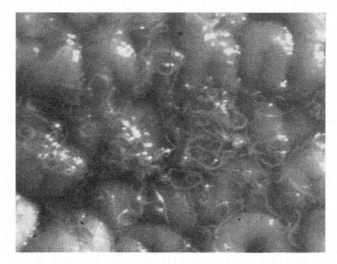

FIGURE 3.74   Adult *Nematodirus* in the small intestine.

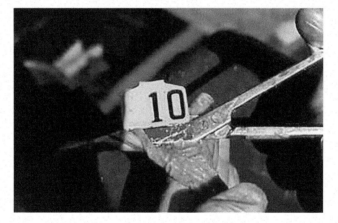

FIGURE 3.75   Adult *Nematodirus* worms on scissors.

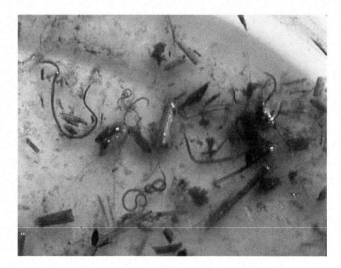

FIGURE 3.76   Adult *Nematodirus* worms in a petri dish.

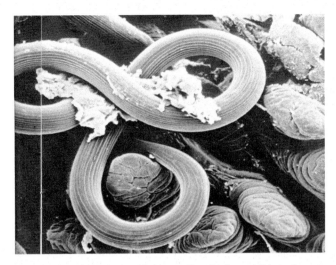

FIGURE 3.77   Electronic microscopic picture of *Nematodirus* in the small intestine.

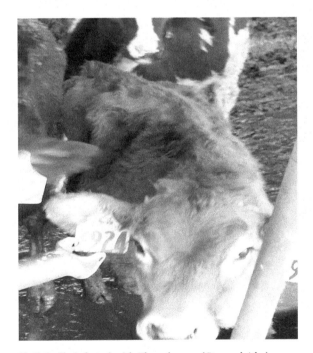

FIGURE 3.78   Dairy calf clinically infected with Threadworm (*Strongyloides*).

Nodular worm (*Oesophagostomum radiatum*) is becoming more important in recent years because intestines are often condemned at slaughter if nodules caused by the nodular worms are found in large numbers (see Figure 3.94). Nodular worm eggs are much larger than Ostertagia and Haemonchus less developed (16–32 cell stage) (see Figure 3.95). Parasites are associated with anorexia, depressed weight gain, and diarrhea. This parasite is most commonly found in adult cows and yearling cattle.

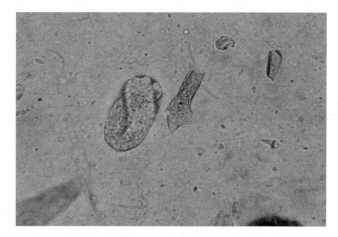

FIGURE 3.79   Threadworm (*Strongyloides papillosus*) egg (40×).

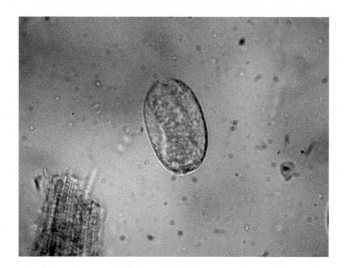

FIGURE 3.80   Threadworm (*Strongyloides*) egg (40×).

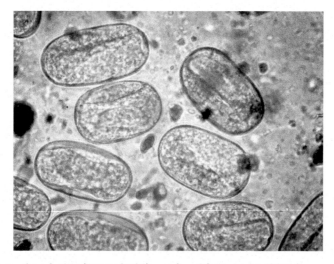

FIGURE 3.81   Heavy threadworm (*Strongyloides*) eggs found from dead calf (10×).

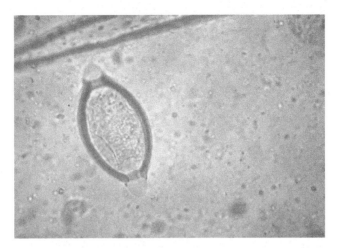

FIGURE 3.82   Whipworm (*Trichuris*) egg (10×).

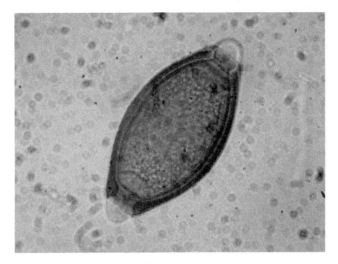

FIGURE 3.83   Dark whipworm (*Trichuris*) egg (40×).

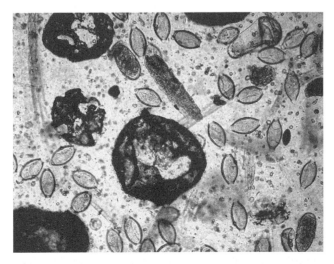

FIGURE 3.84   Heavy whipworm (*Trichuris*) infection.

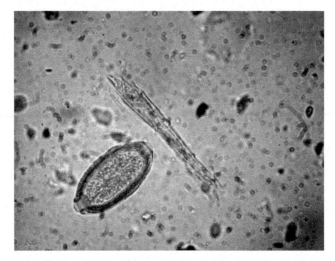

FIGURE 3.85 *Capillaria* egg (10×).

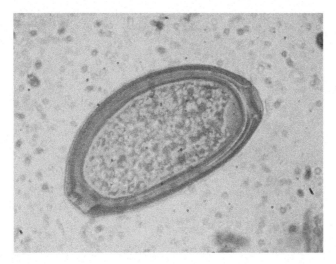

FIGURE 3.86 *Capillaria* egg (40×).

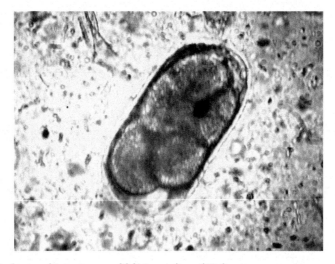

FIGURE 3.87 Hookworm (*Bunostomum phlebotomum*) egg (10×).

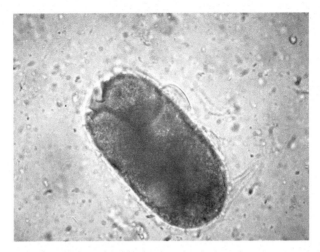

FIGURE 3.88   Hookworm (*Bunostomum phlebotomum*) egg (40×).

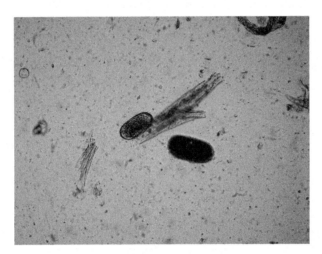

FIGURE 3.89   Hookworm (*Bunostomum*) and *Cooperia* eggs (10×).

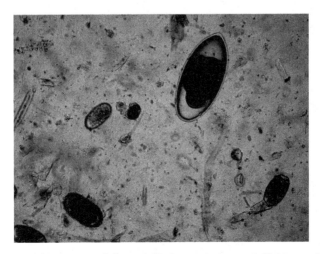

FIGURE 3.90   Hookworm (*Bunostomum*) (lower left), *Ostertagia* (center left), *Nematodirus* (large egg), and Nodular worm (lower right) eggs.

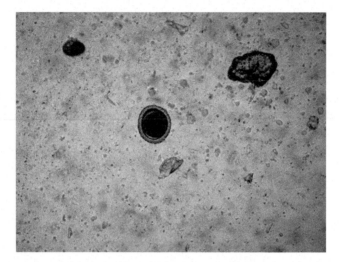

FIGURE 3.91   Cattle roundworm (*Neoascaris*) egg (4×).

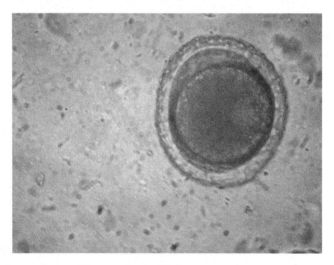

FIGURE 3.92   Cattle roundworm (*Neoascaris*) egg (10×).

INTESTINAL CESTODE PARASITES (CATTLE TAPEWORMS)

The tapeworm (*Monieza expansia*, *Moniezia benedeni*) develops in the soil mite, which is ingested by cattle. The developing time to reach an adult after ingestion is reported to be from six to eight weeks. The adult tapeworm lives in the small intestine and can grow to be 1 in. wide and 6 ft long. They absorb nutrition through their cuticle. In high numbers, tapeworms can block the intestine. Tapeworm eggs are distinct and easily picked up in a fecal exam (see Figures 3.96 and 3.97).

CATTLE LUNGWORM (*DICTYOCAULUS VIVIPAROUS*)

Lungworms are acquired almost exclusive through grazing. Lungworm larvae are not very mobile and, therefore, often require a heavy rain to move out away from the manure pat. Cattle on rotational and intensive grazing systems are often exposed to lungworms. Does not pick up well in a fecal exam but rather the fecal must be subjective to a separate test called a "Baermann test" to find

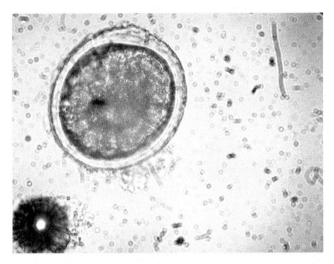

FIGURE 3.93   Cattle roundworm (*Neoascaris*) egg (40×).

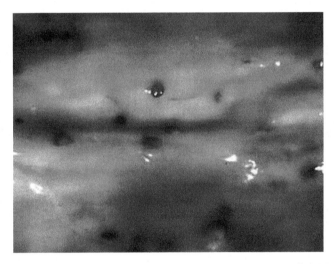

FIGURE 3.94   Nodules found in the large intestine caused by *Oesophagostomum* (Nodular worm).

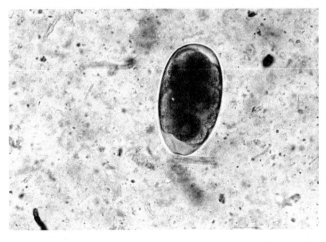

FIGURE 3.95   Nodular worm (*Oesophagostomum radiatum*) egg (40×).

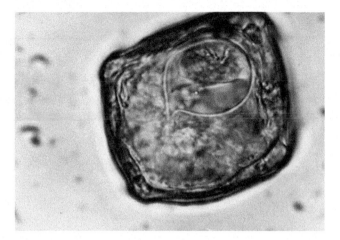

FIGURE 3.96   Tapeworm (*Moniezia*) egg (40×).

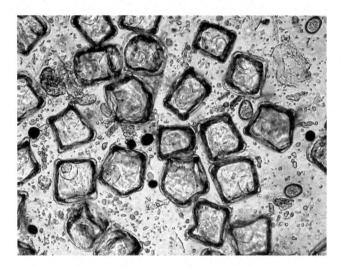

FIGURE 3.97   Multiple tapeworm (*Moniezia expansia*) eggs (10×) plus coccidia.

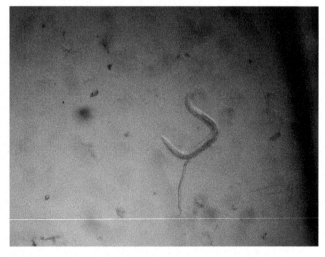

FIGURE 3.98   Lungworm larvae (*Dictyocaulus* spp.) found in fecal sample.

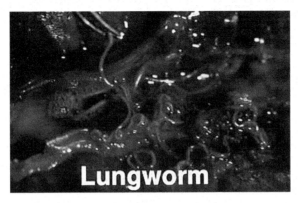

FIGURE 3.99   Adult lungworms (*Dictyocaulus vivipaarous*) in the lung.

lungworm larvae (see Figure 3.98). Postmortem check for lungworms entails removing the lungs and trachea intact, filling with warm water, and pouring the contents on a flat surface; lungworms are easily visible with the naked eye (see Figure 3.99).

TREMATODES PARASITES (LIVER FLUKES)

Fascioloides magna (**deer fluke**) found in the Great Lakes region is relatively untreatable in cattle. Diagnosis can be done accurately only upon necropsy since this fluke is encapsulated in the liver and cannot release its eggs (see Figure 3.100). Infections can be spread with deer with an intermediate snail host. Keeping cattle away from wet areas and streams where deer congregate is currently the only method of control.

Fasciola hepatica (**common liver fluke**) is found in the gulf coast from Florida to Texas and along the Pacific coast regions from California/Nevada to Washington and east to Colorado. Treatment in late summer or early fall is desirable to reduce contamination. Snail can carry the infection through the winter and cattle become reinfected in the spring when grazing wet areas where infected snail habitat. Eggs are recovered from the sediment in the bottom of the test tube after sample is run using the Modified Wisconsin Sugar Flotation Method and collected off a sieve (see Chapter 2). Eggs are easy to identify (see Figures 3.101 and 3.102).

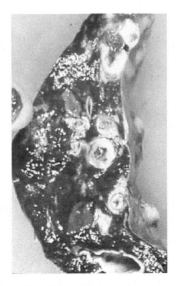

FIGURE 3.100   Beef liver with encapsulated liver flukes.

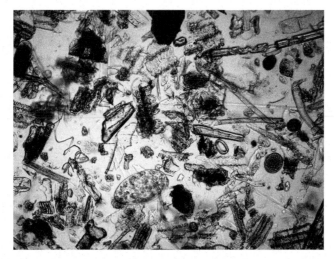

FIGURE 3.101   The common fluke (*Fasciola hepatica*) egg (10×).

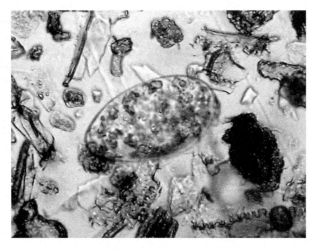

FIGURE 3.102   The common liver fluke (*Fasciola hepatica*) egg (40×).

PROTOZOAN PARASITES OF CATTLE

Coccidia are single-celled protozoan parasites that all cattle are believed to be exposed to sometime in their life (see Figures 3.103, 3.104 and 3.105). Coccidia are very host-specific such that coccidia of swine, dogs, and chickens would not infect cattle. The reverse is also true. Coccidia are ingested through fecal-contaminated feedstuff. Wet muddy conditions usually increase infection levels. Cattle become infected when they ingest oocysts (egg-like structure) containing sporozoites, which escape the oocysts and penetrate the intestinal wall. A disease condition called coccidiosis occurs when coccidia numbers become high and the immune system of the animals becomes challenged. Two species of coccidia in cattle have been blamed for most coccidia outbreaks (*Eimeria bovis* and *E. zurnii*) (see Figures 3.106 and 3.107). Other common coccidia oocyst seen in cattle is *E. bukid-nonsis* and *E. ellipsoidalis* (see Figures 3.108 and 3.109). Coccidiosis often occurs when an animal becomes stressed. Cattle shedding high number of oocysts indicate cell damage is ongoing. Coccidia oocysts can easily be found in a fecal exam.

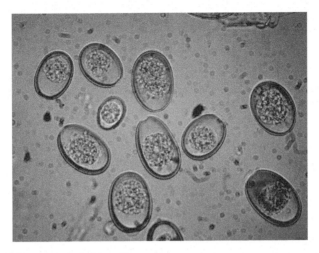

FIGURE 3.103   Coccidia oocysts found in calf samples.

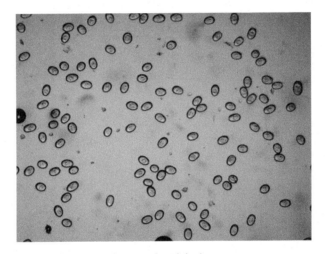

FIGURE 3.104   Multiple coccidia oocysts (*Eimeria bovis*) (4×).

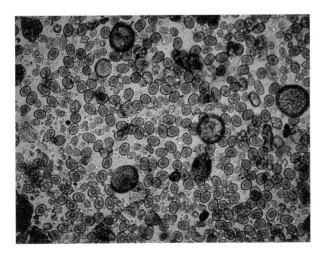

FIGURE 3.105   Heavy *Coccidia* spp. shedding.

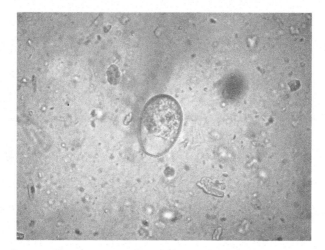

FIGURE 3.106   Coccidia (*Eimeria bovis*) oocysts.

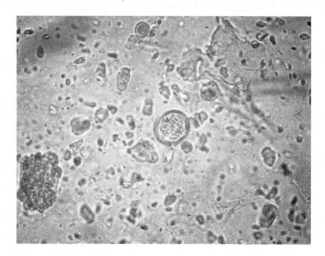

FIGURE 3.107   *Eimeria zuernii* oocysts.

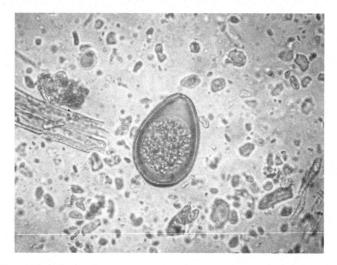

FIGURE 3.108   *Eimeria bukidnonensis.*

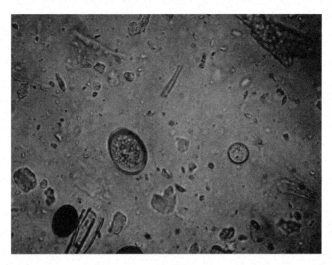

FIGURE 3.109   *E. ellipsoidalis* and *E. zuernii*.

Dung beetles: The residue of a number of anthelmintic products passed in fecal material following treatment have been shown to have an impact on the natural development of parasite fauna in the fecal pats excreted by cattle. This impact may range from destroying fly larvae and the development on these flies to the inhibition of eggs and larval stages of the dung beetle [45]. Most experts agree that the destruction of fly larvae is a good thing; however, the destruction of the eggs or development stages of the dung beetle may not be as universally acceptable for a number of reasons outlined below [18].

The anthelmintic products that have been determined to have a detrimental effect on the dung beetle fauna are ivermectin, doramectin, and eprinomectin [35, 37]. No differences were observed between the injection or pour-on formulations [46]. These avermectins showed larval mortality, mortality of immature adults, reduced egg production, and inhibited ovariole for periods up to one month following treatment. In experiments performed under temperate and tropical conditions, the aging of the dung pat did not lead to significant lowering of the concentrations of ivermectin [46]. There are approximately six months of the year when treatment of cattle with avermectins would affect mortality of newly emerged dung beetles and three months of the year when avermectin would affect dung beetle oviposition or larval survival [33].

Fenbendazole, albendazole, and moxidectin have shown no effect on the dung beetle or its offspring [42, 27]. Even when fenbendazole was administered in a sustained release bolus, no detrimental effect on dung beetles was observed. At 42-days post-treatment, the solid matter of the control and fenbendazole-containing cow pats were reduced to crumbling, granular texture, while the cow pats from the ivermectin-treated animals were solid and compacted.

The dung beetle has been identified as environmental aid for the degradation of the fecal pat, which provides the refertilization of the pastures and aids in the natural destruction of infective parasitic larvae (see Figure 3.110). Recent research has demonstrated that the dung beetle is responsible for the natural destruction of infective larvae present in the fecal pat, which develop from eggs passed from animals infected with gastrointestinal parasites. These studies indicate that these dung beetles naturally destroy from 60% to 80% of these larvae in any given fecal pat (see Figure 3.111). This may turn an out to be an extremely important event that researchers have only just discovered since destruction of the dung beetle could lead to higher levels of parasite contamination on pasture of avermectin-treated cattle (see Figures 3.111 and 3.112) [45].

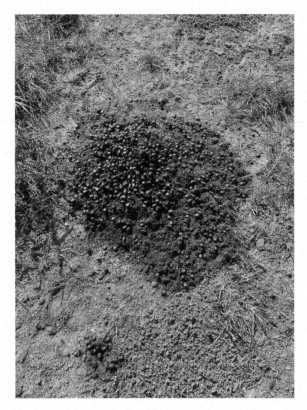

FIGURE 3.110 Dung beetles at work destroying cattle manure pat.

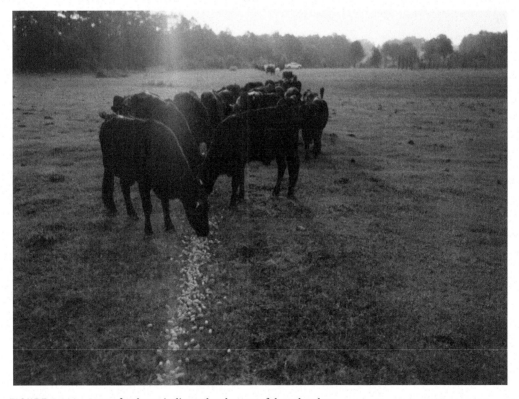

FIGURE 3.111 Intact fecal pats indicate the absence of dung beetles.

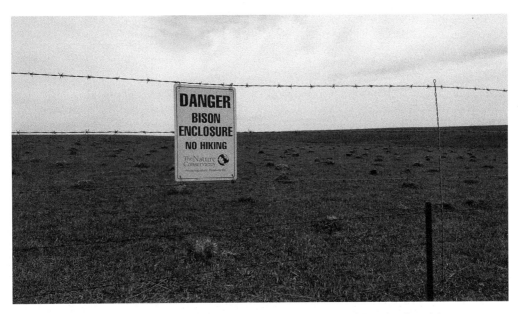

FIGURE 3.112   Bison pastures with intact fecal pats indicating the lack of dung beetle activity.

REFERENCES

1. Armour, J., Bairden, K., Duncan, J.L. et al. (1981). Studies on the control of bovine ostertagiasis using a morantel sustained release bolus. *Vet. Rec.* 108 (25): 532–535.

2. Bisset, S.A. (1990). Efficacy of a topical formulation of ivermectin against naturally acquired gastrointestinal nematodes in weaner cattle. *New Zeal. Vet. J.* 38: 4–6.

3. Blackburn, B.L., Hanrahan, L.A., Hendrix, C.M., and Lindsay, D.S. (1986). Evaluation of three formulations of fenbendazole (10% suspension, 0.5% pellets and 20% premix) against nematode infections in cattle. *Am. J. Vet. Res.* 47: 534–536.

4. Bliss, D.H. (1988). *The Cattle Producer's Handbook for Strategic Parasite Control*. Somerville, NJ: Hoechst-Roussel Agri-Vet Company.

5. Bliss, D.H. and Newby, T.J. (1988). Efficacy of the morantel sustained-release bolus in grazing cattle in North America. *J. Am. Vet. Med. Assn.* 192: 177–181.

6. Bliss, D.H. and Kvasnicka, W.G. (1997). The fecal exam: a missing link in food animal practice. *The Compendium* 4: 104–109.

7. Bliss, D.H. and Kvasnicka, W.G. (2004). Failure of avermectins to control an outbreak of parasitic gastro-enteritis in a cow/calf herd. *49th*

AAVP/*American Association of Veterinary Parasitologists*, Philadelphia (July 24–28) (Abstract 42).

8. Bliss, D.H., Campbell, J., Corwin, R.M. et al. (1993). Strategic deworming of cattle (parts 1-3), roundtable discussion. *Agri-Practice* 14 (5): 34–41, (6):32–37, (7):18–27.

9. Bungarner, S.C., Brauer, M.A., Corwin, R.M. et al. (1986). Strategic deworming for spring-calving beef cow/calf herds. *Am. J. Vet. Res.* 189: 427–431.

10. Campbell, W.C. and Benz, G.W. (1984). Ivermectin: a review of efficacy and safety. *J. Vet. Pharmacol. Ther.* 7: 1–16.

11. Capper, J.L. (2013). The economic and economic impact of withdrawing parasite control (fenbendazole) from U.S beef Product. *ADSA-ASAS Joint Annual Meeting*, Indianapolis, IN.

12. Capper, J.L. (2012). Is the grass always greener? Comparing resource use and carbon footprints on conventional natural, grass-fed beef production systems. *Animals* 2: 127–143.

13. Coles, G.C., Jackson, F., Pomroy, W.E. et al. (2006). The detection of anthelmintic resistance in nematodes of veterinary importance. *Vet. Parasitol.* 136: 167–185.

14. Crowley, J.W., Foreyt, W.J., Bliss, D.H., and Todd, A.C. (1977). Further controlled evaluations of fenbendazole as a bovine anthelmintic. *Am. J. Vet. Res.* 32 (5): 688–692.

15. Davila, G., Irsik, M., and Greiner, E.C. (2010). Toxocara vitulorum in beef calves in North Central Florida. *Vet. Parasitol.* 168: 261–263.

16. Dectomax® (1996). Product Monograph. Pfizer Animal Health.

17. Flincher, G.T. (1981). The potential value of dung beetles in pasture ecosystems. *J. Ga. Entomol. Soc.* 16: 301–316.

18. Floate, K.D., Cotwell, D.C., and Fox, A.S. (2002). Reductions of non-pest insects in dung of cattle treated with endecticides: a comparisons of four products. *Bull. Entomol. Res.*

19. Gasbarre, L.C., Smith, L.L., Lichtenfels, J.R., and Pilitt, P.A. 2004. The identification of cattle nematode parasites resistant to multiple classes of anthelmintics in a commercial cattle population in the US. *49th American Association of Veterinary Parasitologists*, Philadelphia (July 24–28) (Abstract 44).

20. Gaynard, V., Valvinerie, M., and Toutain, P.L. (1999). Comparison of persistent anthelmintic efficacy of doramectin and ivermectin pour-on formulation in cattle. *Vet. Parasitol.* 81: 47–55.

21. Hooke, F.C., Clement, P., Dell'Osa, D. et al. (1997). Therapeutic and protective efficacy of doramectin injectable against gastrointestinal nematodes in cattle in New Zealand: a comparison with moxidectin and ivermectin pour-on formulations. *Vet. Parasit.* 72: 43–51.

22. Hoover, R.C., Lincoln, S.D., Newby, T.J., and Bliss, D.H. (1984). Controlling parasitic gastroenteris in pastured cattle. *Vet. Med.* 79: 1082–1086.

23. Jacobs, D.E., Fox, M.T., Walker, M.J. et al. (1981). Field evaluation of a new method for the prophylaxis of parasitic gastroenteritis in calves. *Vet. Rec.* 108: 274–251.

24. Jones, R.M. (1981). A field study of the morantel sustained release bolus in the seasonal control of parasitic gastroenteritis in grazing calves. *Vet. Parasitol.* 8: 237–245.

25. Keith, E.A. (1992). Utilizing feed-grade formulations of fenbendazole for cattle. *Agri-Practice* 13: 30–33.

26. Kelly, J.D. (1973). Immunity and epidemiology of helminthiasis in grazing animals. *New Zeal. Vet. J.* 21: 183–194.

27. Knutson, A. (2000). Dung beetles – Biological control agents of horn flies (winter). *Texas Biological Control News* (Winter). Texas Agricultural Extension Service, The Texas A & M University System.

28. Kvasnicka, W.G., Krysl, L.J., Torell, R.C., and Bliss, D.H. (1996). Cow/calf herd investigation: fenbendazole in a strategic deworming program. The compendium. *Food Anim. Parasitol.* 41: 113–177.

29. Kvasnicka, B. and Bliss, D. (2002). The efficacy of endectocide pour-ons against national infections in cattle. *AAVP Proceedings from Annual Meeting*, Nashville, TN (July 13–16). Abstract Am Assoc. of Vet Parasit. 47 (2002) 50.

30. Majia, M.F., Fernandez Igartua, B.M., Schmidt, E.E., and Cabaret, J. (2003). Multispecies and multiple anthelmintic resistance on cattle nematodes in a farm in Argentina: the beginning of high resistance? *Vet. Res.* 34: 461–467.

31. Prichard, R.K., Hall, C.A., Kelly, J.D. et al. (1980). The problem of anthelmintic resistance in nematodes. *Aus. Vet. J.* 56: 239–250.

32. Prosl, H., Superer, R., Jones, R.M. et al. (1983). Morantel sustained release bolus: a new approach for the control of trichostrongylosis in Austrian cattle. *Vet. Parasit.* 12: 239–250.

33. Ridsdill-Smith, T.J. (1993). Effects of avermectin residues in cattle dung on dung beetle (Coleoptera: Scarabaeidae) reproduction and survival. *Vet. Parasitol.* 48 (1–4): 127–136.

34. Raynaud, J.B., Jones, R.M., Bliss, D.H. et al. (1983). The control of parasitic gastroenteritis of grazing cattle in Normandy, France, using the morantel sustained release bolus. *Vet. Parasitol.* 12: 261–272.

35. Sallovitz, J.M., Lifschitz, A., Imperiale, F. et al. (2005). Doramectin concentration profiles in the gastrointestinal tract of topically-treated calves: influence of animal licking restrictions. *Vet. Parasitol.* 133: 61–70.

36. von Samson-Himmelstjerna, G. and Blackhall, W. (2005). Will technology provide solutions for drug resistance in veterinary helminths? *Vet. Parasitol.* 132: 223–239.

37. Sommer, C. and Steffansen, B. (1993). Changes with time after treatment in the concentrations of ivermectin in fresh cow dung and in cow pats aged in the field. *Vet. Parasitol.* 48 (1–4): 67–73.

38. Sonstegard, T.S. and Gasbarre, L.C. (2001). Genomic tool to improve parasite resistance. *Vet. Parasitol.* 101: 387–403.

39. Smith, L.L. and Gasbarre, L.C. (2004). The development of cattle nematode parasites resistant to multiple classes of anthelmintic in a commercial cattle

population in the US. *49th American Association of Veterinary Parasitologists*, Philadelphia (July 24–28) (Abstract 43).

40. Smith, R.A., Rogers, K.C., Husae, S. et al. (2000). Pasture deworming and (or) subsequent feedlot performance with fenbendazole. I. Effects on grazing performance, feedlot performance and carcass traits in yearling steers. *Bovine Practitioner* 34: 104–114.

41. Stromberg, B.E., Vatthauer, R.J., Schlotthauer, J.C. et al. (1997). Production responses following strategic parasite control in a beef cow/calf herd. *Vet. Parasitol.* 68: 315–322.

42. Strong, L., Wall, R., Woolford, A., and Djeddour, D. (2000). The effect of fecally excreted ivermectin and fenbendazole on the insect colonization of cattle dung following oral administration of sustained-release boluses. *Vet. Parasitol.* 62 (2–3): 253–266.

43. Todd, A.C., Bliss, D., Scholl, P., and Crowley, J.W. (1976). Controlled evaluation of fenbendazole as a bovine anthelmintic. *Am J. Vet. Res.* 27 (4): 439–441.

44. Vercruysse, J. and Claerebout, E. (2001). Treatment vs non-treatment of helminth infections in cattle: defining the threshold. *Vet. Parasitol.* 98: 195–214.

45. Wardhaugh, K. and Ridsill-Smith, T. (1998). Antiparasitic drugs, the livestock industry and dung beetles – a cause for concern? *Austral. Vet. J.* 76 (4): 259–261.

46. Wardhaugh, K.C., Longstaff, B.C., and Morton, R. (2001). A comparison of the development and survival of the dung beetle, *Onthophagus tarus* (Schreb.) when fed on the feces of cattle treated with pour-on formulations of eprinomectin or moxidectin. *Vet. Parasitol.* 99 (2): 155–168.

47. Williams, J.C., Loyacano, A.F., Broussard, S.D. et al. (1995). Efficacy of a spring strategic fenbendazole treatment program to reduce numbers of *Ostertagia ostertagi* inhibited larvae in beef stocker cattle. *Vet. Parasitol.* 59: 127–137.

48. Williams, J.C., Loyacano, A.F., DeRosa, A. et al. (1999). Comparison of persistent anthelmintic efficacy of topical formulations of doramectin, ivermectin, eprinomectin and moxidectin against naturally acquired nematode infection of beef calves. *Vet. Parasitol.* 85: 277–288.

49. Woods, I.B., Amaral, N.K., Bairden, K. et al. (1995). World Association for the Advancement of veterinary parasitology (W.A.A.V.P.) second edition of guidelines for evaluation the efficacy of anthelmintics in ruminants (bovine, ovine, caprine). *Vet. Parasistol.* 58: 181–213.

Parasites in Dairy Cattle

Due to milk production losses in dairy cows and slow or inefficient growth replacement heifers, dairymen are beginning to understand the overall importance of developing a complete parasite control strategy for their herds [2–6, 9, 12, 13, 14]. Dairy producers are concerned about the cost of production. Economic losses, especially those caused by preventable disease such as parasitism, are a major concern. Knowing how to reduce or prevent these losses from occurring is very valuable to the efficiency of an operation since losses caused by parasites are usually cumulative over a period of time. To make matters worse, parasitisms have been also shown to make animals more susceptible to other disease problems.

Profitability can easily be determined by subtracting the cost of prevention from the potential losses caused by the disease. Deworming dairy cattle is more than just treating the animals after they become infected. For seasonal control, the animal's environmental contamination must be reduced to prevent harmful levels of parasitism from developing in the animals themselves. The buildup of infective larvae in the environment of the animals is damaging even if the ensuing parasitism does not fully develop in the animal because the animals have to give up something in terms of production in order to fight these infections off.

DETECTION IS FOREMOST IN THE ECONOMIC ANALYSIS

Being able to detect and evaluate losses as they occur. The measurement of the actual loss or losses involved within a dairy herd, however, is often difficult to assess because too many economic factors are involved and the proper parameters for measuring the economic loss are lacking or, in many cases, been overlooked. The economic effects of parasitism on cattle production have long been studied in general terms; however, specific losses that might be occurring in any given herd are nearly impossible to be determined. First, the parasite infection must be detected and, second, the damage being done needs to be quantified in terms of economics.

Each dairy herd or dairy operation is a special case in terms of economic losses they might be experiencing because of many influencing factors that are specific to a particular herd (see Figure 4.1). The influence of management, the amount of parasite exposure an individual animal experiences, the age when parasite exposure first occurs, the maximum genetic potential of the individual animal, and the production goals of the overall herd are different for every dairy herd in the country. Some cattle never see pastures and are held in confinement for their entire life, and therefore, parasites are seldom a problem. There are still a lot of dairy cattle, however, that are raised on pastures in conventional old dairy barns (see Figures 4.2 and 4.3).

The most complicated part of developing an efficient deworming program for most dairymen is being able to understand the natural occurrence of these parasites in cattle and to know

Large Animal Parasitology Procedures for Veterinary Technicians, First Edition. Donald H. Bliss.
© 2024 John Wiley & Sons, Inc. Published 2024 by John Wiley & Sons, Inc.

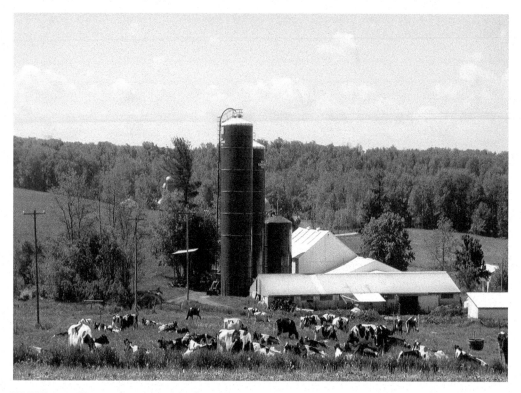

FIGURE 4.1   Picture of Vermont dairy farm.

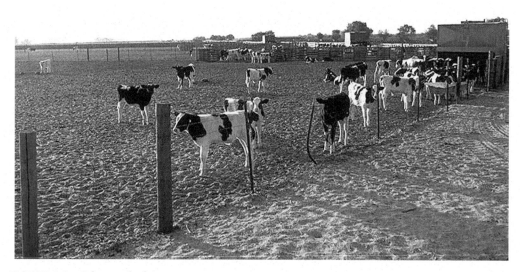

FIGURE 4.2   Calves on dry lot pastures.

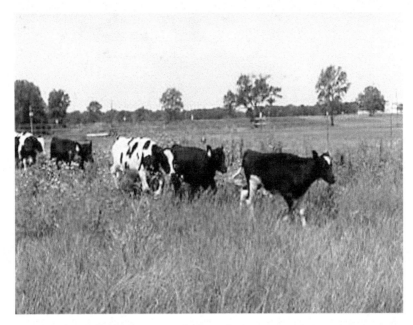

FIGURE 4.3   Dairy calves going out on pasture in the spring.

that differences occur between age groups and management conditions. Difference in developing parasitic burdens will partly depend upon pasture exposure (see Figures 4.4–4.6). Every operation has a different parasite profile. Some dairy operations may have severe parasite problems while

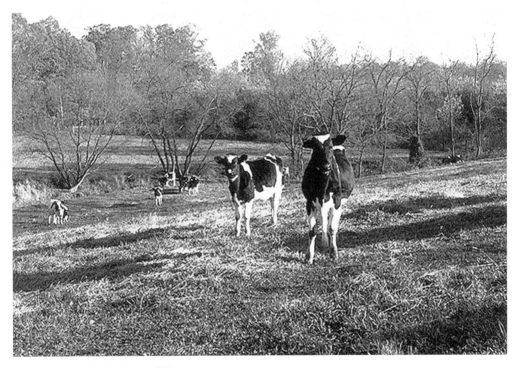

FIGURE 4.4   Dairy heifers on fall pasture.

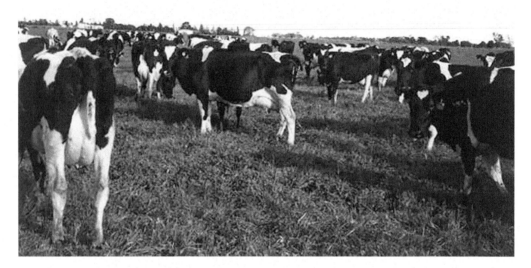

FIGURE 4.5   Dairy cows on pasture.

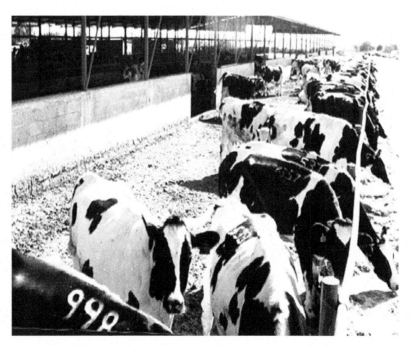

FIGURE 4.6   Cows in total confinement.

Common Dairy Parasites	Commonly Found Parasites										
Production Group	Giardia	Coccidia	Threadworm	Whipworm	Hookworm	Nematodirus	Tapeworm	Stomach Worms	Cooperia	Nodular Worm	Lungworm
Pre-Weaned Calves	X	X	X	X							
Weaning - 3 mo. old		X	X	X	X	X					
3 mo. - 11 mo.			X	X	X	X	X	X	X	X	X
Yearlings/Breeding age heifers					X	X	X	X	X	X	X
Bred Heifers						X	X	X	X	X	X
Fresh Cows							X	X	X	X	X
Lactating Cows							X	X	X	X	X
Dry Cows							X	X	X	X	X

Barnyard Infections - Heavier bedding increases risk (eg. Manure pack)

Both - These parasites can be transmitted in bedding and on grass

Pasture - These parasites usually require grass for transmission.

FIGURE 4.7   Common parasites found by age.

the herd next door may have little or no problems. Herd management and production standards play a big role in influencing the amount of parasite damage or the amount of production loss due to parasites that occurs in a particular operation. Obviously, the higher the production standards are for an animal and the closer an animal is to its maximum potential production, the greater the damage parasites can cause. It takes fewer parasites, therefore, in high-producing cows to cause economic loss than it takes in low-producing animals.

The key to controlling parasitism in a dairy operation is to first identify whether parasites are present in any particular age group of animals. There are two types of parasitism commonly found with dairy animals which can be identified either as "barnyard infections" or pasture infections. The parasites that are commonly found on pasture seldom survive well under barnyard conditions. Parasite infections can often be categorized by age group as well depending upon how the animals are raised (see Figure 4.7). Each parasite will be discussed in detail in the following discussion.

GASTROINTESTINAL AND LUNG PARASITE INFECTIONS FOUND IN DAIRY CATTLE (SEE FIGURE 4.8)

Parasitism in dairy cattle can be broken into five main categories: *Stomach* worms, Intestinal worms, Liver flukes, Lungworms, and Protozoa.

STOMACH WORMS

Haemonchus (the barber's pole worm) is a blood-sucking parasite. This is a very economically damaging parasite in cattle but is especially damaging in sheep and goats, becoming one of the most important causes of death in these animals. *Haemonchus* is considered to be primarily a parasite acquired on pasture. Larval stages have been found in the rumen and abomasal tissues and are extremely hard to kill. *Haemonchus* eggs are easily identified in a fecal exam (see Figure 4.9).

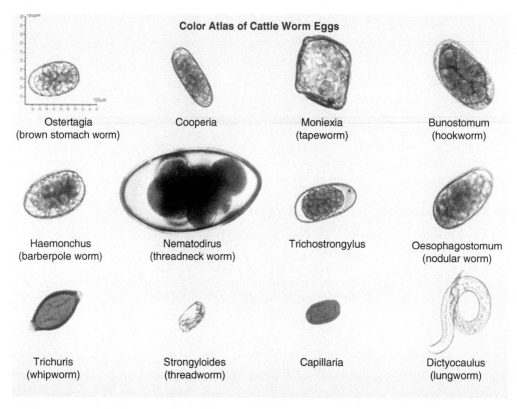

Color Atlas of Cattle Worm Eggs

Ostertagia
(brown stomach worm)

Cooperia

Moniexia
(tapeworm)

Bunostomum
(hookworm)

Haemonchus
(barberpole worm)

Nematodirus
(threadneck worm)

Trichostrongylus

Oesophagostomum
(nodular worm)

Trichuris
(whipworm)

Strongyloides
(threadworm)

Capillaria

Dictyocaulus
(lungworm)

FIGURE 4.8   Color atlas of cattle worm eggs.

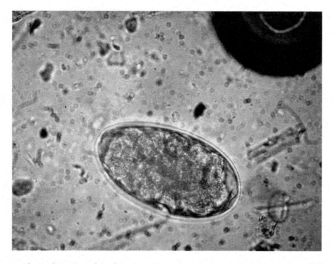

FIGURE 4.9   *Haemonchus placei* egg (40×).

Ostertagia (Brown Stomach Worm) is probably the most studied and most prevalent parasite of cattle. *Ostertagia*, like *Haemonchus*, is considered to be a pasture parasite. Larval stages invade and destroy the gastric glands. Large number of parasites can significantly reduce digestion efficiency. Larval stages can undergo inhibition and remain in the glands for months before emerging into lumen of the abomasum to develop into an adult worm. Eggs are easily identified in a fecal exam (see Figure 4.10).

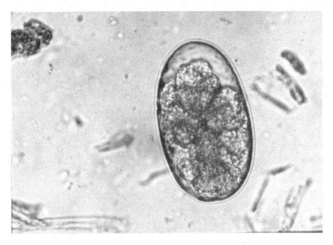

FIGURE 4.10   *Ostertagia ostertagi* egg (40×).

Trichostrongylus (bankrupt worm). There two main species of *Trichostrongylus* found in cattle (*T. columbriformis* and *T. axei*). It sucks gastric fluids from mucosa, causes necrosis of the mucosa, and, therefore, can be very damaging in large numbers. Has a kidney bean-shaped egg (see Figure 4.11), but most parasitology technicians do not distinguish this egg separately from *Ostertagia* and *Haemonchus* but rather group them together under the heading of "stomach worms." *Trichostrongylus* is also considered to be primarily a parasite acquired on pasture only.

INTESTINAL NEMATODE PARASITES

Cooperia spp. (Coopers worm) disrupts digestive functions of the intestine. It is now the second most prevalent parasite of cattle behind *Ostertagia*. The primary species of *Cooperia* found in cattle are *C. punctate, C. pectinate*, and *C. oncophora*. Eggs are easily found in a fecal exam and are distinct because of elongated parallel sides (see Figure 4.12). *Cooperia* is an underrated parasite in terms of damage caused by this worm. Like the stomach worms, *Cooperia* is primarily transmitted on pastures.

Nematodirus (threadneck worm) is most commonly found in young animals and is seldom found in adult cattle. Larvae survive well in cold weather and can live for several years

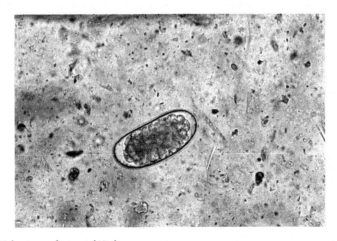

FIGURE 4.11   *Trichostrongylus* spp. (40×).

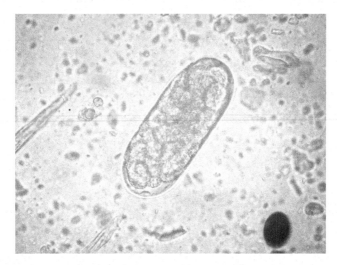

FIGURE 4.12   *Cooperia* spp. egg (40×).

on pasture. This parasite is a common cause of diarrhea [1] and, often times, death in young calves (see Figure 4.13) and yearling cattle when infection levels are high. Because it is very pathogenic, older animals acquired a strong immunity against this parasite. The egg is very large and is easily identified in a fecal exam (see Figures 4.14 and 4.15). *Nematodirus* is a hardy parasite and transmission can take place on pasture as well in barnyards and indoor pens. This parasite can infect calves and yearling cattle during winter conditions.

   Strongyloides papillosus (threadworms) is a very common parasite found in baby calves up to two year old. Threadworm eggs are smaller than stomach worms and are always embryonated when passed in the feces of the host (see Figures 4.16–4.18). Occasionally, mature females containing eggs can be found in the fecal exam (see Figure 4.19). This parasite has a unique life cycle. The infective larvae of the parasitic generation are able to pass through the skin of the host

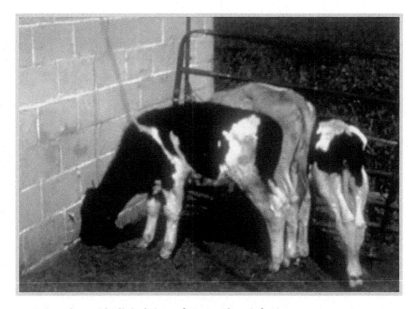

FIGURE 4.13   Dairy calves with clinical signs of *Nematodirus* infection.

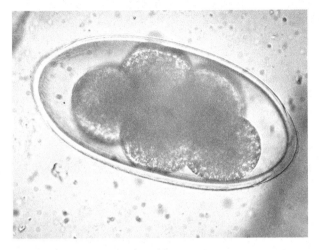

FIGURE 4.14   *Nematodirus helvetianus* egg (40×).

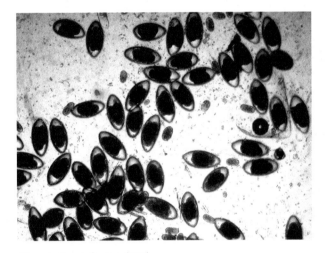

FIGURE 4.15   Heavy *Nematodirus* infection (10×).

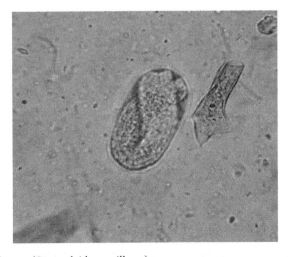

FIGURE 4.16   Threadworm (*Strongyloides papillosus*) egg.

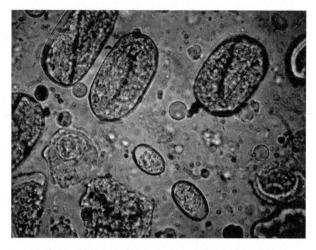

FIGURE 4.17   Threadworm (*Strongyloides papillosus*) eggs with coccidia oocysts.

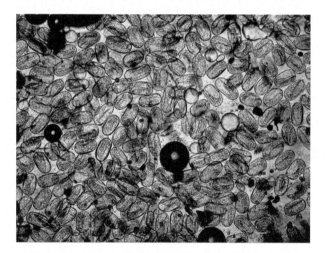

FIGURE 4.18   Extremely heavy threadworm (*Strongyloides*) infection.

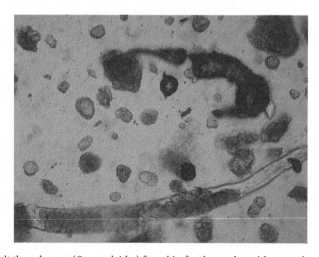

FIGURE 4.19   Adult threadworm (*Strongyloides*) found in fecal samples with several eggs present.

(calves) and pass with the blood to the lungs, then up the trachea to the pharnynx and on to the intestine. Larvae can also pass in the colostrum [16]. It is also not uncommon for calves to become infected through the bedding (see Figures 4.20). This parasite can infect newborn baby calves on pasture, especially if the calving areas have hay or straw bedding areas and become infected with this parasite (see Chapter 3). No other pasture transmission with this parasite is found in dairy cattle. This parasite, however, is commonly found in baby calves in confinement and older calves housed in bedded pens. Since its transmission is possible through the milk [1], we see calves being fed colostrum milk often become infected and then pass this parasite on to older calves (as the infected babies are transferred to new pens as they get older).

Strongyloides lives in the small intestine and can cause very serious disease in very young calves (day old until three to four months of age). Essentially a few infections lead to a marked immunity as proof because only very young animals show signs of severe infections. It is not uncommon to find heavy infections in very young dairy calves, especially if they are housed in a bedded pen(s) (see Figures 4.21 and 4.22). In a New York dairy farm, we recorded infections in day-old calves but it was not until two months later when infections became severe after calves that were housed in bedded pens showed high worm egg counts with threadworm and began to die (see Figure 4.23).

Trichuris (whipworm) is another very damaging parasite that resides in the cecum in young cattle. The adults tunnel into the intestinal mucosa with anterior head ends. Often, symptoms are confused with coccidiosis because of the bloody diarrhea associated with this parasite. Several hundred worms can kill a young calf. The egg is very characteristic and looks like a football with polar caps on each end (see Figure 4.24). The female worm is not prolific and eggs are often missed in the fecal exam unless carefully conducted. We occasionally find this parasite in young pastured

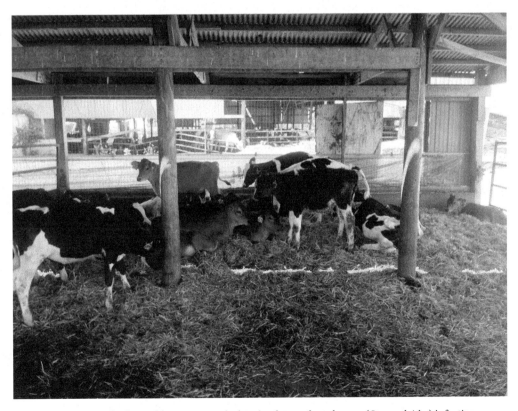

FIGURE 4.20   Pen of calves with manure pack showing heavy threadworm (*Strongyloides*) infection.

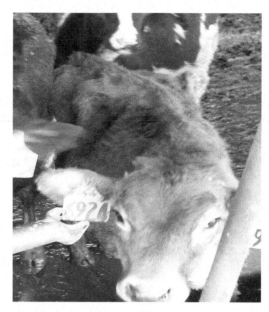

FIGURE 4.21   Dairy calf with fecal showing heavy threadworm (*Strongyloides*) egg count.

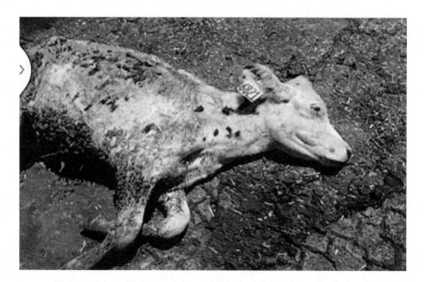

FIGURE 4.22   Dead calf diagnosed with heavy threadworm (*Strongyloides*) infection.

animals but mostly we find it in barnyard calves or from animals housed in older barns and areas where cattle have be housed for years.

Bunostomum (hookworm) adults suck blood, feeding on a plug of mucosa in the intestine. The larvae penetrate the skin and migrate through the lungs causing dermatitis and pneumonia. Calves on manure packs in the winter often become infected with hookworms. Eggs are easily identified in the fecal exam (see Figure 4.25). Often, these large eggs are in the 8- to 16-cell stage when passed.

Oesophagostomum (nodular worm) is becoming more important in recent years because intestines are often condemned at slaughter if nodules caused by the nodular worms are found in large numbers. Eggs are much large than *Haemonchus* and *Ostertagia* plus the embryo is in the

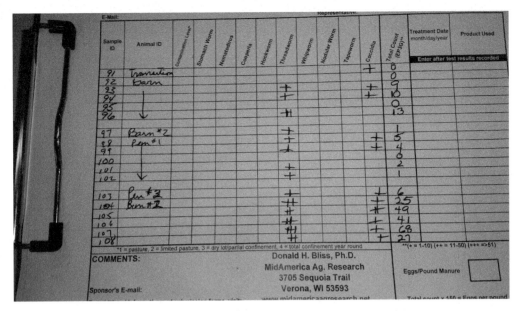

FIGURE 4.23   *Strongyloides* egg count from different age groups leading back to transmission in the milk.

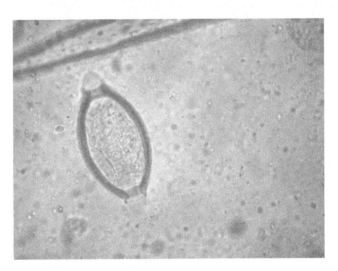

FIGURE 4.24   Whipworm (*Trichuris* spp.) (40×).

16–32 cell stage (see Figure 4.26). Parasites are associated with anorexia, depressed weight gain, and diarrhea. Most commonly found in adult cows and older yearling animals. This parasite is primarily transmitted on pasture.

INTESTINAL CESTODE PARASITES (CATTLE TAPEWORMS)

The tapeworm develops in the soil mite, which is ingested by cattle. The time it takes to develop to reach an adult after ingestion is reported to be from six to eight weeks. The adult tapeworms live in the small intestine and can grow up to 1 in. wide and 6 ft long. They absorb nutrition through their cuticle. In high numbers, tapeworms can block the intestine. Tapeworm eggs are distinct and can be easily picked up in a fecal exam (see Figure 4.27).

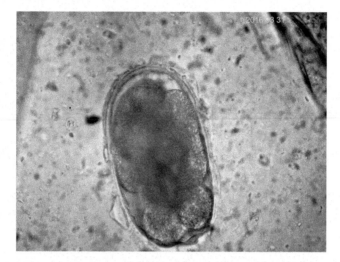

FIGURE 4.25   Hookworm (*Bunostomum phlebotomum*) egg (40×).

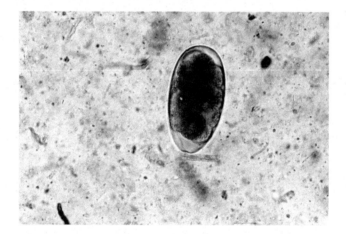

FIGURE 4.26   *Oesophagostomum* spp. (40×).

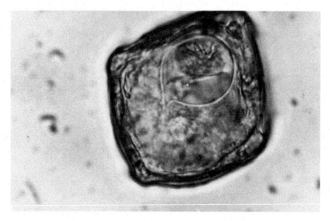

FIGURE 4.27   Tapeworm (*Moniezia expansia*) (40×).

CATTLE LUNGWORM (DICTYOCAULUS VIVIPAROUS)

Lungworms are acquired almost exclusive through grazing [8]. Lungworm larvae are not very mobile and, therefore, often require a heavy rain to move out away from the manure pit. Cattle on rotational and intensive grazing systems are often exposed to lungworms. Does not pick up well in a fecal exam but rather the fecal must be subjective to a separate test called "Baermann test" to find lungworm larvae (see Figure 4.28). Postmortem check for lungworms entails removing the lungs and trachea intact, filling with warm water, and pouring the contents on a flat surface; lungworms are easily visible with the naked eye.

TREMATODES PARASITES (LIVER FLUKES)

***Fascioloides magna* (deer fluke)** found in the Great Lakes region is relatively non-treatable in cattle. Diagnosis can be done accurately only upon necropsy since this fluke is encapsulated in the liver and cannot release its eggs. Infections can spread from deer with an intermediate snail host. Keeping cattle away from wet areas and streams where deer congregate is currently the only method of control.

Fasciola hepatica **(common fluke)** is found in the gulf coast from Florida to Texas and along the Pacific coast regions from California/Nevada to Washington and east to Colorado. Treatment in late summer or early fall is desirable to reduce contamination. Snail can carry the infection through the winter and cattle become reinfected in the spring when grazing in wet areas where infected snail habitat. Eggs are recovered using a Fluke Finder as described in Chapter 2 (See Figure 4.29).

PROTOZOAN PARASITES OF CATTLE

Coccidia are single celled protozoan parasites that all cattle are believed to be exposed to sometime in their life. Coccidia are very host-specific such that coccidia of swine, dogs, and chickens would not infect cattle. The reverse is also true. Coccidia are ingested through fecal-contaminated feedstuff. Wet muddy conditions usually increase infection levels.

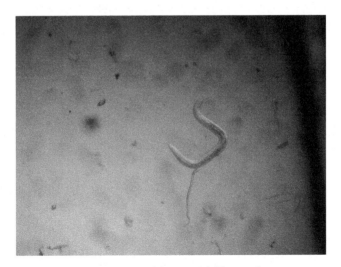

FIGURE 4.28   Lungworm (*Dictyocaulus viviparus*) larvae with blunt ends.

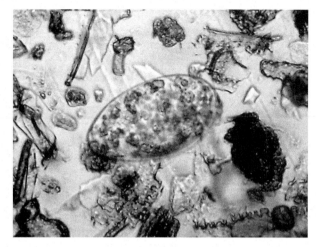

FIGURE 4.29   Common liver fluke (*Fasciola hepatic*) egg.

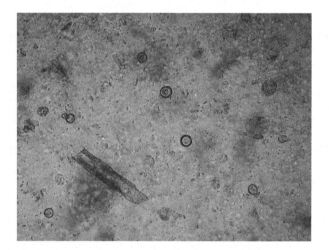

FIGURE 4.30   *Eimeria zuerni* oocysts from calf hutch.

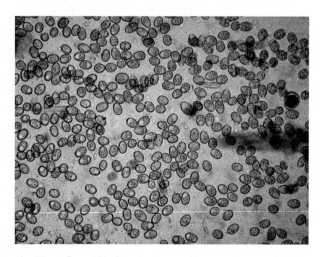

FIGURE 4.31   Heavy shedding of coccidia oocysts.

Cattle become infected when they ingest oocysts (egg-like structure) containing sporozoites, which escape the oocysts and penetrate the intestinal wall. A disease condition called coccidiosis occurs when coccidia numbers become high and the immune system of the animals becomes low. Coccidiosis often occurs when an animal becomes stressed. Cattle shedding high number of oocysts indicate cell damage is ongoing. Coccidia oocysts can easily be found in a fecal exam (see Figures 4.32–4.34).

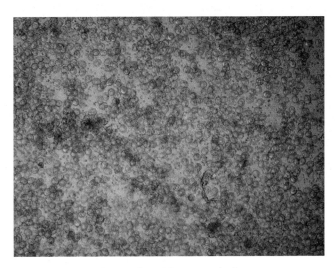

FIGURE 4.32   Calf with a very high number of coccida oocysts (4×).

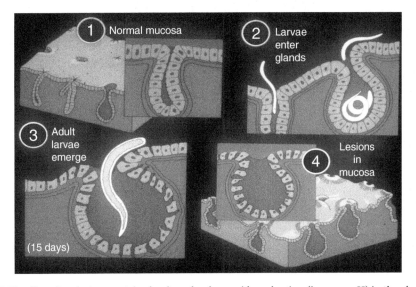

FIGURE 4.33   Parasites destroy gastric glands and reduce acid production (increase pH) in the abomasum.

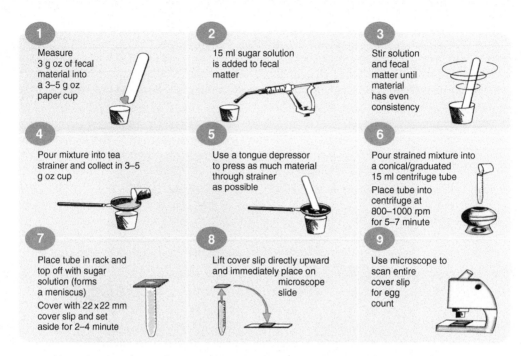

FIGURE 4.34 Modified Wisconsin Sugar Flotation Method.

RISK FACTORS AND PRODUCTION LOSSES CAUSED BY GASTROINTESTINAL PARASITISM

HOW MANY PARASITES ARE NEEDED TO CAUSE CLINICAL DISEASE?

Even a few parasites in a finely tuned lactating dairy cow can be damaging [3]. With internal parasites, it well established that even a few parasites during early lactation could become a detriment to achieving production potential [9]. The presence of parasitism soon after calving is magnifying the stress, which the cow is already undergoing and attacking her immune system [3]. Parasitized cattle are harmed, not only by the parasites themselves but also by the indirect damage the parasites cause to the immune system. A recent feedlot study showed dewormed cattle had significantly fewer health problems compared to non-dewormed cattle [15]. Pastured cattle have the greatest risk since their exposure to parasites is higher than cattle housed on dirt lots or in a confined facility.

Deworming studies conducted in the United States, Canada, and Europe have demonstrated lactating cows may lose anywhere from 100 to 1200 pounds of milk per lactation due to internal parasites [2, 3, 6, 7, 10, 13, 14] (Table 4.1). The greatest responses came from high-producing herds with moderate levels of parasite contamination where the deworming strategy was to keep the lactating animals parasite-free for the first 90–100 days of lactation, i.e., dewormings conducted at freshening and again six weeks later [3, 6, 7]. These studies demonstrated that by removing parasites during the period of greatest stress during the early lactation period, production losses due to internal parasites could be prevented. A separate study conducted at the University of Wisconsin confirmed this premise when parasite-free cows were exposed to infective larvae. Cows that were less than 90 days fresh lost on average 6.5# of milk per head per day [3].

Table 4.1   Published trials measuring parasite effect on milk production in lactating dairy cow following anthelmintic treatment.

Study Location	No. of Herds	No. of Cows	Deworming Strategy	Results
Wisconsin [1]	22	1003	Dewormed once avg 144 DIM [2];	+1.2 lb/day or +366 lb/lactation
Wisconsin [2]	1	48	All cows exposed** to parasites	
			Cows <90 DIM	+6.4 lb/day
			1# = 200 lb/lactation	+1280 lb/lactation
Wisconsin [3]	12	488	Dewormed at freshening	+423 lb/lactation
Vermont [4]	9	267	Parasite-free first 90 days***	+534 lb/lactation
Pennsylvania [5]	9	180	Parasite-free first 90 days	+769 lb/lactation
North Carolina [5]	5	160	Parasite-free first 90 days	+1075 lb/lactation
England [6]	1	210	Parasite-free first 90 days	+827.2 lb/lactation
Australia [7]	1	58	Parasite-free first 90 days	+338.8 lb/lactation
Netherlands [8]	81	2025	Dewormed prior to freshening	+292.4 lb/lactation
England [9]	9	268	Dewormed prior to freshening	+380.6 lb/lactation
Overall	150 herds	4707 cows	One to three dewormings in early lactation +628.6 lb/lactation	

*   DIM, days in milk.
**   Artificially exposed to parasite larvae.
*** First 90 days of lactation.

The process whereby a 1600 lb Holstein cow can be harmed by a few tiny parasites is complicated. Damage caused by parasites in the abomasum changes the physiology of the digestive system. One, worm, *Ostertagia*, for example, completes it life cycle by spending time in a gastric gland. While this larva is in the gland, it undergoes a molt growing and expanding within the gland (see Figure 4.35). The parasite temporarily and mechanically destroys the gland, shutting down acid production and causing blood leakage back into the gastrointestinal tract. When acid production is reduced by the parasites in the gland, the pH rises and digestion efficiency is reduced.

LEVEL OF EFFICIENCY CAN AFFECT PRODUCTION LOSSES

The more efficient an operation is, the fewer parasites it takes to cause a problem. Further complicating the picture is that the parasite contamination levels may be less that what they were just 20 years ago because of increased usage of better and more efficient dewormers; however, economic loss caused by the parasitism is greater now because of increases in efficiency and higher production standards than was present just a few years ago.

Production standards have increased greatly over the past few years due to new technology such as the use of hormones, improved nutrition, improved genetics, and numerous other management changes. A few parasites in a cow producing 25,000 pounds annually will cause more problems to her health, reproduction, and production levels than a higher worm burden in a low-producing cow. Therefore, as dairy technology improves, and animals move closer and closer toward their maximum genetic potential, it becomes increasingly important for these high-producing herds to monitor their herd for parasites and maintain a strategic deworming program for all animals in the herd that needs protection.

Dairy and Beef Cattle Parasite Evaluation Form

PEC ☐   Mail In ☐   Page____ of____

Collection Date:	Consultant: Dr. Don Bliss
Name of Farm:	Sponsor:
Producer's Name:	Sponsor Contact:
Producer's Address:	Sponsor Address:
City Phone	City Phone
State Zip Fax	State Zip Fax
E-Mail:	Representative:

Sample ID	Animal ID	Contamination Level*	Stomach Worm	Nematodirus	Cooperia	Hookworm	Threadworm	Whipworm	Nodular Worm	Tapeworm	Coccidia	Total Count (EP3G)**	Treatment Date month/day/year	Product Used
													Enter after test results recorded	

*1 = pasture, 2 = limited pasture, 3 = dry lot/partial confinement, 4 = total confinement year round   **(+ = 1-10) (++ = 11-50) (+++ =>51)

COMMENTS:

Donald H. Bliss, Ph.D.
MidAmerica Ag. Research
3705 Sequoia Trail
Verona, WI 53593

Sponsor's E-mail:

For additional information and submission forms, visit: www.midamericaagresearch.net

Eggs/Pound Manure ☐

Total count x 150 = Eggs per pound

FIGURE 4.35   Dairy and beef cattle parasite evaluation form.

VARIATION IN PARASITES NUMBERS AND LEVELS OF CONTAMINATION RATES EXISTS

Changes in weather, nutrition, management, immune status of the animals, and the amount of exposure each animal has within a parasite-contaminated area, such as a pasture, affect the type of parasites present, the numbers of parasites present, and the numbers of parasites that are picked up by an animal and that develop within such animal. Each type or species of parasite is different in terms of where it lives within the animals and how it survives during the part of its life cycle that is spent outside the animals.

Shifts in parasite populations are common, where the predominate parasites found early in the year may be different than that those found later in the year. Dairy calves and heifers tend to have different parasite makeup than adult cows and develop higher numbers of parasites than adult cows (see Figure 4.7). In addition, the susceptibility of animals to parasites varies according to season of the year, age, and immune status of the animals.

Seasonal variation becomes a factor in northern climates where cattle are exposed to parasite infection from early spring to late fall, but during winter months have no opportunity to ingest infective larvae and thus immunity to parasites decreased until spring when exposure begins again. This is reflected in fecal worm egg counts when non-treated adult cows have higher eggs in late winter to early spring than they do in summer to late fall when the immune status of the animals is the highest. The true is the same for the lactation cycle when cows seem to be more refractory to parasites late in the lactation cycle, whereas during the first few weeks after calving when the cows undergo a "peri-parturient relaxation of resistance," worm egg counts appear to be the highest.

AGE AND MANAGEMENT VARIATIONS AFFECT PARASITE BUILDUP IN ANIMALS

Parasites buildup in the animals is strongly related to management practices as to how the animals are handled; if on pasture, stocking rate and grazing management play a large role in total parasite burden. Where the animals are housed is also important. Young animals housed on a "manure pack" can develop heavy infections during cold winter months with a number of intestinal parasites. These infections are called "barnyard" infections (see Figure 4.7) and are seldom ever seen in adult cows but can be very harmful to young cattle. These barnyard infections include *Trichuris* (whipworm), *Nematodirus* (threadneck worm), *Moniezia* (tapeworm), *Bunostomum* (hookworm), and *Strongyloides* (threadworm).

The actual numbers of parasites found in adult cows is small in comparison to young cattle with the same exposure to parasites. A survey of cull cows from 54 Wisconsin herds [11] demonstrated from 0 to 12,000 parasites were found, while in a similar survey at 10 locations across the United States and Canada in 120 yearling cattle, from 0 to 265,000 parasites were recovered [9]. The reason for this large difference between mature cattle and young animals is not fully known. Certainly, age resistance plays a role but whether it is due to an activated immune system of the cow due to parasite exposure or due to mechanical damage to tissues caused by parasites at an earlier age preventing larval development later on. Parasites number found in an animal may not be as important to production loss as is the immune status of the animal, production levels of the animal, stage of lactation, and degree of exposure to parasites.

UNDERSTANDING HOW GASTROINTESTINAL PARASITES AFFECT LACTATING DAIRY COWS

A. **Parasites can stress an already stressed animal:** Many milk production studies have been conducted over the years measuring the effect of deworming with varying results. The results of these studies often depended upon how the studies were designed and how the studies were conducted. Since milk production is a highly variable trait greatly influenced by many environmental conditions as well as genetic, it is a very difficult trait to accurately measure when conducting deworming trials under natural field conditions with commercial cattle.

The early studies identified that the period following calving when the dairy cow is under the greatest stress is the period when parasites exert their greatest damage. It appears that several things transpire at the same time when calving occurs. In a high-producing cow, the calving period is one of "negative energy balance" where dry intake cannot meet production needs and, therefore, the animals have to draw off their stored energy to meet this high demand. An average cow may lose up to 200 lb or more soon after calving. If parasites are present in the animal or if she is being exposed to infective larvae during this period, another physiological stress is being added to an already stressed animal [3].

B. **Internal parasites can adversely affect the immune system:** One benefit to deworming, that is often overlooked, is its impact on the effectiveness of vaccinations. Cows that are infected by parasites have compromised immune systems caused by the negative nutritional impact gastro-intestinal parasites have on the immune system [11]. In addition to this indirect impact, some parasites have a direct impact on the immune system through mechanical damage they cause to the animal itself.

Immunosuppression occurs when parasites actively hinder one or more of the host's defense mechanism. For example, *Ostertagia* secrete substances that suppress the host's immune system. Because the *Ostertagia* larvae damage the glands of the abomasum during development (see Figure 4.33), they disrupt metabolism and are thought to affect development of immunity simply by reducing the necessary substances such as protein and trace minerals.

It has been shown that some parasites can cause cows to create immune cells that shut down the production of antibodies and macrophages, key components in a functioning immune system. Such measures ensure that the parasite will survive and be able to reproduce in the cow. These immune-suppressive tactics that protect the parasite leave the cow susceptible to other invaders such as bacteria and viruses. As noted previously, immunosuppression interferes with the host's ability to respond to a vaccination, our most effective tool for preventing infectious disease.

MONITORING DAIRY HERDS FOR GASTROINTESTINAL PARASITE INFECTIONS

EVERY HERD IS DIFFERENT WHEN IT COMES TO INTERNAL PARASITIC INFECTIONS

A need exists, therefore, for specific and adequately sensitive tests to detect the existence of a known subclinical disease as well as to measure the adverse effects of the subclinical disease. A highly sensitive test for detecting internal parasites in dairy cattle is the Modified Wisconsin Sugar Flotation Technique. It is proven to be an excellent test to determine the presence or absence of parasitism within a herd. Once the presence of parasitism and the location within a herd is established, a specific control strategy can be implemented.

One key element for many dairymen is to first determine what the parasite contamination level is for their herd. One method to determine contamination level is to use the general guideline for determining parasite exposure under different types of herd management. The key issue is that the more the cattle are exposed to outdoor pasture-type conditions, the more parasite exposure that occurs.

THE FOLLOWING ARE GUIDELINES TO DETERMINE PARASITE EXPOSURE OF A DAIRY HERD BASED ON ANIMAL MANAGEMENT

High parasite contamination levels
 Cows rotationally grazed during lactation.
 Cows exposed to pasture during lactation.
Moderate parasite contamination level
 Cows exposed to pasture during the dry period.
 Cows with access to an exercise lot with grass (at least part of the year).
Low parasite contamination level
 Cows with access to dirt dry lot only.
Extremely low parasite contamination level
 Cows in total confinement housed on a concrete dry lot.

To scientifically determine where infections exist on an operation, the fecal exam is the most reliable and least expensive way to accomplish this task. Lactating dairy cows can produce close to 100 pounds of manure each day. Looking for worm egg in the feces is therefore like looking for a needle in the haystack and so a sensitive test must be used. The most sensitive fecal exam method developed to use with adult dairy cows is the "Modified Wisconsin Sugar Flotation Method." The type of exam conducted is very important because the Wisconsin Sugar Flotation Method is the only exam sensitive enough to accurately detect parasitism in lactation dairy cows (see Figures 4.34 and 4.35).

OBTAINING A COMPREHENSIVE "PARASITE FECAL CHECK" OF THE HERD CAN BE IMPORTANT

Fecal checks help provide scientific information about parasite levels within a certain category of animals on the operation and find out exactly where the parasite infections are within the herd. They can determine whether the cows, heifers, or calves are harboring internal parasites as well as the type of parasites present and then make an accurate assessment about the deworming strategy for each category of animal checked. Sampling approximately 5% of the herd is adequate. Samples should be taken from every major age group or category of animals on an operation. A "zip locked" baggie is the best collection devise to use by inverting baggie over the hand to pick up a golf ball-size sample from a fresh fecal pad. Make sure the sample bag is properly marked to identify where the samples were collected. Samples should be refrigerated or otherwise kept cool to prevent worm eggs from hatching before examination.

PRODUCTION LOSSES DUE TO GASTROINTESTINAL PARASITES

SEASONAL CONTROL OF GASTROINTESTINAL PARASITIC INFECTIONS IN DAIRY OPERATIONS

Establishing a Strategic Deworming Program

The economics of parasitism not only involves the development of parasites under pasture and confined systems of management but also the prevalence of parasitism in these systems. Knowing whether parasites are present on the operation is the first step to establishing a control strategy. Once the parasite presence is established, a control strategy can be implemented.

Parasite development is usually seasonal, depending upon location of the operation. Seasonal treatment is compromised slightly with lactating cows because their lactation cycles seldom match seasonal weather conditions. Strategic use of fenbendazole on a seasonal basis will reduce parasite challenge for the entire year by as much as 85%. The problem with lactating cows, keeping them parasite-free during the first trimester of lactation may require a slightly different program. Maybe the best program for lactating dairy cows is a combination of seasonal treatment with individual treatment (see below).

Steps Necessary to Develop A Successful Control Program for the Prevention of Parasitism on an Operation

Select the Correct Product A deworming product must have FDA approval for use in lactating dairy cows without milk withdrawal and should be highly efficacious with a 98% efficacy against all-important internal parasites (including lungworm) and all stages of the parasite within the animal. This feature is important because a late fall deworming should remove all parasites in the animal at the time of treatment so that the cattle remain relatively parasite-free until the following spring. The other feature is that the dewormer should work quickly, especially with lungworm infections because, if it takes two or three days to work, animals may die from the infection before it is completely removed.

Fenbendazole (Safe-Guard®/Panacur® – Merck Animal Health) has been shown to be the safest and most efficacious gastrointestinal and lungworm dewormer on the market. It has been to shown to destroy the worms within the first 12 hours after treatment. It can be used at any stage of lactation or gestation with no health problems and no milk withdrawal. It can be given in a single oral dose as a drench or paste (see Figure 4.36). So, you do not have to chase animal (see Figure 4.37)

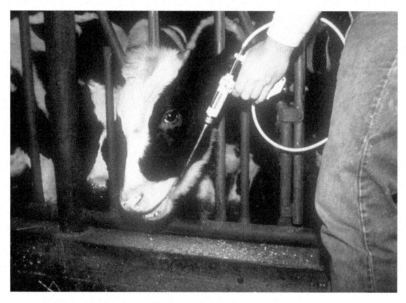

FIGURE 4.36   Dairy calf deworming treatment with a drench.

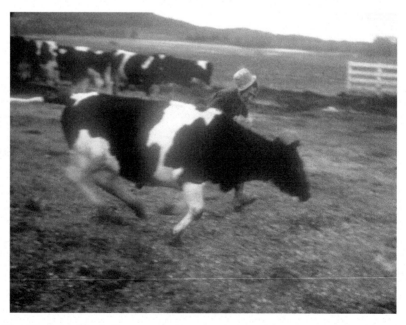

FIGURE 4.37   Chasing a dairy heifer.

and catch them to treat. Safe-Guard can also be top-dressed, mixed in the ration or mixed in the total mixed ration (TMR), and given free-choice (see Figure 4.38). For non-lactating animals such as replacement heifers, fenbendazole can be administered in a medicated block or medicated mineral, which can be given free-choice to be eaten over a three- to six-day period to make sure all animals have time to come to the source and receive an adequate deworming dose (see Figure 4.39).

Oral deworming with fenbendazole has been shown to be much more efficient in removing both immature and mature stages of the parasites than the pour-on dewormers. Deworming through the feed places the dewormer directly into the gastrointestinal tract exactly where the parasites live, thus providing the most effective method. For feed-choice deworming with fenbendazole, the product is cumulative in the parasite, so when the animal has consumed enough

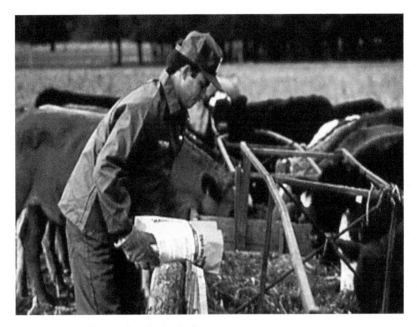

FIGURE 4.38   Deworming dairy calves in the feed.

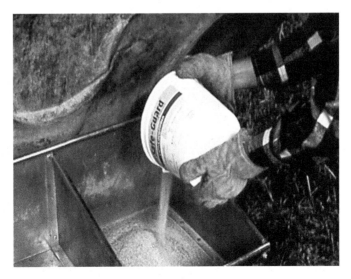

FIGURE 4.39   Deworming dairy heifers in the mineral.

product to be lethal, the parasites are destroyed since it may take several days for the animals to receive adequate dose.

Pour-ons are only effective if sufficient product is absorbed in the blood, which must then travel to the gastrointestinal tract to kill the parasites living there.

Recent studies demonstrate that most pour-on dewormers lack adequate absorption into the bloodstream to be fully effective. Blood level studies show that only one-third the amount of pour-on product reaches the blood when compared to injectable formulations of the same product.

Select the Correct Treatment Time for Adult Dairy Cows The best dewormer in the world used at the wrong time is a wasted resource. Treatment can be given on herd basis or individual basis or a combination thereof.

Herd treatment: This treatment regime should be initiated in late fall with a follow-up deworming given four to six weeks into spring grazing. The late fall deworming should be given after a hard frost or after the pastures are dormant. The goal is to render the animal's parasite-free going into the winter. Feeding wormy animals during the winter is highly inefficient. The overall goal is twofold, first, to create a parasite-free animal for maximum over-wintering ability and, second, to create an animal that remains parasite-free until it returns to spring pasture so that this animal will not be shedding parasite eggs or recontaminating the pasture at the beginning of spring but rather will not contribute to the recontamination of the pasture until this animal becomes reinfected by consuming infective larvae which have grown over winter on the pasture and until these parasites are mature egg-laying adult parasites.

Individual or group treatment: Treat individual cows or use a feed through dewormer every two to three weeks in the pre-fresh group or individually at the time of calving. Ideally, deworming should be repeated six weeks postpartum or at breeding time when moderate or high levels of parasite contamination are often found. The most important part of this strategy is to have the pregnant cows deworming just prior or at freshening to make sure these cows are parasite-free at the beginning of the lactation period.

Combination treatment: All cows and young stock are dewormed in the fall as a whole herd deworming and then beginning the following spring and early summer as cows and bred heifers come into the milk line, an individual deworming is given to each animal just prior to or at the time of freshening.

Select the Correct Treatment Time for Replacement Heifers and Other Youngstock

Replacement heifer treatment: Replacement heifers and other youngstock on the operation should be treated on a season basis depending upon whether they are turned out to pasture or not.
Pastured youngstock: Treat all animals four and eight weeks after turnout onto pasture or paddocks. Young cattle will begin worm eggs in the feces 25–30 days after turnout onto spring pastures. Deworming the youngstock twice four weeks apart in the spring eliminates pasture contamination by a high percentage for the entire summer grazing season (see Figure 4.40). Deworm all animals at the end of the season in late fall or early winter to maintain parasite-free status.

Confined youngstock: Most calves raised in confinement or concrete yards are parasite-free unless housed on a manure pack or have access to dirt lots. If these animals are raised in total confinement, they should be checked for parasites at every six months. Otherwise, deworming should be given at breeding time and again just prior to the time they are entering the milk herd, i.e., just prior to freshening. Occasional fecal checks are important to make sure animals are

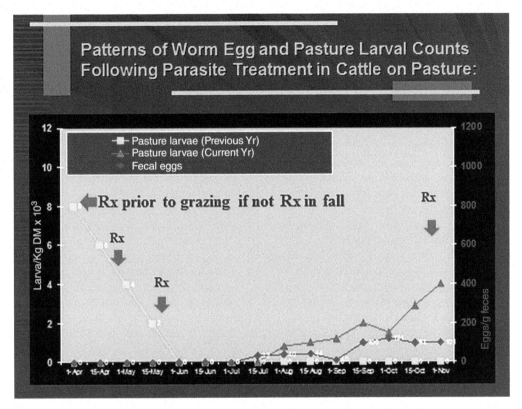

FIGURE 4.40   Spring treatment reduces parasite challenge for the summer grazing season.

parasite-free. Deworm all animals if any parasite eggs are found. Animals in confinement can pick up "barnyard" infections (see Figure 4.7), which include whipworm, threadworms, tape-worms, hookworms, and threadneck worm (*Nematodirus*).

Maintaining an Annual Treatment Program   The economic benefits from strategic timed deworm-ing in dairy cattle improves each year because as parasite contamination is reduced in the cows' environment, parasite control is easier to achieve. Strategic deworming is a management tool that when producers follow the steps given above and make sure their cattle are treated at the proper time each year they can be assured that parasites are not interfering with their animals production efficiency. The second year on a strategic deworming program is usually better than the first year because environmental contamination gets less each year the program is in place.

CONCLUSION

Deworming dairy cattle is a venture beyond treating clinical disease; the treatment of parasitism should be aimed first at the elimination of the threat of economic loss and later at the reduction or elimination of the parasites as a potential future risk within an operation itself. Parasitism contrib-utes nothing good to the animals they parasitize; even if the animals are 1600 lb dairy cows, they need to be eliminated to prevent unseen production losses.

REFERENCES

1. Dickinson, E.O., Armstrong, D.A., Schafer, J.H., and Bliss, D.H. (1991). Nematodirus helvetianus: an overlooked and underestimated parasite of calves. *Topics Vet. Med.* 2: 12–19.

2. Bliss, D.H. and Todd, A.C. (1973). Milk production by Wisconsin dairy cows after deworming with Baymix. *Vet. Med. Small Anim. Clin.* 68: 1034.

3. Bliss, D.H. and Todd, A.C. (1977). Milk losses in dairy cows after exposure to infective trichostrongylid larvae. *Vet. Med. Small Anim. Clin.* 72: 1612–1617.

4. Bliss, D.H. and Todd, A.C. (1974). Milk production by Wisconsin dairy cattle after deworming with Thiabendazole. *Vet. Med. Small Anim. Clin.* 69: 638–640.

5. Bliss, D.H. and Todd, A.C. (1976). Milk production by Vermont dairy cattle after deworming (two deworming during the first 90-days of lactation). *Vet. Med. Small Anim. Clin.* 71: 1251–1254.

6. Todd, A.C., Bliss, D.H., Grisi, L., and Crowley, J.W. (1978). Milk production by dairy cattle in Pennsylvania and North Carolina after deworming (treatment at freshening and systemically over the first three months of lactation). *Vet. Med. Small Anim. Clin.* 73: 614–619.

7. Bliss, D.H., Jones, R.M., and Condor, D.R. (1982). Epidemiology and control of gastrointestinal7parasitism in lactating, grazing adult dairy cows using a morantel sustained release bolus. *Vet. Rec.* 110: 141–144.

8. Bliss, D.H. and Myers, G.H. (1998). Lungworm (Dictyocaulus) outbreak in lactating cows. *Large Pract.* 19: 20–23.

9. Bliss, D.H. and Newby, T.J. (1988). Efficacy of the morantel sustained release bolus in grazing cattle in North America. *JAVMA 192* 172 (2): 177–181.

10. Mathews, G.L., Gray, R.M., and McGowan, A.A. (1983). Effects of anthelmintic treatment immediately after calving on milk production. *Aust. Vet. J.* 60 (4): 116–119.

11. Gutierres, V., Todd, A.C., and Crowley, J.W. (1979). Natural populations of helminths in Wisconsin dairy cows. *VM/SAC* 74: 69–374.

12. Kelly, J.D. (1973). Immunity and epidemiology of helminthiasis in grazing animals. *New Zeal. Vet J.* 21: 183–194.

13. Ploeger, H.W., Koosterman, A., Bargeman, G. et al. (1990). Milk yield increase after anthelmintic treatment of dairy cattle related to some parameters estimating helminth infection. *Vet. Parasitol.* 35: 103–116.

14. Mcbeath, D.G., Dean, S.P., and Preston, N.K. (1979). The effect of preparturient fenbendazole treatment on lactation yield in dairy cows. *Vet. Rec.* 105: 507–509.

15. Smith, R.A., Rogers, K.C., Husae, S. et al. (2000). Pasture deworming and (or) subsequent feedlot performance with fenbendazole. I. Effects on grazing performance, feedlot performance and carcass traits in yearling steers. *Bovine Practitioner* 34: 104–114.

16. Stone, W.M. and Smith, F.W. (1973). Infection of mammalian hosts by milk-borne nematode larvae. *A review. Exp. Parasit.* 34: 306–312.

Parasites in Equine

Cattle, raised in total confinement often exist free of gastrointestinal nematode parasites: however, regardless of how they are raised, horses rarely, if ever, escape parasite exposure. Horses are said to have the largest collection of parasites of all domestic livestock. It is not unusual for a seemingly healthy horse to harbor over one-half million gastrointestinal nematode parasites. The largest parasite group that causes the overall biggest problem for horses are the strongyles. Equine strongyles are characterized as both "small strongyles" and "large strongyles" which are all located in the large intestine. Small strongyles are often called as cyathostomes and there exist about 40 species, while the large strongyles include just a three or four species. Together this group has become the nemesis for equine parasitologist for the past 40 years because successful control has seldom been accomplished. We will discuss this problem in detail within this chapter on parasites of equine [1–3].

Gastrointestinal parasites cause damage to the animals both during the infection phase when the invading larvae are undergoing early development in the tissues of the gastrointestinal tract and then again after these organisms have emerged and developed fully to adult parasites living in their final or predilection sites laying eggs back into the environment.

In the development phase, tissues are damaged and the immune system of the horse is negatively affected causing a cellular response directly proportional to the number of invading larvae. With daily exposure, the effect on the immune system can be very strong, limiting the horse's ability to fight off other disease problems at the same time attempting to ward off a continuous stream of invading larvae. Random therapeutic treatments unless carefully timed have little or no effect on controlling the source of the infections or in preventing damage to the horse caused by the developing infections. Worm eggs shed early in the season develop into infective larvae at an increasing rate as the temperature warms and summer approaches. A large number of larvae living free in the environment can become infective over a short period, re-exposing the horse to high levels of parasitism. These free-living parasitic infective larvae present in the horse's environment are the foremost problem because they serve as the source for all new infections.

Overall, millions of dollars are spent every year for internal parasite control in horses; however, internal parasites remain one of the most important problems affecting the health and well-being of horses. The reason for this is that parasite control measures recommended and practiced over the past 25 years have provided limited protection to the horse by simply treating the infections after they have already developed with little or no effect on preventing environmental contamination [4–6]. Once horse owners develop a basic understanding of the infection process for small strongyles and change the way treatments are administered, the ability to reduce environmental contamination with infective larvae can be reversed [7].

Large Animal Parasitology Procedures for Veterinary Technicians, First Edition. Donald H. Bliss.
© 2024 John Wiley & Sons, Inc. Published 2024 by John Wiley & Sons, Inc.

GASTROINTESTINAL NEMATODE PARASITES AFFECT HORSES IN MANY WAYS

A. **Clinical Parasitism** is a condition where the number of invading parasites have reached a point that the negative effects of parasitism become visible. Animals with rough hair coat, potbelly, poor body condition, and colic are examples of problems due to clinical parasitism. Clinical parasitism is complicated because it is interrelated to a number of variables including nutrition and immune status of the animals. Horses carrying heavy worm burdens can appear normal if nutrition levels are adequate to "feed the animal past the parasitism." If nutrition is inadequate or an animal is stressed from hard work or maybe even overworked, the animal may begin to develop signs of clinical parasitism more rapidly than in animals that receive adequate nutrition (see Figure 5.1).

Animal that are allowed to overgraze the pasture are at greatest risk for developing clinical parasitism because late in the season when the parasitic free-living larval populations on the pastures are at their greatest numbers, the nutrition of the pastures are usually at their lowest level. If left untreated, it is not uncommon for clinically affected horses to colic and die from a heavy level of parasitism. Also, because of the coprophagic nature of horses, it is a very difficult task to maintain horses totally free of parasites without first reducing or eliminating environmental contamination by infective larval stages.

Most clinically infected horses harbor high numbers of adult parasites but also are carrying high numbers of encysted or inhibited larvae imbedded in the wall of the colon. As worm burdens build throughout the summer months, it appears that the physiology of the gastrointestinal tract changes and conditions are no longer ideal for larval development. New incoming infective larvae then undergo a period of arrested development waiting in the tissues until the physiological condition of the gastrointestinal tract returns to normal at which time these larvae resume development again. Since it is not in the best interest of the parasites to kill their host, the arrested development of larvae protects the host from being overwhelmed which also protects the parasites because if the host dies, the parasites also perish.

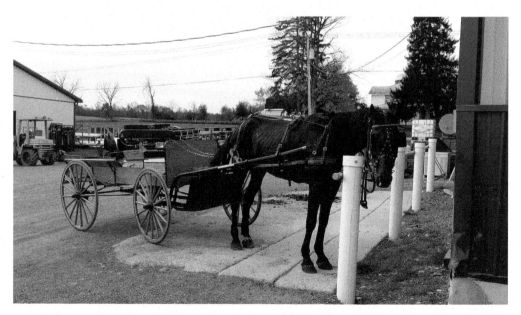

FIGURE 5.1   Clinically infected horse carrying heavy strongyle infections with an worm egg count over 1000 eggs per 3 g sample.

The actions that triggers the release and redevelopment of encysted larvae into adult worms occur when older worms die off naturally and are not rapidly replaced by new larvae, especially during winter months or hot dry periods. The administration of a dewormer can also trigger the development of encysted larvae.

Once these larvae become encysted, their metabolism slows down and they become difficult to kill with conventional treatment because they are protected in the tissues. Since these larvae are in an inhibited state, their uptake of chemical dewormers intended to kill them is also reduced depending upon chemical makeup of the deworming compound. Once encysted larvae begin development and emerge into the lumen of the colon, clinical disease can develop if high numbers of larvae emerge all at the same time. This is often called cyathastomiasis. It is not unusually for some clinically infected horses to harbor over 1,000,000 encysted larvae at one time.

B.   **Subclinical parasitism** is hard to see and measure. Subclinically infected animals appear normal but these parasitisms are responsible for reduced growth rates in foals; reduced reproductive rates in mares, reduced milk production for the young, and a reduced ability of the infected animal's immune system to fight off other disease conditions. In performance horses, subclinical levels of parasitism can be very important because even slightly reduced performance may be very important. It only takes a few parasites to significantly reduce performance in a finely tuned animal.

Subclinical parasitism can be very costly because the owner is often unaware of the damage that is taking place since the parasites are not visible and lost performance can occur unknowingly (see Figure 5.2). The most important aspect of subclinical parasitism, however, is the ability of subclinical infected animals to shed worm eggs into the environment producing future infections. Subclinically infected animals, even with low worm egg counts, may be shedding thousands of eggs back in the horse's environment every day A horse with an egg count of only 30 eggs per 3 g sample (30 eggs × 150 = 4500 eggs per pound of manure)

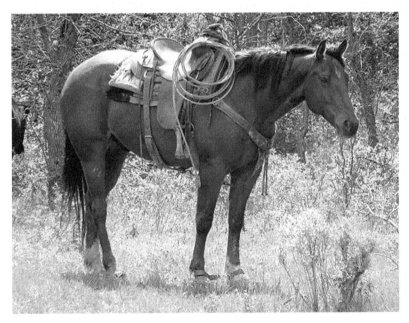

FIGURE 5.2   Subclinically infected working ranch horse as confirmed though a positive fecal worm egg count.

is shedding 4500 eggs in a pound of manure. If a horse excretes 60 lb of manure per day, the daily worm egg output in this case would 270,000 eggs excreted per day back into its environment.

Monitoring fecal worm egg counts is the best way to detect subclinical levels of parasitism. Using the "Modified Wisconsin Sugar Flotation Method" for monitoring parasite infections in horses is the most sensitive and accurate of all fecal exams (see Figure 5.3). Positive results indicate a parasitic worm burden is present and contamination of the environment is taking place. High egg counts indicate a high level of contamination is already occurring. Also, fecal worm egg counts in horses often correlate better with numbers of adult parasites present than fecal worm egg counts in most other species. Equine parasite evaluation forms allow veterinary technicians to record parasite worm egg counts according to a worm egg atlas (see Figures 5.4 and 5.5). Horses with fecal worm egg counts conducted by the "Modified Wisconsin Sugar Flotation Technique" in excess of 300 eggs/3 g sample are considered to be heavily infected while animals with egg counts over 1000 eggs/3 g (150,000 eggs/pound of manure) sample are often showing signs of clinical parasitism.

PARASITES DEVELOP DIFFERENTLY IN HORSES THAN IN CATTLE

A. **Parasitism in horses is most often an individual problem** while parasitism in cattle is considered a herd disease because cattle often graze together in designated groups on the same pastures, are all exposed to the same infection level and subsequently develop similar parasite burdens. Domestic horses are different because they are seldom herded or handled in large groups. Many horses across the country are raised in isolation or semi-isolation where contact with other horses is limited to just a few animals. Even in equine operations with multiple numbers of horses, the animals are usually either maintained separately or in small

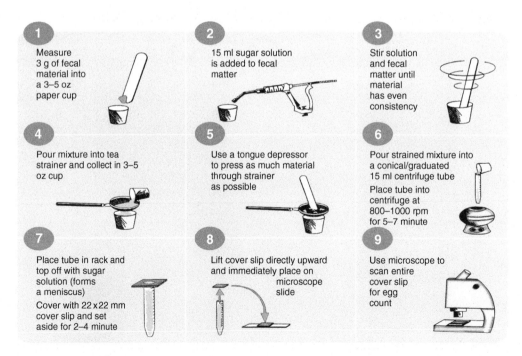

FIGURE 5.3   Modified Wisconsin Sugar Flotation Method.

Equine Parasite Evaluation Form

PEC ☐   Mail In ☐

Page____ of____

Collection Date: _____

Name of Farm: _____

Producer's Name: _____

Producer's Address: _____

City _____ Phone _____

State _____ Zip _____ Fax _____

E-Mail:

Consultant: Dr. Don Bliss

Sponsor: _____

Sponsor Contact: _____

Sponsor Address: _____

City _____ Phone _____

State _____ Zip _____ Fax _____

Representative:

Lab ID No.	Animal ID	Age/Gender *	Contamination**	Strongyles	Roundworm	Threadworm	Tapeworm	Pinworm	Coccidia	Total Count (EP3G)***	Treatment Date month/day/year	Product Used
											Enter after test results recorded	

* 1 = Mare, 2 = Stallion, 3 = Gelding, 4 = Yearling, 5 = Weanling, 6 = Foal, 7 = Other

**1 = pasture, 2 = limited pasture, 3 = dry lot/partial confinement, 4 = total confinement year round

***(+ = 1-10) (++ = 11-50) (+++ =>51)

COMMENTS:

Donald H. Bliss, Ph.D.
MidAmerica Ag. Research
3705 Sequoia Trail
Verona, WI 53593

Eggs/Pound Manure [   ]

Sponsor's E-mail:

For additional information and submission forms, visit: www.midamericaagresearch.net

Total count x 150 = Eggs per pound

FIGURE 5.4   Equine parasite evaluation form.

groups with little cross-contamination between animals. In both cases, cumulative worm burdens are generated from exposure to the infective offspring found in the environment which developed from eggs shed by the horses themselves. Because of this autoinfection, parasitism in horses is a disease problem requiring special attention to individual animals and their immediate environment.

B. **Horses routinely develop higher worm burdens than cattle especially under confined conditions.** Grazing cattle can develop extremely high levels of parasitism depending upon their environment; however, unless cattle are overstocked on heavily contamination pastures, parasitism in cattle is usually subclinical in nature and can easily be controlled with strategic timed dewormings. The primary way cattle become infected is by eating forages contaminated with infective larvae. Feedlot cattle or mature dairy cattle on "full feed" seldom become reinfected while held in confinement although calves can develop a "barnyard infection" with certain species of parasites while held in confinement especially when housed on a manure pack or in a crowded pen.

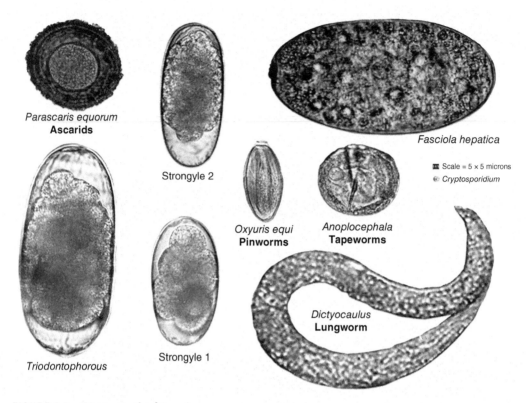

FIGURE 5.5 Worm egg atlas for equine.

Horses tend to bit, chew, or nibble at their surroundings often consuming parasite-infected bedding and, therefore, can develop relatively high levels of parasitism even while in confinement. Also, horses normally graze closer to the ground than cattle easily picking up large numbers of infective larvae while they graze. Because of these factors, horses can develop significant worm burdens depending upon environmental contamination whether they are housed in the stall, pen, or on pasture.

C. **Fecal worm egg output in parasitized horses is often much higher than parasitized cattle of similar age.** Horses have higher average worm egg counts than cattle for a number of reasons. One reason is that horse manure is more concentrated and contains less moisture than cattle manure so the concentration of worm eggs shed per gram of manure is often much greater in horses. A second reason that horses tend to have much higher worm egg counts than cattle of similar age is that certain species of parasites such as the small strongyles are identified as more prolific egg layers than the common gastrointestinal parasites (*Ostertagia*, *Haemonchus*, and *Trichostrongylus*) found in cattle. Overall, the most important aspect of high egg shedding is recontamination of the environment leading to continued parasite exposure.

The number of worm eggs shed per gram of feces influences the contamination rate of the environment surrounding the animals. The more eggs that are shed into the environment, the greater the chance for reinfection to occur. Using the "Modified Wisconsin Sugar Flotation Fecal Technique" for floating worm eggs out of fecal material, it is not uncommon for a mature horse to have a fecal worm egg count greater than 1000 eggs/3 g sample (150,000 eggs/pound of manure) whereas a count of greater than 100 eggs/3 g sample (15,000 eggs/pound of manure) is rare in mature cattle. As a general statement, the average fecal worm egg counts from horses routinely produce a 10-fold higher contamination rate when compared to cattle and is notably one of the main reasons for the ongoing failure to adequately control parasites in horses across the country.

D. **The economic value of deworming or cost of treatment is often less important with horse owners than with cattle producers.** Cattle dewormers are often purchased and administered to the animals based on perceived economic benefit in terms of increased feed efficiency or growth whereas most horses are handled individually with personal care so treatments are given based on perceived need with less concern about cost versus benefit of the treatment given. Deworming costs for adult horses are also regularly more expensive that the cost for deworming cattle. Horse dewormers can cost from several dollars per dose to as high as $60.00/treatment with an average cost of treatment around $8.00–$19.00/horse while treatment cost for adult cattle run from $1.80 per dose to as high as $7.00/treatment with average costs of around $3.50/mature animal.

Many horse owners alternate dewormers to help prevent parasite resistance from developing, whereas, cattle producers often use products that are convenient, products that work well with their type of operation and products that match the season, i.e., cattle producers may use an endectocide pour-on in late fall for lice and grub control while administering a medicated mineral or dewormer block in the spring. Because horse owners generally have lower concerns over product cost than cattlemen, the need to create a "least-cost most-effective" treatment program for horses has not been one of great concern for the horse industry. Because of this lack of economic concern, strategic deworming programs designed to reduce or eliminate environmental contamination by gastrointestinal internal parasites has not been widely researched or recommended.

E. **The lack of scientific evidence that strategic deworming strategies are effective is a problem for horse owners when compared to cattle producers.** Most cattle deworming programs are based on economic use data generated from carefully conducted trials measuring such parameters as growth rate, reproductive efficiency, and feed efficiency. These types of studies are seldom conducted with horses but rather horse owners are exposed to numerous treatment recommendations from a multitude of sources of which few provide scientific evidence that seasonal parasite control can be achieved by following the recommended program. Most of these deworming recommendations are confusing where one author recommends product rotation to prevent "resistance" while another author suggests that product rotation promotes "resistance" to all products used. Neither author provides any scientific evidence but rather provides their recommendations because it sounds like a "good recommendation." Horses all across the country are meanwhile suffering from unnecessary parasitism and parasite resistance has now become widespread such that horses can be exposed to increased levels of parasite exposure while their owners believe they are using an effective deworming strategy.

Equine dewormers are also easily available to horse owners where the owner purchases dewormers without knowing which products will work for their horses and which will not. The problem here is that if a particular product provides inadequate control due to the presence of parasite resistance, for example, a high number of worm eggs can be shed into the environment before another deworming is given. A second deworming product may also not work. The only way owners can determine whether the products they are using are successful in their horses is to have fecal worm egg count exams conducted on a regular basis.

Another problem facing the horse industry is that many horses are purchased and moved to new locations every year immediately contaminating the new location because care is seldom taken to confirm that animals are parasite-free before being moved. These horses usually have health records that outline deworming treatment history dewormings but animals can still be shedding worm eggs despite a recent deworming since parasite resistance could be present in the animals or sufficient time has elapsed allowing the animals to become reinfected since their last treatment. Two fecal checks should be conducted several weeks apart to determine parasite-free status prior to moving the horse to the new environment.

PARASITE RESISTANCE TO DEWORMERS HAS BECOME A MAJOR PROBLEM

A. **Although horses throughout North America receive routine dewormings, serious parasite problems have developed over the past 25 years and continue to exist.** The cause of parasite resistance to dewormers is not fully known. In fact, questions exist as to whether "parasite resistance to dewormers" is true resistance in the horse or that maybe it is "product tolerance" where many of the products used are unable to kill certain stages of the parasite, especially while these parasites are encysted in the wall of the intestine. "Parasite resistance" is defined in the literature as determined by the extent to which parasites that survive drug treatment contribute their genes to future generation. This contribution is influenced by the frequency and timing of treatment, drug efficacy, life expectancy and fecundity of the adult worms, rate of larval intake, egg deposition, grazing management, and weather.

Control programs are numerous and recommendations vary from one expert to another. Most experts agree that "parasite resistance" is a serious problem that is not going to go away on its own. However, little is being done to help the horse owner to prevent parasite resistance or to help solve the problem of resistance if it already occurs on an operation. Not only are programs not designed to eliminate environmental parasite contamination as the source of the problem, the widely recommended concept of repeated treatments given every 60–90 days to horses has caused and promoted the development of parasite resistance to many of the currently available deworming products. If, for example, a horse is not shedding eggs for approximately 30 days following treatment and then sheds for next 30–60 days before retreatment is given, the horse's environment is continually being recontaminated with parasites and treatment, therefore, has very little impact on keeping the horse's environment free from parasites.

B. **Deworming horses often triggers the development of inhibited or arrested larvae in the wall of the colon making it appear as though "parasite resistance" is present.** Most products have poor efficacy against encysted larvae (pyrantel pamoate, levamisole, oxibendazole, and fenbendazole) which means that the encysted larvae which survive treatment can emerge (see Figure 5.6) and develop to adult worms soon after the drug is gone from the horse's system. These newly developed adult parasites begin shedding eggs immediately and can give the appearance that "parasite resistance" had developed, instead, the egg are coming from adults worms that developed from encysted larvae missed during the time of treatment. Depending upon the time of the year, the level of parasite infection present and the dewormer used, adult parasites and some developing larvae may be killed; however, a population of inhibited larvae may be left in the animal (see Figure 5.7). Within the population of arrested larvae that remain intact following treatment, some of these larvae will begin development immediately following treatment such that in just a few days worm eggs can be detected in the feces of treated horses.

A recent investigation by the author for a possible "parasite resistance" to fenbendazole in horses located in Ontario, Canada, revealed a case where 100 yearling horses were housed in an outdoor snow-covered facility that experienced parasite problems despite treatment in early February with fenbendazole. Upon investigation, the horses had been on snow-covered

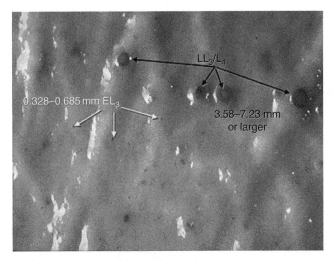

FIGURE 5.6   Encysted Strongyle larvae in the large intestine of the horse.

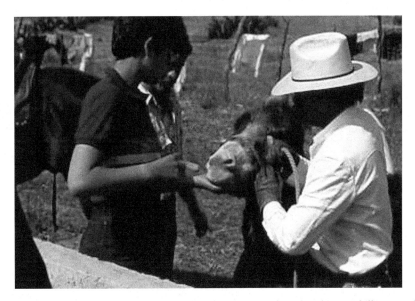

FIGURE 5.7   Deworming a Mexican donkey with a deworming product that does not kill encysted larvae.

ground since early November the previous fall. On December 1, all horses received ivermectin oral paste, on January 1, all horses received pyrantel paste at double dose and then on February 1, all horses received fenbendazole paste. Fecal samples taken several weeks following the fenbendazole treatment were positive for worm eggs showing incomplete parasite removal indicating "parasite resistance to the fenbendazole treatment." In this case, however, parasite transmission had not occurred since early November when the ground was frozen and first covered with snow. The parasites found in February, therefore, must have survived treatment with ivermectin (December 1), pyrantel (January 1), and fenbendazole (February 1) because the chance of the horses developing heavy infection between the time of the January treatment with pyrantel and the February treatment with fenbendazole is highly unlikely.

This information indicates that the mature infections probably developed from encysted larvae which survived the various treatments and emerged in February as adult parasites after the final treatment with fenbendazole rather than the horses suddenly became "resistant" to three different classes of dewormers all at once.

C. **Parasite control strategies recommended by manufacturers for equine dewormers are not designed to prevent or to reduce environmental contamination.** If the environment of an animal is heavily contaminated with infective larvae and treatment is given to an animal while exposed to daily ingestion of larvae, the administered drug treatment will kill those larvae susceptible to treatment and leave those that are not susceptible. For example, most dewormers will not kill infective larvae or even early developing larvae, so if these parasite stages are present at the time of treatment, they will survive treatment and continue development. Random treatment given to horses living in a heavily contaminated environment, therefore, accomplishes little in terms of controlling the existing parasitism but rather only temporarily removes a percentage of parasites present and increases the risk of causing resistance to those present but not killed at the time of treatment.

A parasite resistance study was conducted by the author with horse known to be harboring "parasite resistance" to fenbendazole. This study was conducted in four separate geographical regions of the country and demonstrated that when "parasite resistant" animals were removed from the source of parasite contamination and treated serially with the recommended dose of fenbendazole every 30 days, fecal worm egg counts were reduced to negative levels in 95% of the animals by the third treatment.

The question raised by this study was whether the parasites developed true resistance or whether the treatments removed only adult and late developing parasites allowing the encysted parasites to develop into adult egg-laying parasites soon after treatment making it appear like "parasite resistance" was present. Parasites resistant to a dewormer should be able to withstand continued exposure to the compound and not be killed. In this case, the animals were moved away from their original contaminated environment, thus no new parasites were ingested during the study. It is assumed, therefore, that the supply of encysted larvae in the colon was depleted by the third treatment, thus worm egg counts dropped to negative levels in 95% of the animals following the third treatment.

THE SEASONAL TRANSMISSION OF PARASITES IN THE HORSE

A. **Parasite infections come from the ingestion of infective larvae which develop in the environment of the horse.** Most of the economically important gastrointestinal parasites of horses have a direct life cycle as follows: adult parasites living within the horse lay eggs which are excreted in the manure; a larva develops within each egg, which then hatches, growing and molting twice until it reaches the infective third-stage (L_3) larva (see Figure 5.8). Egg development occurs outside the animal when weather conditions are warm and moisture is present. The development of eggs to infective larvae is slowed down or even stopped once temperatures fall below 45° or when temperatures exceed 90°. Development from the egg stage to an infective L_3 larva can take just a few days under optimal conditions or many months under suboptimal conditions. Once infective, the larva needs to be consumed by a horse to re-establish a new infection in the gastrointestinal tract. In the horse, the ingested larvae undergo two additional molts going from the infective L_3 stage to an L_4 larva and then to an L_5 or early adult stage. Male and female adult worms must both be present to produce viable eggs which then pass out with the feces starting the cycle over again. The time from

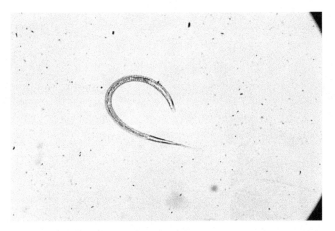

FIGURE 5.8   Infective larvae with protective outer sheath.

when an infective larva is consumed until an adult worm is present in the gastrointestinal tract depends on the worm species but can be anywhere from four weeks to eight months.

The first (L_1)- and second (L_2)-stage larvae are not mobile but stay in the fecal material feeding off bacteria and fecal debris. These larval stages appear to be sensitive to adverse weather conditions; however, once the larva reaches the L_3 infective stage, it becomes more resistant to adverse weather condition and also becomes mobile, moving away from the fecal material by following moisture trails to reach nearby vegetation where it can be consumed by foraging animals. Infective larvae are encased with a sheath they acquire from the molt as L_2 larvae. This encasement protects the larvae from environmental conditions and immediately after ingestion (from stomach acids) before the outer coat is shed in the colon where the new infection is initiated. The encasement covers the entire larva including the mouth parts and prevents the infective L_3 larvae from feeding. The infective L_3 larva must live off stored food material in the body of the larvae and, therefore, have a finite life span, once the stored material is gone, the larvae die. This especially is important in the spring of the year when larvae which have overwintered become active in the spring, looking for a host animal. If a host is not found, these larvae will soon die because of limited energy from stored food material.

Once infective, these L_3 larvae are mobile following moisture trails moving from the fecal matter onto the vegetation in order to reinfect the animals. The larvae that are consumed on a daily basis develop within the animals to mature adult worms releasing eggs back in the environment. These eggs develop into infective larvae which accumulate in the pastures often building up to very high levels by late summer or early fall (see Figure 5.9). When the temperatures are cool, it takes longer for the infective larvae to develop than it does when the temperature is warm and moist. Often, the eggs that are deposited in the environment of the horse in early spring develop into infective at the same time as the eggs deposited on the pasture later when the temperature is more favorable. Many times, larval buildup can reach as high as 10,000 larvae per square meters of grass collected. Once frost or freezing temperatures arrive, the larvae intake drops off as the larvae become immobile and are either killed or remain protected in the soil or under the vegetation. At this point, reinfection drops to low or negative levels.

Under heavy larval contamination of the environment, infective larvae can be found almost everywhere horses are present. Larvae can be found in the dirt, in bedding, around water troughs, on the animals themselves, and throughout the horses surroundings wherever

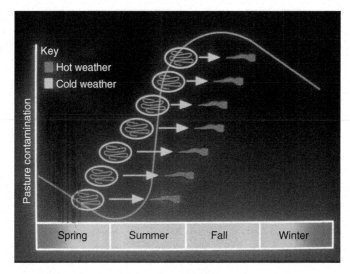

FIGURE 5.9   Seasonal pattern of eggs and larval distribution on pasture showing contamination levels for equine.

the larvae can find protection from sunlight, desiccation, cold temperatures, and other adverse environmental conditions. The infective L_3 stage survives in a protected microclimate in the soil, in fecal pats, or under layers of herbage. These free-living infective larvae can live for an entire year in the environment if well protected from extreme heat, cold, or drying. During periods of extreme cold or when conditions are very dry, the larvae become immobile waiting for warm moist conditions to return when it begins to become mobile again trying to find a host. Animals that are exposed to mild winter conditions or housed in heated barns can become exposed to parasitic larvae and develop active infections throughout the year.

B. **Parasites can survive winter or hot summer conditions either as adult, inhibited larvae or infective larvae in the environment.** The adult parasite within the horse have a finite life span; however, as the older parasites die off, they are replenished by the new incoming larvae or larvae that have emerged from the gut wall (in the case of the small strongyles), from the lungs (in the case of roundworms), and from the mesentery arteries (in the case of *Strongylus vulgaris*). Infected horses then reseed the pastures with parasite eggs which develop into infective larvae contaminating spring pastures. Animals that enter the spring months harboring parasites begin shedding worm eggs immediately while those which begin the spring season parasite-free will not recontaminate their environment until a new infection has developed from newly acquired infection off spring pastures. As temperature increases with spring developing, these eggs hatch and develop into infective larvae. In the eggs that have been lying in the environment waiting for warm weather, many of these eggs will develop around the same time depending upon the weather causing high levels of contamination to occur once.

Pastures not grazed by horses from the beginning of the spring season for the first three months (90 days) will become "parasite safe" pastures since the overwintered larvae have expired and died off while no new worm eggs have been released on the pastures (since there were no horses on the pasture to replenish larval contamination of the pasture). Any animal going on to "parasite safe" pastures should be dewormed prior to being to the pasture. Treating horses strategically to make sure they are not shedding eggs during the first three months

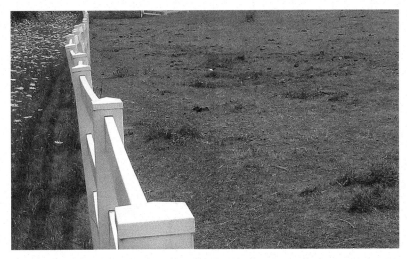

FIGURE 5.10   Overgrazed horse pasture showing intact fecal pats as possible lack of dung beetle activity.

of the season will achieve the same goal: the existing larvae will be gone by late June or early July and the pastures will be safe from parasites until fall.

Pasture contamination by infective larvae maybe influenced by dung beetle populations. Studies have shown that an active beetle population will bury both fly and worm eggs into the soil as well as by breaking the manure pats down exposing fly and worm larvae to sunlight which can be lethal. A healthy beetle population can help reduce parasite exposure to the animals grazing these pastures [8–10]. On the negative side, these beetle populations can be reduced by anthelmintic treatment with products that are lethal to beetles. The main culprit is ivermectin and its effect on removing dung beetle populations can be seen wherever intact fecal pats are evident on horse pastures (see Figure 5.10).

C. **Larval transmission to the horse:** Transmission is the phase when infective larvae are consumed by animals and the infection process begins. The key transmission times are often in early morning or late evening when dew is on the vegetation and the animals are grazing. When the sun comes out it in the morning, the dew dries up and the larvae move back to the base of the grass. Rain also moves the larvae onto the vegetation where they can be consumed. When conditions are right for vegetation growth, conditions are also right for parasite development and infective larvae that survive the winters become active once temperatures warm up in the spring and move onto the vegetation where they are consumed by grazing animals. If the larvae are not consumed, they will eventually deplete their food supply and die. If the pastures are not replenished with new eggs by early summer, the larvae from the previous year will have expired.

SEASONAL CONTROL OF PARASITES IN HORSES CAN BE ACHIEVED BY REDUCING PARASITE CONTAMINATION FROM THE ENVIRONMENT

A. **Environmental contamination by infective larvae** is the main deterrent to effective parasite control. If environmental contamination is not controlled, animals immediately become reinfected following treatment. Current deworming practices are unsuccessful in the long term because dewormers are used to purge parasitic worm burdens only after they have developed and the damage to the animals and the environment has already occurred.

Fecal worm egg counts taken weekly following treatment show that horses treated every eight weeks have little impact on reducing environmental contamination. Monitoring fecal worm egg counts following treatment also shows that many of these treatments are ineffective. This means on an eight week treatment cycle, the treated animals are free from shedding eggs for approximately four weeks and then shed eggs for four weeks every cycle. Even with a low egg count, the environment is quickly contaminated.

B. **The concept of preventing parasite contamination of the environment** can be accomplished by eliminating egg shedding back into the environment by strategically timed dewormings. Internal nematode parasites of horses can be controlled and, in some cases, eliminated with current deworming products by using these products at strategic times to prevent horses from reinfecting themselves or other horses that share the same environment. Autoinfection or reinfection comes from the environmental contamination of housing facilities, exercise areas, or pasture environment with infective larvae. Many times the environment of the horse, even in total confinement, can become highly contaminated with infective larvae such that dangerous levels of parasitism can develop within the horse unknowingly. Current recommended deworming practices only temporarily elevate the problem by removing worm burdens in the animals but have little effect on reducing the numbers of infective larvae in the environment, thus the animals become reinfected immediately after treatment.

The most important part of keeping fecal worm egg counts at negative levels during the early part of the season is to monitor treatment to make sure the animals are not shedding eggs into the environment. Whether a dewormer works in a particular horse depends on the species of parasites present, the number of parasite present, the number of inhibited small strongyle larvae present in the colon, and whether a particular infection is resistant to the dewormer used.

GENERAL RECOMMENDATIONS FOR STRATEGIC TIMED DEWORMING FOR THE SEASON CONTROL OF GASTROINTESTINAL PARASITES IN HORSES

A. **Successful deworming requires a seasonal program** with multiple treatments given at strategic times to prevent the buildup of parasite contamination in the environment. A successful program is one that is designed to reduce both the number of parasites in the animal as well as subsequent parasite contamination of the environment. Strategic treatments need to be timed with the season when transmission is most likely to occur to be successful. Except for areas of the country where year-around grazing is practiced, parasite transmission is limited during winter months. In most parts of the country, therefore, transmission occurs most successfully during the spring and again in the fall of the year. In parts of the country where year-around grazing is practiced, all horses should be worm-free during the hot dry months with repeated strategic dewormings during the rainy months.

B. **Phase I: All animals should be parasite-free during the winter months.** To begin the program, all horses should be parasite-free throughout the winter months and prior to the start of the transmission season in the spring. This includes making sure all animals are free from harboring encysted larvae acquired during the previous grazing season. The goal has multiple benefits, the first is to make sure the animals are free from harmful parasitism during the winter months, the second, is to make sure the animals are not shedding worm eggs at the beginning of the grazing season in the spring and, the third, is to make all mares are parasite-free at the time of foaling. The last treatment of the season should take place after pastures are dormant (late November to December). If post-treatment fecal exams indicate infections are still present after the December treatment, repeated treatment may be necessary including the use of the larvicidal dose of fenbendazole (10 mg/kg daily for five days) followed by a ivermectin treatment if required. A fecal sample should be taken in late winter to make sure all horses are parasite-free to start the grazing season. All horses that are heavily parasitized (when fecal worm egg counts are over 300 eggs/3 g sample) or horses that have not been dewormed on a regular basis should be dewormed with a larvicidal of fenbendazole to remove inhibited larval stages.

C. **Fall deworming does not mean that all horses will stay worm**-free during the winter since inhibited larvae present in the fall will begin to mature during the winter months and emerge to begin laying eggs contaminating the spring pastures to start the infection-cycle all over again. Late Feburary and March (possible April in northern climate) are the best time to fecal-check horses to make sure they are worm-free when grazing begins in the spring.

D. **Phase II: Strategic timed spring dewormings:** In the horse, treatment should be timed with the seasonal parasite life cycle on pasture where parasite development in the environment in most parts of the country is the greatest in the spring and the fall. To reduce the overall parasite contamination of the environment, three spring dewormings should be given approximately 30 days apart in the spring and again once in the fall (see Figures 5.11 and 5.12). If the animals are parasite-free at the beginning of the spring season, the first treatment should be given approximately 30 days after the start of spring grazing (see Figure 5.13). The repeated treatment works because as animals pick up infective larvae in early spring, these larvae are killed with the first treatment before they can mature and begin laying eggs back in the environment of the horse. The horses continue to pick up more larvae, which are killed by the second and then the third treatment before they can shed eggs again. By preventing eggs from being shed for the first three to four months in the beginning of the grazing season significantly reduces parasite contamination for the following three months.

Where grazing exists year-round, strategic timed deworming treatment should be given three times in the spring and three times in fall approximately one month apart as shown (see Figure 5.14). These repeated dewormings are designed to reduce the seasonal parasite challenge throughout the summer and maintain the horses relatively parasite-free throughout the winter months. The last treatment should be given in late November or early December and may include both bot and tapeworm treatment if needed. Each "three treatment regime" provides approximately six months control, thus the spring treatment protects the horses until fall and the fall regime protects the horses until spring. These repeated treatments also help remove encysted larvae which may have survived in the horse through the winter months while preventing more from establishing throughout the entire grazing season by reducing the overall buildup of infective larvae in the environment of the treated animals.

A TWO-YEAR STUDY DEMONSTRATING THE VALUE OF STRATEGIC DEWORMING TO REDUCE ENVIRONMENT CONTAMINATION WAS CONDUCTED IN NEVADA

A two-year study was conducted with the University of Nevada to determine if strategic timed dewormings with fenbendazole (Safe-Guard®) given at three monthly intervals in the spring starting in March and three monthly intervals in the fall starting in October could be used to reduce

"Strategic Deworming Protocol for the Seasonal Control of Gastro-intestinal Parasites of Equine"
Overall summary assessment of parasitism in equine:

(1) The number one problem in controlling parasites in horses begins with environment contamination with infective larvae during summer months.

(2) Contamination leads to heavy infections in the horse.

(3) Heavy infections lead to inhibition of the strongyle parasites. It is not in the best interest of the parasite to kill its host, so when parasite loads reach high levels, the parasites stop development and undergo arrested development until conditions in the gastrointestinal tract improve.

(4) High levels of inhibition leads to ineffective treatment (thus resistance to dewormers become evident) especially in the fall.

(5) As winter approaches and ingestion of infective larvae stops, the gut begins to return to normal and the inhibited begin to continue development to adult egg-laying parasites.

(6) Fecal worm egg counts taken in later winter tell the entire story [7]. Very high counts (500–1000 eggs/3 g) indicate heavy parasite challenge from the previous season and indicates that inhibition is probably likely occurring.

Treatment timing:

1. **Fall deworming regime:** At the end of the grazing season (best after a hard frost), feed Safe-Guard Pellets during morning feed at the rate of 1.0 lb per 1000 lb of body weight (Safe-Guard 0.5%) or 4 oz per 1000 lb body weight (Safe-Guard 1.96%) spread total dose over three days. On the fourth day, give ivermectin paste according to label directions.

2. **Winter deworming:** Conduct a fecal exam in late February to early March. If positive, repeat fall treatment regime to prevent worm eggs at the beginning of the grazing season.

3. **Spring–early summer strategic timed dewormings:** Give (3) treatments 30 days apart beginning 30 days after turn out or 30 days after first spring grass growth (e.g., May 1, June 1, and July 1):

   First deworming = 3-day Safe-Guard given 30 days after beginning of grazing season.
   Second deworming = 3-day Safe-Guard given 30 days after the first treatment.
   Third deworming = 3-day Safe-Guard (plus ivermectin paste given on the fourth day) given 30 days after the second treatment.

4. **Fall deworming:** Repeat fall program listed above.

Note: Multiple days of Safe-Guard activates encysted larvae which are then killed by ivermectin.

FIGURE 5.11   Strategic deworming protocol for seasonal parasite control for equine.

environmental parasite contamination and to maintain horses safe from harmful levels of parasitism throughout an entire year (see Figure 5.15). A total of 200 horses from local cooperating horse owners were used in the study. These horses were selected based on treatment history divided into five categories as follows: non-treated, infrequent treatment (two to four treatments a year), treatment every eight weeks (six treatments per year), and strategic treatment with Safe-Guard (six treatments per year) as describe above. The non-treated horses and the infrequent treated horses demonstrated a high parasite challenge throughout the year.

When fecal worm egg counts from strategically dewormed horses were compared with horses receiving no treatment, infrequent treatments and treatment every eight weeks, the difference was

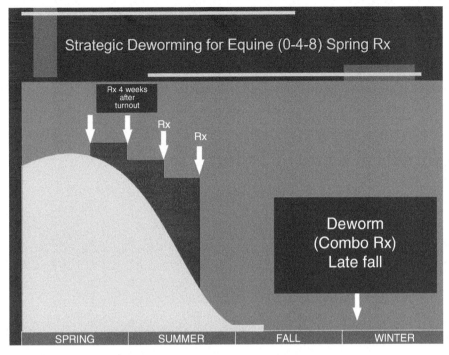

FIGURE 5.12   Strategic timed deworming strategy for seasonal control of parasites in horses.

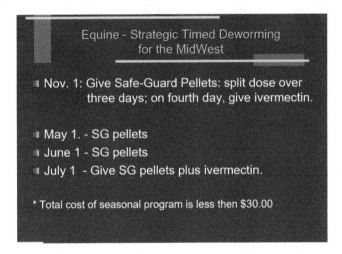

FIGURE 5.13   Suggested deworming dates for strategic timed control strategy for horses in the Midwest.

showing that worm egg counts stayed below 10 eggs per 3 g sample for eight months of the year increasing to a high of 36 eggs per 3 g sample in October but falling back below 20 eggs per gram by November. When comparing all treatments in the same figure, the strategic deworming group maintained low levels throughout the year when compared to all animals including those treated every eight weeks.

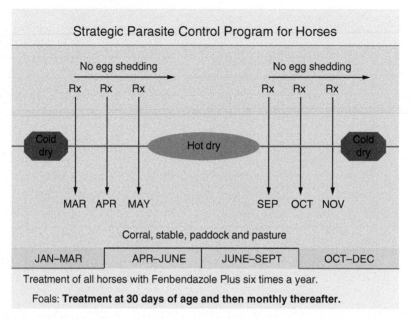

FIGURE 5.14   Seasonal deworming strategies for horses raised in southern US.

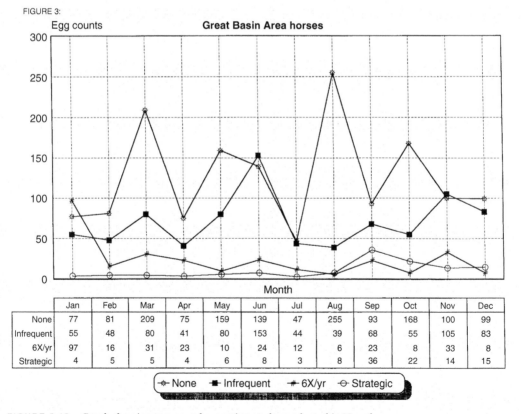

	Jan	Feb	Mar	Apr	May	Jun	Jul	Aug	Sep	Oct	Nov	Dec
None	77	81	209	75	159	139	47	255	93	168	100	99
Infrequent	55	48	80	41	80	153	44	39	68	55	105	83
6X/yr	97	16	31	23	10	24	12	6	23	8	33	8
Strategic	4	5	5	4	6	8	3	8	36	22	14	15

FIGURE 5.15   Graph showing two-year deworming study conducted in Nevada.

The non-treated horses average 125 eggs per 3 g sample throughout the two-year study period. The infrequently treated horses averaged 66 eggs per 3 g sample throughout the year while the horses treated every eight weeks averaged 24 egg per 3 g samples and the strategically dewormed horses treated three times in the spring and again in the fall average 11 eggs per 3 g sample. The fecal worm egg output in the strategically dewormed horses was reduced by 91.2% compared to the non-treated horses, by 83.3% in the infrequent treated horses, and 57.6% in the horses treated every eight weeks (see Figure 5.15).

EQUINE DEWORMERS

Equine dewormers currently on the market in the United States can be classified into three separate classes based on the mode of action): These three major classes are: the benzimidazoles and pre-benzimidazoles (febantel, fenbendazole, oxibendazole, mebendazole, and oxfendazole), the macrocyclic lactones (avermectin and moxidectin families), and the tetrahydropyrimidines (pyrantel). The mode of action is different for each class of compounds. The benzimidizoles are nonsoluble compounds that destroy the metabolism of the parasites by interfering with the cell functions in the parasites and by preventing the uptake of food starving the worms to death. The macrocyclic lactones are very soluble compounds and affect the nervous system killing the parasites causing a non-spastic paralysis while the pyrimidines kill the parasites by acting on the nervous receptors causing a spastic paralysis.

All three classes of compounds have excellent efficacy against the adult parasites, but since each dewormer class has a defined mode of action, each class exhibits its own level of activity against encysted larvae. Because of this efficacy difference, the time it takes for larvae missed by treatment to develop into an adult parasite following treatment depends on the compound used and at what larval stage the product is efficacious [4–6]. It takes longer for early L_4 larvae to develop into an adult parasite than it will for a late L_4 larva. This difference can be measured in the time it takes for worm eggs to reappear in the feces following treatment. With some products, it only takes a couple of days following treatment before worm eggs reappear in the feces while other products may take weeks before eggs are observed in the feces. The longer it takes for eggs to reappear the more effective the product is against the developing and encysted larvae.

Using products correctly and understanding their characteristics has helped keep this class of products viable. Fenbendazole, for example, is an excellent product when used in a strategic deworming schedule [7]. However, if parasite contamination is allowed to develop in the environment and parasite levels increase in the animals until a high population of encysted larvae are present in high numbers, the efficacy of fenbendazole at the recommended dose is drastically decreased. Two key issues have been identified with fenbendazole that can affect its efficacy. The first issue is that this compound is not very soluble in liquids such as gastric juices or blood. The second issue is that it kills the parasite by destroying its ability to metabolize food. Encysted larvae are in an arrested state with reduced metabolism. For fenbendazole to kill these encysted parasites, the product needs direct physical contact. When fenbendazole is given at 10 times the normal dose spread over a five-day period, it is successful (10 mg/kg given daily for five days). By flooding the gastrointestinal tract with molecules of fenbendazole, direct contact is made with the encysted larvae successfully killing them.

FECAL MONITORING IS THE BEST WAY TO DETERMINE WHETHER TREATMENT IS EFFECTIVE

A. **The Modified Wisconsin Sugar Flotation Technique is a fecal exam that is conducted by floating worm eggs out of fecal material.** This technique is highly sensitive (0.3 egg/1 g sample) for use with horses. Efficient use of a dewormer requires the knowledge of whether a particular dewormer is effective in a particular animal. Fecal worm egg counts, if conducted correctly, can determine the general type of parasites present such as pinworms, threadworms, roundworms (*Parascaris*), strongyles, and tapeworms. A fecal worm egg count can also provide accurate information on total numbers of worm eggs shed per pound of feces which determines the rate by which an animal is recontaminating its environment.

  The Fecal Exam is a simple and effective way to check whether an animal is infected with gastrointestinal parasites or whether parasite control has been successful to conduct a fecal worm egg count analysis. Adult parasites living in the gastrointestinal tract lay eggs which pass out of the animals in the feces. Fecal worm egg counts conducted using the "Modified Wisconsin Sugar Flotation Technique" simply floats the worm eggs out of the fecal material so they can be found and identified under a microscope (see Figure 5.13).

B. **The best way to determine whether a dewormer is effective is to conduct a Fecal Worm Egg Reduction Test (FECRT).** This test is accomplished by conducting a fecal exam before treatment and again 14 days following dewormer administration [7]. Percent reduction in fecal worm egg counts due to treatment is calculated by subtracting the post-treatment egg count from the pre-treatment egg count divided by the pre-treatment egg count. If the percent reduction is not 90% or greater, "parasite resistance" is a possibility and the animals in question should be monitored regularly to make sure products used are working properly. Conducting a single fecal exam following treatment is also effective but knowing the level of egg shedding prior to treatment helps determine whether or not a dewormer is effective in the treated animal. Efficacy calculations are conducted by taking the pre-treatment count minus the post-treatment count divided by the pre-treatment count. To be effective, the final calculations should show an efficacy value of 90% or greater.

C. **Taking fecal worm egg counts should be an important part of the standard procedure for all equine operations.** Monitoring fecals should be conducted at least semiannually to monitor treatment progress. One of the best time to take samples is during the winter months to make sure the animals are parasite-free when environmental contamination is at its lowest point and to make sure the animals are not recontaminating their environment immediately when grazing returns. The second best time to take fecals is in late summer or early fall in order to monitor whether the annual treatment program is successful. If average worm egg counts taken in late fall are greater than 100 eggs/3 g sample, adjustment in the treatment program should be made.

  The Modified Wisconsin Sugar Fecal Method: A 3-g fecal sample is mixed with a saturated sugar solution designed to float the eggs out of the fecal matter. The samples are strained to remove large debris, then poured into a 15 ml taper test tube, and centrifuged at a low RPM (<1000) for five minutes which increases the egg recovery rate by a significant amount. After centrifuging, a few drops of sugar are added to form a meniscus on top of the tube. A cover slip is placed on the top of the tube for two minutes, removed, and examined under the microscope at 40× magnification. Eggs are identified to type and counted (see Figures 5.3 and 5.5).

  The collection process is conducted using a sealable bag or baggie, invert the bag like a glove, and pick up freshly dropped fecal material the size of a golf ball from each horse to check for parasites. Keep each individual sample separate. Seal each bag and write on the bag to identify the horse and date of collection. Keep samples cool after collection since heat causes the eggs to hatch and freezing distorts the eggs.

THE MAJOR GASTROINTESTINAL NEMATODE PARASITES OF HORSES ARE

1. **Large strongyles** (*Strongylus vulgaris, Strongylus edentatus, Strongylus equinus,* and *Triodontophorus*)

2. **Small strongyles** (Cyathostomes, Cylicocyclus, Cylicostephanus, and Gyalacephalus) Cyathostomes is most commonly used to identify small strongyles.

3. **Large roundworms** (*Parascaris equorum*)

4. **Pinworms** (*Oxyuris equi*)

5. **Threadworm** (*Strongyloides westeri*)

6. **Stomach worms** (*Trichostrongylus axei, Draschia megastoma,* and *Habronema musca, Habronema majus*)

OTHER NOTABLE INTERNAL PARASITES OF THE HORSE

1. Lungworms (*Dictyocaulus arnfieldi*)

2. Tapeworms (*Anoplocephala magna, Anoplocephala perfoliata,* and *Paranoplocephala mamillana*)

3. Eyeworms (*Thelazia lacrimalis*)

4. Body Cavity Worms (*Setaria equina*)

5. Bots (*Gasterophilus intestinalis*)

REVIEW OF INTERNAL NEMATODE PARASITE OF HORSES

A. **Large strongyles** (*Strongylus vulgaris, Strongylus edentatus,* and *Strongylus equinus*) are reportedly the most damaging parasites in horses throughout the world, of which, *Strongylus vulgaris* is the most notorious of these parasites. Their life cycle is direct where the adults live in the large intestine (colon) and cecum and reproduce by laying eggs that pass back into the environment of the animals via the feces (see Figure 5.16). As adults, these parasites are all plug feeders on the intestinal wall and are bloodsuckers. The prepatent period, which is the time it takes for an infective larva once ingested by a horse to reach an egg-laying adult parasite, can take over six months.

   The reason it takes so long for these parasites to mature is because the immature stages undergo a period of migration through the body of the horse. These immature parasites cause considerable damage during the migration through the body on their way to the large intestine. Part of their migration is through the mesentery artery where excessive numbers can cause obstruction, fever, and shock-like symptoms. The larvae can remain in the artery for three to four months causing severe problems including restricted blood flow resulting in diarrhea, aneurysm, and colic, which may result in the death of the horse.

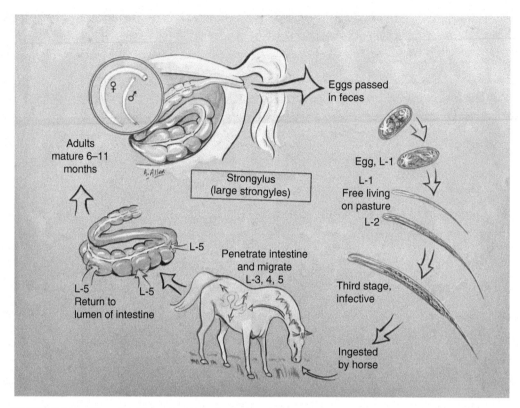

FIGURE 5.16   Life cycle of large strongyles in the horse.

B. **Small strongyles:** There are many small strongyle species but most common belong to the Cyanthostome family. These parasites are non-migrating parasites that live in the large intestine. The immature larval stages of this parasite develop in the walls of the intestine where they are protected until they emerge as early adult parasites (see Figure 5.17). While they are in the walls of the intestine, there are several stages of development when the larvae can encyst and undergo a period of inhibition or arrested development that is called hypobiosis; first, as newly arrived third-stage larvae and second, as a late third-stage larvae or early fourth-stage larvae. When these larvae are encysted, they go through a period of arrested development or hypobiosis that can last from several months to as long as three years.

The physiological mechanism that causes hypobiosis to occur is unknown but it is seasonal and occurs only when parasite populations or parasite density in the gastrointestinal tract is the greatest. It has become obvious that the greater the parasite population, the more changes that occur in the physiology of the gastrointestinal tract and the higher the percentage of incoming larvae that become encysted and undergo hypobiosis. The small strongyles as a group are the primary parasites of horses that are considered to the greatest "drug resistance" problems.

The problems for the horse come when these encysted cyanthostome larvae begin development again and emerge, rupturing through the intestinal wall. Usually this is a dynamic process with older worms dying off and new larvae replacing them. However, due a parasitic purge by a dewormer where a large number of worms are removed at the same time, mass emergence of encysted larvae can often occur causing severe gastrointestinal problems called cyathostomiasis. Clinical cyathostomiasis is often associated with the mass emergence of inhibited larvae from the mucosa of the cecum and colon which is a prominent cause of diarrhea in horses. Clinically, it is characterized by sudden onset of diarrhea, weight loss,

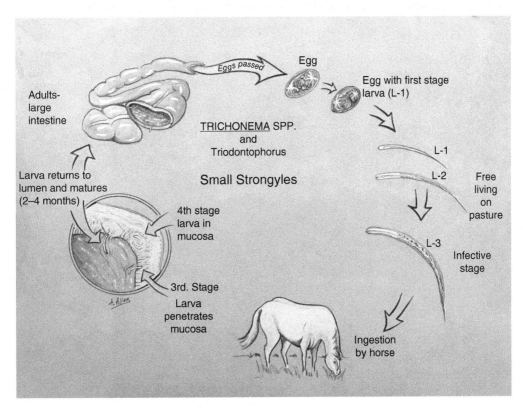

FIGURE 5.17   Life cycle of small strongyles in the horse.

subcutaneous edema, and death [11]. It is reported to be seasonal in occurrence and younger animals tend to be the most affected.

C. Worm eggs that belong to both small strongyles and large strongylus are not differentiated separately when observed upon a fecal exam with the "Modified Wisconsin Sugar Flotation technique." Size differences are visible with this technique; however, the work of identifying which species excretes the larger eggs have never differentiated (see Figures 5.18–5.20).

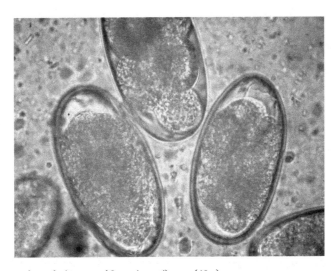

FIGURE 5.18   Strongyle and pinworm (*Oxyuris equi*) eggs (40×).

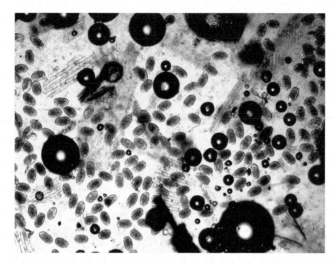

FIGURE 5.19   Multiple strongyle eggs (4×).

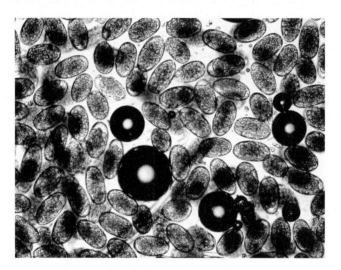

FIGURE 5.20   Heavy *Strongyle* spp. infection with multiple eggs (10×).

D. **The large roundworm** (*P. equorum*) is a very important parasite of horses especially for young foals. The infective larva remains within the egg and can survive for years in the environment. The prepatent period which is from the time on infection until an adult worm is present for *Parascaris* is reported to be between 1 and 12 weeks (see Figure 5.21). Adult roundworms are very prolific worms that can lay thousands of eggs, which pass back into the environment (see Figures 5.22–5.25). The transmission of this parasite is the result of foals ingesting the eggs from previously infected animals that have contaminated the environment where the foals are kept. The larvae hatch from the eggs soon after ingestion and migrate from the intestine through the liver to the lungs and then are coughed up and swallowed back into the small intestine where they grow into an adult parasite. Coughing and the development of pneumonia are common. Also, blockage of the small intestine by these very large adult parasites can be a problem in the young foal.

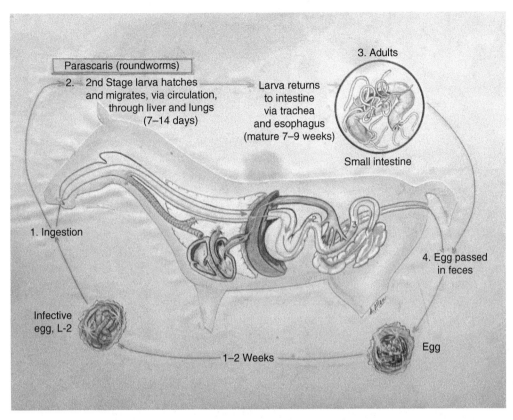

FIGURE 5.21   Life cycle of *Parascaris* (roundworm) in the horse.

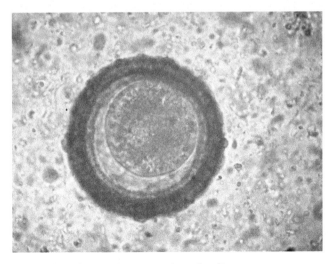

FIGURE 5.22   Large roundworm (*Parascaris equorum*) egg (40×).

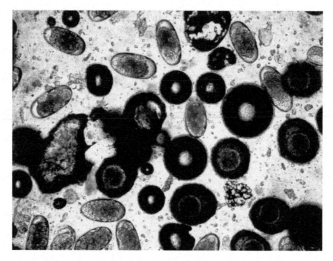

FIGURE 5.23   Roundworm (*Parascaris equorum*) and strongyle eggs (10×).

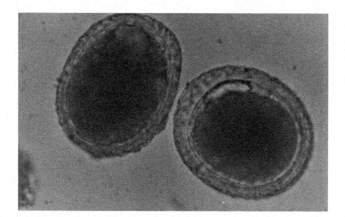

FIGURE 5.24   Two large roundworms eggs (40×).

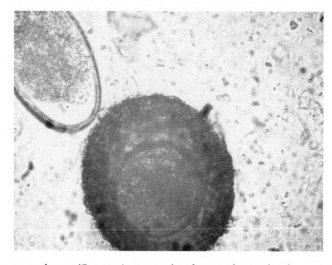

FIGURE 5.25   Large roundworm (*Parascaris equorum*) and strongyle eggs (40×).

E. **Pinworms** (*Oxyuris equi*) are an annoying but not life-threatening parasite of the horse. Visual evidence of this parasite is seen when infected horses continually rub their backsides against fence posts or other solid structures for relief (see Figure 5.26). The female worm lives in the large intestine and rectum area and lays eggs in the skin of the perineal region, which can cause pruritus associated with this infection. Since this parasite seems to be nocturnal in nature, some parasitologist suggest taking fecal samples in the morning if a pinworm infection is suspected. Some parasitologist even suggest using transparent adhesive tape for a more accurate positive or negative diagnosis (Figures 5.27–5.32). The visual irritation and rubbing

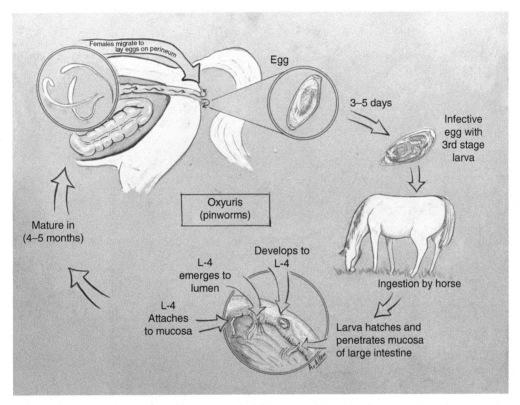

FIGURE 5.26   Life cycle of pinworms (*Oxyuris*) in the horse.

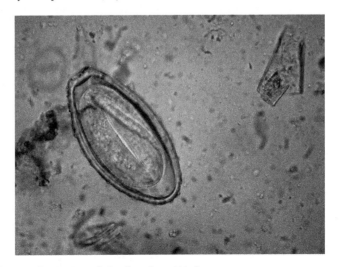

FIGURE 5.27   Pinworm (*Oxyuris equi*) developed egg (40×).

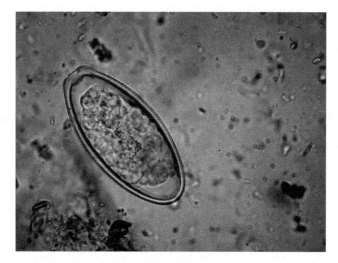

FIGURE 5.28   Pinworm (*Oxyuris equi*) undeveloped egg (40×).

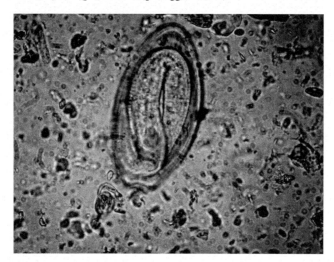

FIGURE 5.29   Embryonated pinworm (*Oxyuris equi*) egg (40×).

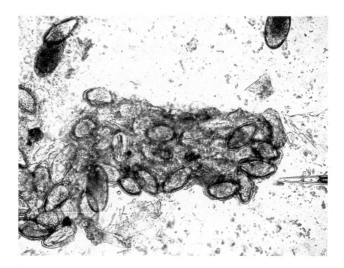

FIGURE 5.30   Pinworm (*Oxyuris equi*) eggs in tissue (10×).

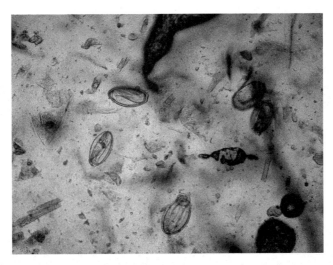

FIGURE 5.31   Pinworms (*Oxyuris equi*) eggs (10×).

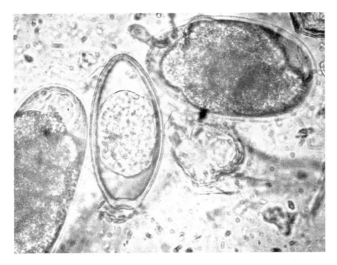

FIGURE 5.32   Pinworm (*Oxyuris equi*) and strongyle eggs (40×).

of the rear quarters on any available object found in their environment with characteristic loss of hair about the tail head is considered as a sign of infection. When these observations regarding rubbing by a horse or horses are made by the owner, it makes pinworms a very important parasite. Dewormers that fail to control this parasite are obvious because owners consider continual rubbing by the horse a failed treatment.

F.   **Threadworm** (*Strongyloides westeri*) is found in the small intestine of foals, usually less than six months of age. The parasite is transmitted either when suckling through larval transmission in the mother's milk or by skin penetration from larvae living in the bedding from eggs passed in the mare's feces (see Figures 5.33 and 5.34). Foals can become infected during the first day of life and begin shedding eggs in the feces as early as 6–10 days later. Young animals with unexplained diarrhea are often found to be infected with this parasite. Infections can be

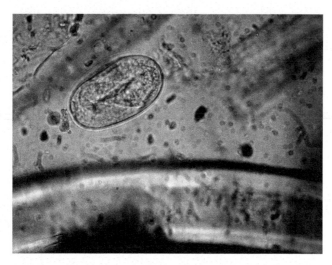

FIGURE 5.33   Threadworm (*Strongyloides westeri*) egg (40×).

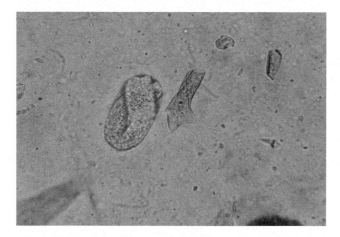

FIGURE 5.34   Threadworm (*Strongyloides papillosus*) egg (40×).

severe enough to require treatment, after which recovery will be rapid as the animals develop immunity against this parasite.

G. **Stomach worms** (*Habronema muscae*, *Habronema microstoma*, and *Draschia megastoma*) live in the horse stomach. Habronema species live under a thick mucus coat on the surface of the stomach while Draschia live in large nodules in the stomach wall. The housefly transmits both parasites.

OTHER PARASITES

A. **Tapeworms** (*Anoplocephala magna*, *Anoplocephala perfoliata*, and *Paranoplocephala mamillana*) are all acquired by the ingestion of orbit mites that live on pastures and in infested grain. Damage caused by tapeworms is limited to the attachment site causing thickening of the gut wall with some ulceration and enteritis. Tapeworms eggs can be found in the stool samples (see Figures 5.35–5.37). Tapeworms in horses are reportedly more common in

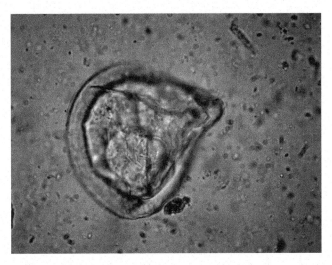

FIGURE 5.35   Tapeworm (*Anoplocephala* spp.) egg (40×).

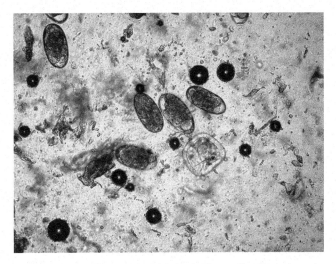

FIGURE 5.36   Tapeworm (*Anoplocephala* spp.) and 5 strongyle eggs (10×).

northern parts of the country and in Canada than they are in southern parts of the country. Tapeworm presence is reported between 2% and 15% of the horses found infected.

B. **Lungworms** (*Dictyocaulus arnfieldi*) are more commonly found in donkeys and mules than in horses. Lungworms lay eggs that are coughed up and pass out of the gastrointestinal tract as embryonated eggs in the feces. The eggs hatch soon after passing and the larvae develop into an infective free-living stage outside of the animals; move onto the vegetation with the aid of moisture (rainfall) to reinfect the horse. Young horses are somewhat most susceptible to this parasite and can show signs of respiratory stress which do not usually occur until two weeks after the onset of the infection.

C. **Bots** (*Gasterophilus intestinalis* and *Gasterophilus nasalis*) are the larval stages of the non-feeding adult bot fly or nit fly (see Figure 5.38). The adult fly deposits her eggs on the hairs of the legs, mane, or body, and under the chin of the horses. Horses ingest the larvae that

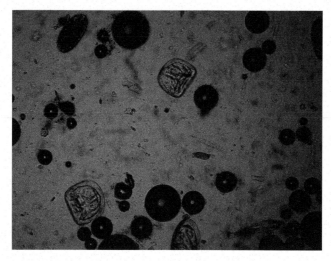

FIGURE 5.37   Three tapeworm (*Anoploclephala*) and one strongyle eggs.

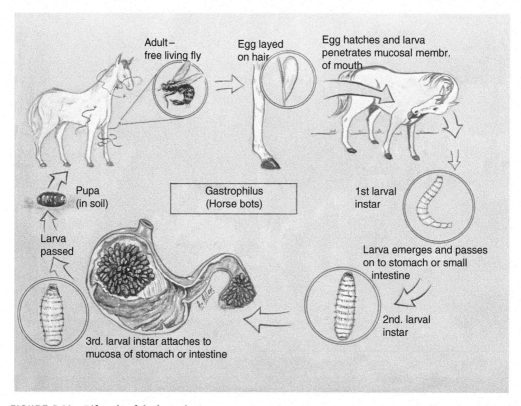

FIGURE 5.38   Lifecycle of the horse bot.

develop from the eggs when licking their legs and then the fly bots eventually develop in the stomach of the horse. To complete the cycle, the bot larvae pass out in the feces and develop into the bot fly that starts the cycle over again.

D. **Eye worms** (*Thelazia lacrymalis*) are transmitted by the face fly. Some reports indicate that conjunctivitis or keratitis is caused by this parasite. Necropsy reports prevalence as high as 30%.

GUIDE FOR INTERPRETATION OF FECAL WORM EGG COUNTS IN HORSES USING "THE MODIFIED WISCONSIN SUGAR FLOTATION TECHNIQUE"

Understanding the meaning of worm egg counts will provide the necessary insight needed to help equine owners build a seasonal deworming strategy for their animals. Factors that affect fecal worm egg shedding are numerous, so a number of these factors need to be considered every time an analysis is made and a fair assessment of the worm egg counts generated. The age of the animal, the season of the year, the amount of exposure to pasture, and the stocking rate of the animals on pasture all affect worm egg counts. The amount of rainfall or moisture on the pasture and the number of degree days with temperatures sufficient to promote parasite develop on pasture is also very important to future infections. Furthermore, the health of the animals, the stage of gestation, stage of lactation, and the numbers and type of parasites present at each examination must be considered. Post-foaling worm egg counts in a mare, for example, are almost always higher than pre-foaling worm egg counts. These factors all directly affect worm egg count interpretations.

Horses have five major types of internal parasites that are commonly diagnosed present in routine fecal exams: threadworms (*Strongyloides* sp.), pinworms (*Oxyuris* sp.), roundworms (*Parascarus* sp.), strongyles (30+ different species of large and small strongyles), and tapeworms (*Anaplocephia* sp.). All eggs are counted and included in the worm egg count total except for tapeworms. Tapeworms are listed simply as positive at a low level (+) 1–10 eggs, medium level (++) 11–50 eggs, or high level (+++) 50 eggs or greater.

1 egg/3 g equals 150 eggs/lb of manure. A worm egg count of 10 translates to 1500 egg/lb of manure. A worm egg of 300/3 g means 45,000 eggs/lb of manure or 2,950,000 eggs (in 65 lb of manure) excreted daily per horse back into their environment (see Chapter 1 on daily manure output per animal species).

QUICK ASSESSMENT FOR EQUINE BASED ON FECAL WORM EGG COUNTS

	Eggs/3 g	Estimated Parasite Level
Strongyle egg count	1–10	Low
	11–50	Moderate
	51–300	High
	301+	Very high*

*At this level, it appears that parasites begin to undergo inhibition in tissues.

A unique feature about horses is that some horses are consistently "low" or "none" shedders. This means that if an animal continually has a low (1–10 eggs) or zero worm egg count, it is impossible to relate this count to worm burden. We find on average 10% of the horses are "low or none shedders" even though they are comingled with heavy shedding horses.

INHIBITED SMALL STRONGYLES CAUSE PROBLEMS WITH WORM EGG COUNT INTERPRETATIONS

Another confounding issue with equine is that once a small strongyle infection grows in numbers and reaches a certain point within the horse (it appears that every horse is different), the physiology of the gut changes negatively which, in turn, tells the parasites that they are operating in a danger zone such that if the horse dies so will the parasites. The solution for the parasite is to stop development and remain in the tissues until conditions within the gut improve at which time development can begin again. In many cases, a large percentage of newly ingested larvae must undergo an arrested development period or they will, in turn, kill the horse. The most common time for inhibited larvae to begin development is 60–90 days into the grazing in mid-summer or in parts of the country where horses are on pasture all year, inhibition usually occurs about 60–90 days after continual grass growth or during the raining season, along as temperatures range from 70 to 95 °F. This is usually the period when pasture contamination is at its highest level.

The worm egg count for horses, therefore, only indicates the presence of adult parasites within a particular horse. It is impossible to know how many parasites are inhibited at any given time although high egg counts (>300 eggs/3 g) indicate a high worm burden which in turn means inhibited larvae are probably present. Most often, when a horse is dewormed, the dewormer kills the adult and late-developing larvae but leave the inhibited larvae in the tissues. Following treatment, some of these larvae come out the tissues and quickly develop into egg-laying adult parasites. In many parts of the country, winter is the most common time for the larvae to come out of the tissues. The reason for this is, as the horse goes into winter, grazing stops, the old worms are either killed by deworming or a natural process where the old worms die off and new worms come out of the tissues. It is not common for a heavily infected horse to have their highest counts in late winter or early spring before grazing begins [11].

Phase 1: An infected horse is put out to graze in the spring. This horse begins to ingest infective larvae that has survived from the previous grazing season, while at the same time, this horse is excreting worm eggs from an existing infection (first generation acquired from the previous grazing season), recontaminating the pasture for the new year.

Phase 2: Depending upon temperature and moisture, these new eggs hatch, develop into infective larvae, and move away from the manure pats onto the vegetation where the reinfection process begins. In the meantime (approximately 30 days after turnout), the newly ingested larvae mature into second-generation egg-laying adult parasites which begin laying eggs back on the pasture (causing an ever increasing buildup of larvae on the pasture).

Phase 3: As the contamination of the pasture builds for the season, so does the infection within the horse. So, now as the season progresses, high numbers of eggs are shed daily on the pasture, which means the grazing horse is also exposed to high numbers of infective larvae. This is when the physiological trouble starts internally, incoming larvae begin to undergo inhibition or arrested development, worm egg counts lose their meaning and, of course, treatment is no longer effective.

REFERENCES

1. Lyons, E.T., Swerczek, T.W., Tolliver, S. et al. (1994). A study of natural infections of encysted small strongyles in a horse herd in Kentucky. *Vet. Med.* 1: 1146–1155.

2. Drudge, J.H. and Lyons, E.T. (1986). *Internal Parasites of Equids with Emphasis on Treatment and Control.* Somerville, NJ: Hoechst-Roussel.

3. Duncan, J.L. (1985). Internal parasites of the horse and their control. *Equine Vet. J.* 17 (2): 79–82.

4. Stratford, C., Lester, H.E., Pickles, K.J. et al. (2013). An investigation of anthelmintic efficacy against strongyles on equine yards in Scotland. *Equine Vet. J.* 44: 1–8.

5. Lyons, E.T., Drudge, J.H., and Tolliver, S.C. (1983). Controlled tests with fenbendazole in equids: special interest on activity of multiple dose against natural infections of migrating stages of strongyles. *Am. J. Vet. Res.* 44 (6): 1057–1063.

6. Von Samson-Himmelstjerna, J.G., Fritzen, B., Demeler, J. et al. (2007). Cases of reduced cyathostomin egg-reappearance period and failure of *Parascaris equorum* egg count reduction following ivermectin treatment as well as survey on Pyrantel efficacy on German horse farms. *Vet. Parasit.* 144 (1–2): 74–80.

7. Brady, H.A., Nichols, W.T., Blanek, M., and Hutcheson, D.P. (2008). Parasite resistance and the effects of rotational deworming regimens in horses. *AAEP Proc.* 54: 1–6.

8. Knutson, A. (2000). Dung beetles – biological control agents of horn flies. *Texas Biological Control News.* Winter. Texas Agricultural Extension Service. The Texas A & M University System.

9. Floate, K.D., Cotwell, D.C., and Fox, A.S. (2002). Reductions of non-pest insects in dung of cattle treated with endectocides: a comparisons of four products. *Bull. Entomol. Res.* 92: 471–481.

10. Wardhaugh, K. and Ridsill-Smith, T. (1998). Antiparasitic drugs, the livestock industry and dung beetles – a cause for concern? *Aust. Vet. J.* 76 (4): 259–261.

11. Love, S., Murphy, D., and Mellor, D. (1999). Pathogenicity of cyathostome infections. *Vet. Parasit.* 85: 113–122.

Parasites of Swine

Parasite diagnosis is a very important service to all swine operations since the prevalence of parasites is directly related to the production standards of each operation or swine units within an operation. The "Modified Wisconsin Sugar Flotation Method" is the most sensitive fecal method available for swine (see Figure 6.1). Most techniques will show positive results when Ascaris worm egg counts are high, but detecting low counts are very important. Also, the swine whipworm tends to be a low egg shedder not detected by other techniques. A fecal worm egg count evaluation form for swine is shown in Figure 6.2. An example of an actual evaluation form already fill out by our lab is shown in Figure 6.3.

With improvement in genetics, nutrition, animal health drugs, and vaccines, controlling parasites becomes a very important management tool to reduce or eliminate losses occurring within an operation and to prevent future infections from developing. Even swine operations with an

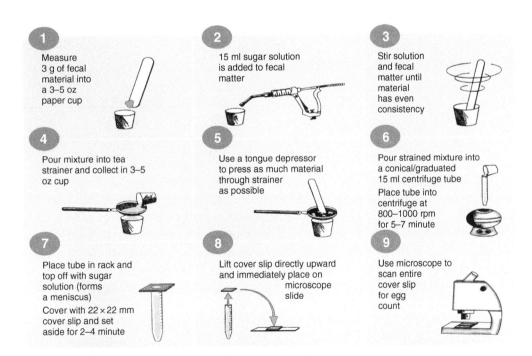

1. Measure 3 g of fecal material into a 3–5 oz paper cup

2. 15 ml sugar solution is added to fecal matter

3. Stir solution and fecal matter until material has even consistency

4. Pour mixture into tea strainer and collect in 3–5 oz cup

5. Use a tongue depressor to press as much material through strainer as possible

6. Pour strained mixture into a conical/graduated 15 ml centrifuge tube. Place tube into centrifuge at 800–1000 rpm for 5–7 minute

7. Place tube in rack and top off with sugar solution (forms a meniscus). Cover with 22 × 22 mm cover slip and set aside for 2–4 minute

8. Lift cover slip directly upward and immediately place on microscope slide

9. Use microscope to scan entire cover slip for egg count

FIGURE 6.1 Modified Wisconsin Sugar Flotation Method.

Large Animal Parasitology Procedures for Veterinary Technicians, First Edition. Donald H. Bliss.
© 2024 John Wiley & Sons, Inc. Published 2024 by John Wiley & Sons, Inc.

Swine Parasite Evaluation Form

PEC ☐   Mail In ☐   Page____of____

Collection Date: _____   Consultant: _____

Corporate Name: _____   Sponsor: _____

Name of Farm: _____   Sponsor Contact: _____

Producer's Address: _____   Sponsor Address: _____

City: _____ Phone: _____   City: _____ Phone: _____

State: _____ Zip: _____ Fax: _____   State: _____ Zip: _____ Fax: _____

E-Mail: _____   Representative: _____

Lab ID No.	Animal ID/ Pen #	Management*	Large Roundworm	Whipworm	Nodular Worm	Threadworm	Coccidia	Total Count** (EPзG)	Treatment Date month/day/year	Product Used
									Enter after test results recorded	

COMMENTS:

*Management:
1 = Nursery, 2 = Grower, 3 = Finisher,
4 = Lactating Sow, 5 = Gestation Sow,
6 = Gilt, 7 = Boar

**(+ = 1-10) (++ = 11-50) (+++ =>51)

FIGURE 6.2   Swine parasite evaluation form.

excellent nutritional program soon realize that leaving parasites untreated greatly reduces the benefit of their nutritional program [1–3]. The best swine feed in the world is wasted on "wormy" hogs.

Many factors determine the level of economic loss caused by parasitism to a swine operation. Economic loss will depend upon the age of the animals at the time they are exposed to an infection, whether an animal is being exposed to parasites for the first time, the level of environmental parasitic contamination present within a facility, the infection levels developing within the animals, and the production level or production efficiency of the operation. Sometimes the most efficient operations have the most to lose from parasite-infected facilities. The risk of an infection spreading throughout an operation and whether other disease problems are related to the parasitism present are also economic factors to be considered. The problem that exists today for the consulting veterinarian is locating where an infection might exists within an operation, then attacking and eliminating the infection through continual monitoring.

During the past 20 years, the way swine are raised for breeding and meat production has changed to where nearly all major swine operations (of all age groups) are raised in total confined or semi-confined facilities (see Figures 6.4–6.7). Most farrowing crates restrict the sow's head from turning around in the crate and, therefore, helps prevent her from contact with excreted worm eggs

| State: | OK | Zip: 73048 | Fax: | | | State: | IL | Zip: 61853 | Fax: |
| E-Mail: | | | | | | Representative: | | | |

Lab ID No. FARM #SAMPLE	Animal ID/ Pen #	Management*	Large Roundworm	Whipworm	Nodular Worm	Threadworm	Coccidia	Total Count** (EP3G)	Treatment Date month/day/year	Product Used
										Enter after test results recorded
91 1	48166 (P2)							0		
92 2	48979 (P1)		‖‖‖					291		
93 3	47470 (P3)		‖‖					27		
94 4	48061 (P2)							2		
95 5	48125 (P2)		‖‖					32		
96 6	45559 (P5)		‖					2		
97 7	45885 (P4)							2		
98 8	49587 (P1)		‖‖					270		
99 9	49624 (P6)		‖‖					397		
100 10	47086 (P1)							0		
101 11	49203 (P1)		‖‖‖					511		
102 12	47305 (P3)		‖‖					1576		
103 13	48240 (P3)		‖					2		
104 14	49279 (P1)									
105 15	49422 (P1)		‖‖‖‖					978		

COMMENTS:

Sponsor's E-mail:

For additional information and submission forms, visit: **www.midamericaagresearch.net**

Donald H. Bliss, Ph.D.
MidAmerica Ag. Research
3705 Sequoia Trail
Verona, WI 53593

*Management:
1=Nursery, 2= Grower, 3= Finisher,
4= Lactating Sow, 5= Gestation Sow,
6= Gilt, 7= Boar

**(+ = 1-10) (++ = 11-50) (+++ =>51)

FIGURE 6.3   Samples results from *Ascaris* parasitized facility.

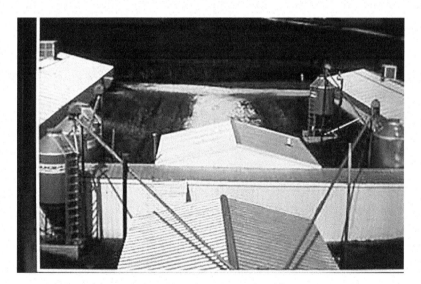

FIGURE 6.4   Swine confinement barn in Iowa.

so the earliest she can reinfect is when weaned and moved to the breeding area. The move to confinement buildings nationwide, which occurred in the mid-1990s has totally changed the numbers and types of parasites that can affect swine production [4–6]. The large roundworm (*Ascaris suum*) is now primarily the only gastrointestinal parasite consistently found in confinement swine operations today. Whipworm (*Trichuris suis*), threadworm (*Strongyloides ramsoni*), and the nodular

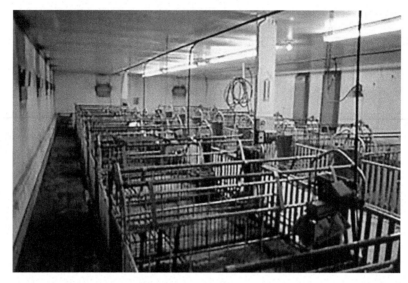

FIGURE 6.5   Sow crates in confines farrowing facility.

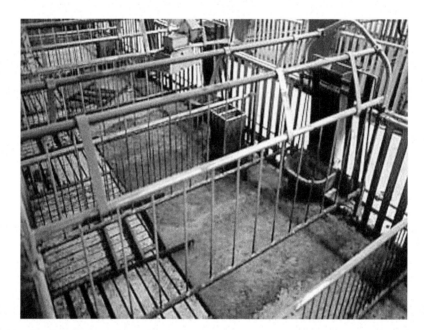

FIGURE 6.6   Total confinement farrowing crate.

worm (*Oesophagostomum* spp.) can on occasion be found in confinement swine operations, but these parasites do not survive well under confinement conditions and often disappear after a short period of time. Because of this, many operations have stopped deworming their animals once they moved their animals to confinement buildings, thereby, allowing the large roundworm to gain a strong foothold in many of these confinement buildings. The large roundworm, therefore, remains the most prevalent parasite found in swine (of all ages) today. Also, because of this, the presence of roundworms in these facilities appears to have become more prevalent as the swine barns age. I have found that many of these buildings are slowly become heavily contaminated over time.

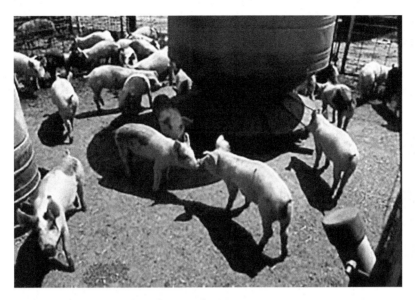

FIGURE 6.7   Grower pigs at feeder in confinement facility.

All other parasites such as kidney worms (*Stephanurus dentatus*), lungworms (*Metastrongylus* spp.), and the red stomach worm (*Hyostrongylus rubidus*) have all but disappeared in domestic swine raised in confinement and are only found, for the most part, in swine raised outside on dirt lots (see Figures 6.8 and 6.9). Nodular worms (*Oesophagostomum* spp.) and threadworms

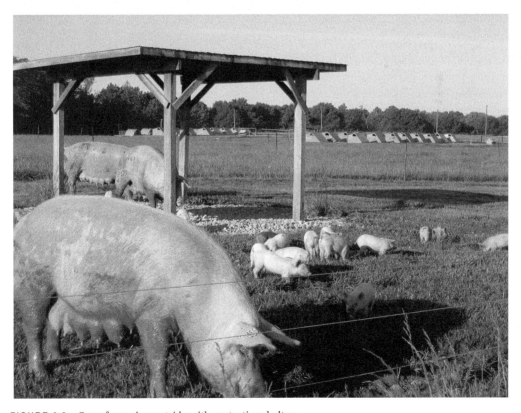

FIGURE 6.8   Sows farrowing outside with protective shelters.

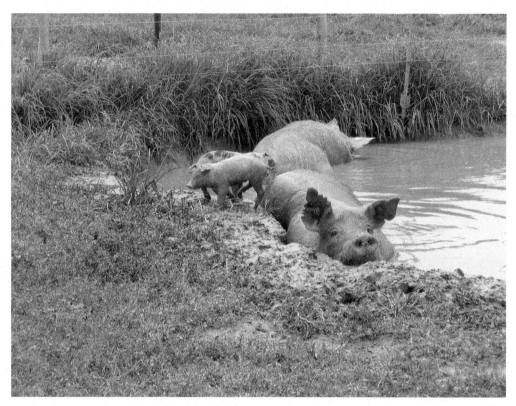

FIGURE 6.9   Sows and pigs enjoying mud pond.

(*Strongyloides* spp.) can be found in confined hogs only where sows are bedded which allows this parasite to survive and reinfect its host. One final internal parasite, the coccidian (*Isospora suis*), a protozoan parasite of the small intestine of swine, can be found especially in young pigs. It can be present in confinement swine but is by far the most prevalent in swine of all ages raised on dirt lots.

Even through parasite population shifts have occurred, *Ascaris* remains a tough opponent in raising swine and has adapted to surviving in all types of confinement situations. This parasite is a major deterrent to efficient production and its control is an important part of the health and well-being concerns of swine regardless of where they are raised. The more efficient an animal's performance is in terms of growth, feed conversion, or health status, the more important parasites become. It takes fewer parasites in a highly efficient animal to disrupt this efficiency that it does in in an inefficient animal. *Ascaris* has also been shown to depress the immune system and, therefore, predisposes animals to other diseases as well as reducing its ability to fight off disease problems which they may be exposed to.

Once roundworm infections developed inside a confinement facility, for example, it is extremely difficult to get rid of them. The Ascaris egg is very resistant to environmental conditions and can survive harsh environmental conditions. The infective larva develops inside the egg and does not hatch until ingested by swine. The egg is covered with a gelatinous protein matter which helps the egg stick to surfaces such as concrete floors and walls. The Ascaris egg can survive a number of years in the environment and still be viable. There are numerous reports where pigs are placed on old swine facilities where animals have not been present for as long as 30 years and yet the pigs become infected immediately upon being placed in these abandoned units. Since most swine are now raised in total confinement buildings and often have a carefully controlled environment, it is possible that *Ascaris* eggs could live and reproduce for many years within these buildings before being detected, thus negatively affecting thousands and possibly millions of hogs nationwide.

Parasites cause liver, lungs, and intestinal damage, interfere with digestion, and disrupt nutrient absorption in the intestine which reduces the efficiency of growth, interferes with breeding efficiency, and reduce immune response to other disease such as coccidiosis [1–3]. Direct losses to a producer can be from condemned livers or carcasses at slaughter, increased feed costs due to losses in feed efficiency, reduced rate of gain, and losses caused by disease outbreaks directly linked to parasitism. These parasites also cause "mechanical" damage to the intestinal lining and lungs and reduced immune status of the infected animals, which may predispose the animal to bacterial, viral, and other disease agents or conditions.

LARGE ROUNDWORMS (*ASCARIS SUUM*)

BACKGROUND

The large roundworm is the most common internal parasite found in US swine operations today (see Figures 6.10 and 6.11). It is also the largest exceeding 8 in. in length. This parasite is a very important pathogen because it causes damage at every stage of its development in the animal. The life cycle of the roundworm begins in an animal when it consumes embroynated eggs present in the environment (see Figure 6.12). This egg hatches in the gastrointestinal tract and the emerged larva penetrates the mucosal wall and travels via the blood stream where it migrates to the liver (see Figures 6.13 and 6.14).

The larvae then move from the liver to the lungs within three or four days after invading the liver (see Figure 6.15). Most often, the livers that are damaged by the Ascaris migration are condemned at slaughter (Figure 6.16). These larvae continue their development and stay in the lungs for another 4–10 days before they are coughed up and swallowed back to the intestine. Livers from noninfected hogs should be free of liver spots (see Figure 6.17). Several weeks after an infection occurs, many of the larvae, which develop from ingested eggs, are back in the intestinal tract,

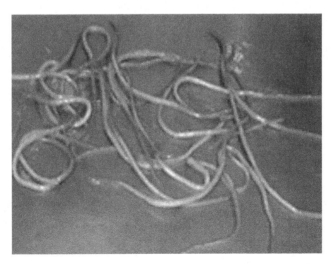

FIGURE 6.10   Adult *Ascaris suum* worms.

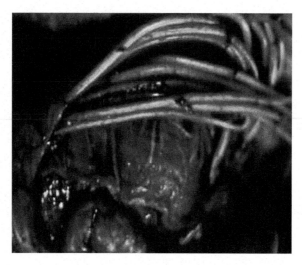

FIGURE 6.11 Large round worms (*Ascaris suum*) found at necropsy in the small intestine.

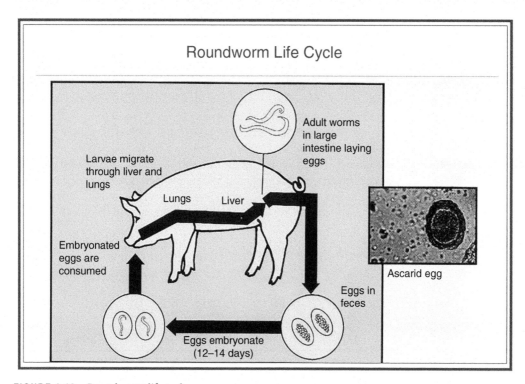

FIGURE 6.12 Roundworm life cycle.

which then develop into adult worms. The female worm begins laying eggs back into the intestinal tract that are passed out of the animal in the feces. The total development time in the animal is approximately 6 weeks (35–45 days) depending upon the age of the animal and previous exposure to *Ascaris* infections.

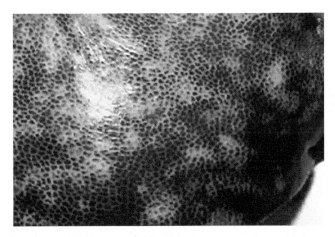

FIGURE 6.13   Liver spots indicating larvae migration of the large roundworm (*Ascaris suum*).

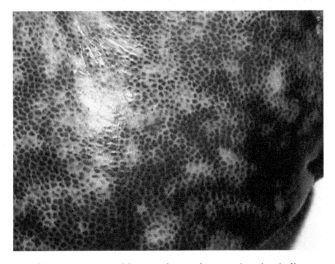

FIGURE 6.14   Closeup of liver spots caused by roundworm larvae migration in liver.

The large roundworm lives off nutrient contents of the intestinal tract. The adult female worms then begin excreting eggs, which pass out in the fecal material. One female roundworm can reportedly lay hundreds of eggs a day. These eggs can remain viable for many years. These microscopic eggs are coated with a protein-like material, which allows these eggs to stick in the rough edges of concrete material and are not easily removed even with high-pressure sprayers. The only known method to remove these eggs is by torching with fire. Numerous reports exist where heavy roundworm infections developed in young pigs placed in swine facilities, which have not had animals present for as many as 20 years.

DIAGNOSIS IN LUNGS

Visual signs of a roundworm infection in swine begin with coughing followed by labored breathing. Coughing usually begins about 7–10 days after animals are placed in a roundworm-contaminated

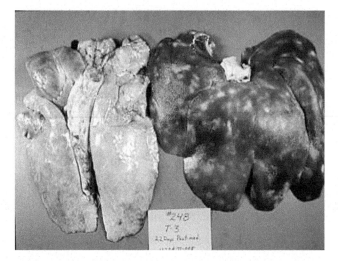

FIGURE 6.15   Liver and lungs affected by migrating roundworm (*Ascaris suum*) larvae.

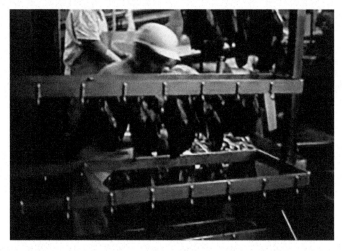

FIGURE 6.16   Livers being condemned due to liver spots caused by migrating roundworm (*Ascaris suum*) larvae.

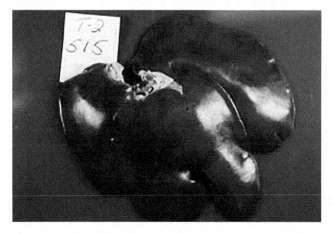

FIGURE 6.17   Roundworm-free liver as found at necropsy.

facility. At necropsy, lung tissue can be examined, and larvae found. Also, lung tissue can be cut into small pieces and wrapped in cheese cloth or double layer of gauze and then put in a Baermann apparatus (glass funnel with a stopcock or clamp on a rubber hose at the end of the funnel) filled with warm water. Roundworm larvae can be found in the fluid at the bottom of the Baermann funnel after three to eight hours. Draw the bottom 10–15 ml to examine for roundworm larvae (fourth stage).

DIAGNOSIS IN LIVER

Where the animal's immunity to parasite challenge is low and infection levels are high, animals will become moribund within 7–10 days after arriving in the contaminated area. It is not uncommon for heavily infected animals to succumb to the infection by the third week after arrival, if not treated. The major damage caused by large roundworms is due to larval migration through the liver and lungs. At slaughter, liver damage is evident as white scars termed "milk spots." Large roundworm damage to the lungs may cause a soft moist cough in animals 7–10 days after embroynated eggs are ingested. Additionally, pigs become more susceptible to mycoplasma pneumonia, flu virus, and bacteria-related problems as a result of damage caused by larval migration.

Liver "milk spots" have been shown to heal and disappear approximately 30–35 days after an animal is moved away from the infection. Therefore, finding liver "milk spots" at slaughter indicates an infection is occurring within 30 days of slaughter. Infections occurring on the grower floor, for example, may not be indicated as occurring either by the presence or the lack of "milk spots" found at slaughter.

DIAGNOSIS IN THE FECES

Fecal exams are the best nonintrusive way to detect roundworm infections in swine. One single female worm can lay thousands of eggs and the environment can be come heavily contaminated. The newly laid egg can become infective under ideal conditions in about 10 days after passing out into the environment. The roundworm egg is very distinct, so it is easily to find even in dense fecal material (see Figures 6.18–6.22). Often, numerous eggs will be present in a small 3 g sample (see Figure 6.23).

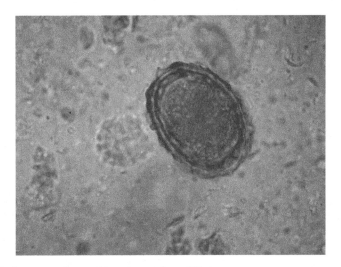

FIGURE 6.18   The large roundworm (*Ascaris suum*) egg (40×).

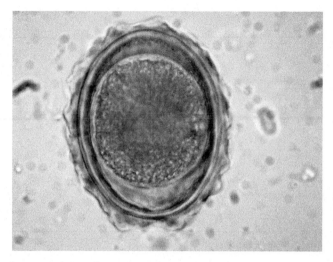

FIGURE 6.19   The large roundworm (*Ascaris suum*) egg showing lipoprotein vitelline outer layer (40×).

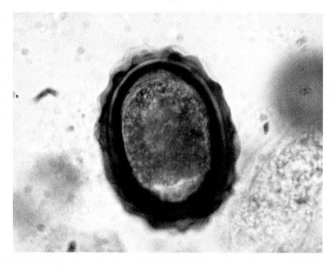

FIGURE 6.20   The large roundworm (*Ascaris suum*) egg with well-developed outer vitelline layer (40×).

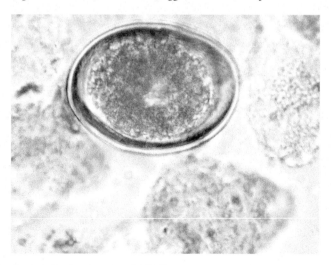

FIGURE 6.21   *Ascaris suum* (undeveloped egg) (40×).

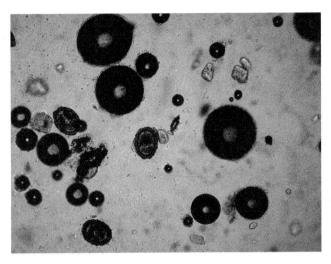

FIGURE 6.22   Three *Ascaris suum* eggs (10×).

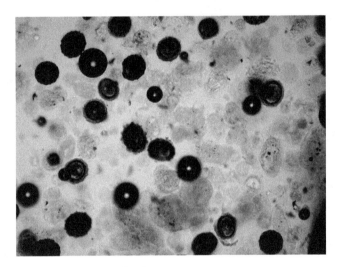

FIGURE 6.23   Multiple *Ascaris suum* eggs (10×).

WHIPWORMS (*TRICHURIS SUIS*)

BACKGROUND

Whipworms are probably the most damaging parasite in swine. It only takes a few whipworms to cause severe problems. Scour problems are almost always indicated when these parasites are present on a swine operation. The most common problems with this parasite occur in young growing hogs (40–100 lb). Whipworms are very pathogenic and it is not uncommon for producers to experience a high death loss in growing pigs exposed to high levels of whipworm infections.

DIAGNOSIS IN THE CECUM

Whipworms live in the cecum which is the junction between the small and large intestines. Adult whipworms are approximately 2 in. in length (see Figures 6.24 and 6.25). Adults whipworms can

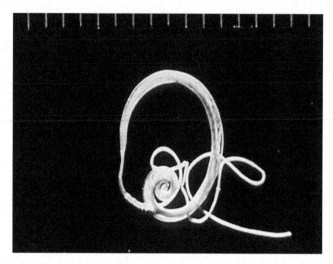

FIGURE 6.24 Whipworm (*Trichuris suis*) adult worm.

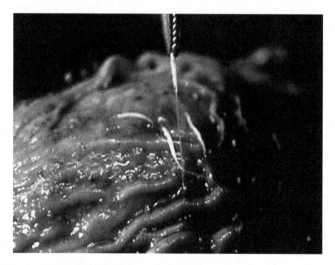

FIGURE 6.25 Whipworm (*Trichuris suis*) attached to the cecum.

be seen with the naked eye when examining an infected animal upon postmortem examination (see Figure 6.26).Visually, the worms are white in color and are shaped like a whip with the head end the smallest part of the worm. The adult worms tunnel into the intestinal mucosal lining burying their heads in the tissue. Whipworms are reportedly intermediate feeders releasing their grip with their heads in the tissue and then reburying their heads in a new location on the surface of the mucosa. Looking at cross sections of the mucosa, it is possible to find the anterior end of the parasites are embedded in the tissues (see Figures 6.27 and 6.28). With heavy infections, it is possible to see the entire cecum inflamed from whipworm larval infections and to find larval stages embedded in the tissues (Figures 6.29 and 6.30).

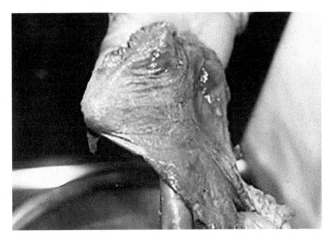

FIGURE 6.26   Whipworms (*Trichuris suis*) attached to the cecum found at slaughter.

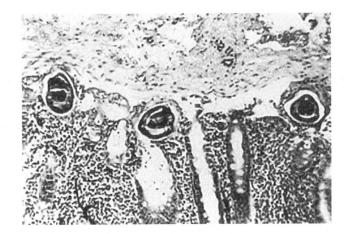

FIGURE 6.27   Whipworm (*Trichuris suis*) embedded in folds of the cecum.

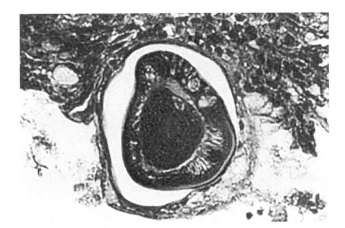

FIGURE 6.28   Whipworm (*Trichuris suis*) in tissue cross-section of cecum.

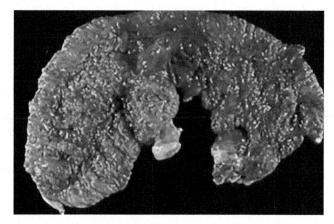

FIGURE 6.29   Whipworm (*Trichuris suis*) inflamed cecum.

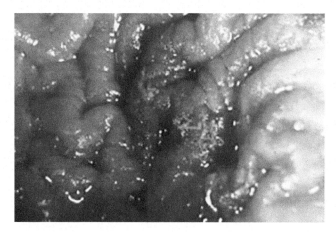

FIGURE 6.30   Whipworm (*Trichuris suis*) larvae in cecum wall.

DIAGNOSIS IN THE FECES

Females lay eggs, which require about approximately three weeks to become infective larvae encased in the egg under ideal conditions. Whipworm eggs are very hardy and even under adverse conditions can remain viable for as long as 10 years (see Figures 6.31–6.34). The female worm is not a very prolific egg layer like the large roundworm female and, therefore, contamination levels are generally much lower for whipworms. Also, when using fecal exams to find whipworm eggs, care has to be taken since these eggs are more difficult to find because often only a small number of eggs can be found even with severely infected animals (see Figure 6.32).

Once swallowed, the eggs hatch and larvae move to the small intestine and cecum to continue their developmental cycle. Both larvae and adult worms burrow into intestinal walls and severely damage the lining and disrupt the absorption of nutrients. The development time from an invading larva until an egg-laying adult is present in approximately six weeks.

Even moderate whipworm infections can result in serious losses from scours, reduced appetite, reduced weight gain or weight loss, and even death. Because the parasite burrows into the mucosal lining and apparently is not a bloodsucker, it is refractory to most dewormers.

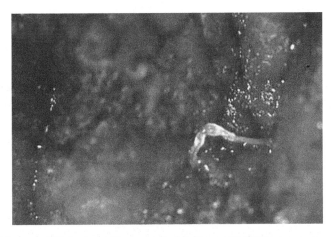

FIGURE 6.31   Whipworm (*Trichuris suis*) larvae embedded in cecum tissue.

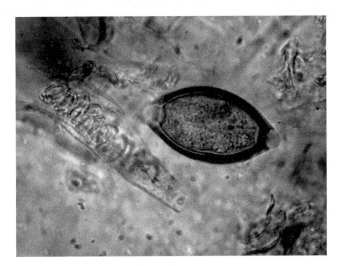

FIGURE 6.32   Whipworm (*Trichuris suis*) egg (10×).

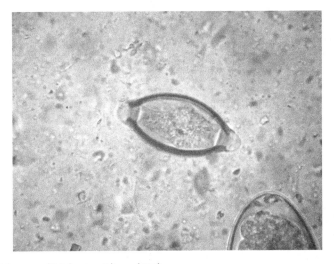

FIGURE 6.33   Whipworm (*Trichuris suis*) egg (10×).

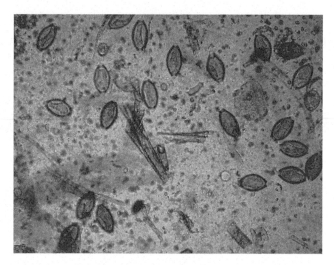

FIGURE 6.34   Multiple whipworm (*Trichuris suis*) eggs (10×).

THREADWORMS (*STRONGYLOIDES RAMSONI*)

BACKGROUND

Threadworms are mainly a problem for pigs raised on dirt or in bedded pens. Occasionally, thread-worm eggs will be found upon fecal exam in confinement pigs. Threadworms, when present, are most severe in very young pigs. This unusual parasite has a free-living stage that lives in the environment which can multiply outside the host. Occasionally, adult worms can be found in a fecal float (see Figure 6.34). Baby pigs become infected from skin penetration by larvae, ingestion of infected larvae, and migration of larvae through fetal tissue or by ingestion of milk from infected sows. Sours, dehydration, stunting, and unthriftiness are the most common signs of infection. Death can be a result of heavy infection.

DIAGNOSIS IN THE FECES

Diagnosis of threadworm problems is best accomplished by finding the characteristic threadworm eggs in the feces of very young pigs or in gestating or lactating sows (see Figures 6.35 and 6.36).

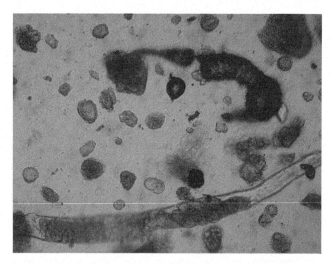

FIGURE 6.35   Female threadworm (*Srongyloides ransoni*) in fecal sample with eggs.

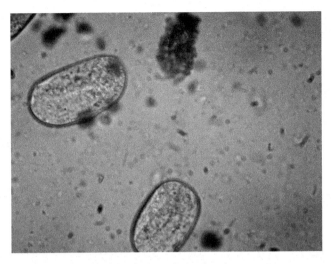

FIGURE 6.36   Two threadworm (*Srongyloides ransomi*) eggs (40×).

TREATMENT GUIDELINES

Treatment of the sows prior to farrowing will help but if nursery area is contaminated, pigs need to be treated from two to four weeks of age with possible retreatment two to three weeks later. Pigs will self-cure after two to three months of age.

NODULAR WORMS (*OESOPHAGOSTOMUM DENTATUM*)

BACKGROUND

Nodular worms are reported to follow a normal trichostrongylid life cycle where eggs are passed by the female worms living in the host back into the environment through the feces (see Figure 6.37). Adult worms are found in the lumen of the large intestine, their eggs reaching the external environment in the host's feces. No intermediate host is involved in the life cycle, the pig becoming infected by the ingestion of the third-stage larva. These eggs hatch into a first-, second-, and third-stage larvae

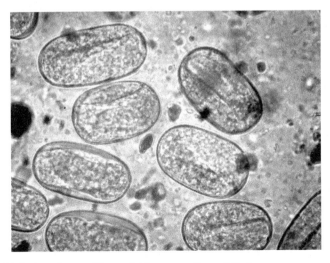

FIGURE 6.37   Multiple threadworm (*Strongyloides ransomi*) eggs (40×).

and then upon ingestion by swine, spend several weeks encysted in the tissues of the wall of the large intestine before these larvae emerge and grow into an adult worm and begin the cycle over again.

Nodular worm is most commonly found in adult swine and baby pigs. These worms measure about 1 in. long when adults and live in the large intestine and the eggs are passed in the animal's feces. Under favorable weather conditions, eggs will develop infective larvae in just a few days. Nursing pigs can pick up infective larvae from the sows. Sows held outdoors with access to dirt lots during the gestation period are the most likely to become infected with nodular worms. Sows gestating in confinement seldom become infective with nodular worm unless the gestating area contains bedding where infective larvae can remain protected. After being swallowed by pigs, larvae migrate to the large intestine where they mature and the cycle continues. Nodular worm larvae burrow into intestinal walls, forming abscesses or nodules.

DIAGNOSIS IN THE LARGE INTESTINE

Upon postmortem examination, these nodules are visible grossly and will lead to visceral and carcass condemnations at slaughter if present (see Figures 6.38 and 6.39). Baby pigs born to sows carrying heavy infections of nodular worms will often develop a gray or white sticky diarrhea two

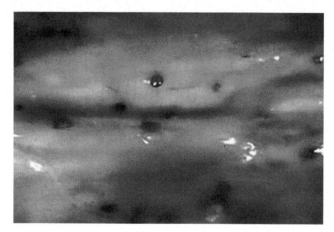

FIGURE 6.38 Nodules found in the large intestine caused by the nodular worm (*Oesophagostomum dentatium*).

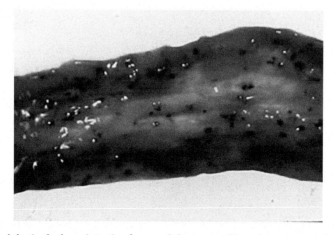

FIGURE 6.39 Nodules in the large intestine from nodular worms (*Oesophagostomum dentatium*).

to three weeks old. Often times, where nodular worms are found, several pigs out each litter will succumb to nodular worms and the rest will demonstrate uneven growth rates for several months. Reinfection on the grower or finisher floor is not common for young pigs. Nodular worm is mostly only found where animals are raised on dirt or where bedding is used since this parasite requires protection from external conditions such as sunlight and direct exposure to external conditions.

DIAGNOSIS IN THE FECES

Nodular worm eggs are distinct and easy to identify (see Figure 6.40). The best time to find eggs are in late gestating sows held on dirt or outside lots. Many samples will have hundreds of eggs present. If high numbers of eggs are found, it is predictable that the baby pigs are becoming infected during nursing and will exhibit gastrointestinal problems just a few weeks of age. As a cautionary note, with nodular worm egg identification make sure there is no confusion with mite eggs (see Figures 6.41 and 6.42) as well as other spurious rodent tapeworm eggs which are commonly found in swine feces (see Figures 6.43 and 6.44).

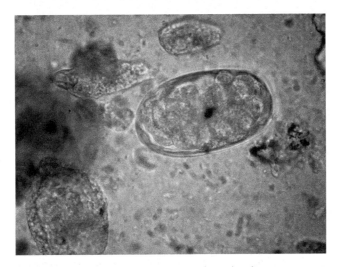

FIGURE 6.40   Nodular worm (*Oesophagostomum dentatium*) egg (10×).

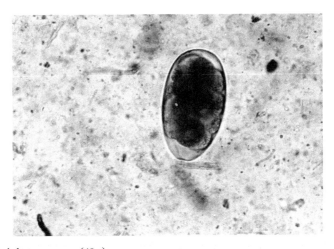

FIGURE 6.41   Nodular worm egg (40×).

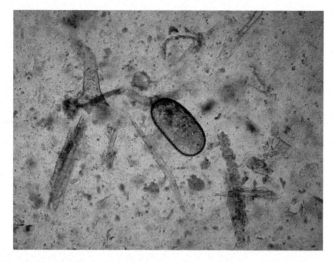

FIGURE 6.42   Oribatid mite eggs (4×).

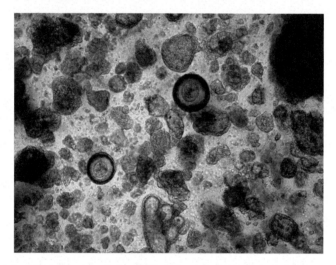

FIGURE 6.43   Spurious tapeworm eggs in hogs (10×).

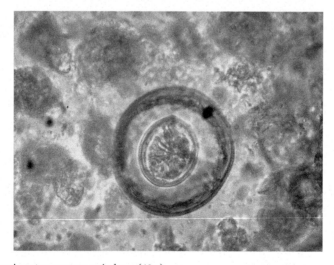

FIGURE 6.44   Spurious tapeworm egg in hogs (40×).

TREATMENT GUIDELINES

Treatment of the sows prior to farrowing with an appropriate dewormer will prevent the baby pig syndrome describe above.

THE DEVELOPMENT AND BUILDUP OF PARASITISM WITHIN A SWINE OPERATION DEPENDS ON MANY FACTORS

- **Indirect transmission:** Once a pen or area is contaminated with worm eggs, the level of parasite contamination continues to increase as time goes on. Both the roundworm and whipworm egg has been shown to live for many years in the environment. The process of contaminating a pen or facility follows a set pattern. As facilities become contaminated from infected animals, and the infected animals are treated or moved out of the facility, the infection remains in the facility; therefore, when new animals are placed in the pen or facility where infected hogs have been previously housed, the new animals become infected and the process of contamination continues. Once contaminated, it may take years to clean up a contaminated pen or facility.

- **Favorable development:** If environmental conditions are favorable for the survival of parasites, a continuous parasite buildup will most likely occur in this facility over a period of years. Obviously, the age of the facility is important because the older the facility the greater the chance for parasite contamination levels to reach significant levels.

- **Type of parasite present:** If the dewormer used in an operation misses one or more parasite specie(s) or stage of parasite present in an animal, then that parasite can thrive and multiply. The whipworm (*T. suis*) is a good example, since both pyrantel and avermectins have been shown poor efficacy against this parasite, operations that deworm extensively with these products can still have production losses due to whipworm despite the fact they are using a dewormer.

- **Direct transmission:** If a sow is infected and is shedding eggs during the farrowing period, the chances are high that this infection will pass on directly to her offspring through contact during nursing contaminating the grower/finisher floor later on in the production cycle.

Internal parasites may be found in many different ways. Infections may be limited to a few pens or to a certain location within an operation. The infection may be isolated to particular building or facility such as a grower floor, or to a certain group of animals such as the gestating sows, or incoming gilts. Identifying where these parasite "hot spots" are can save the operation money and time and allow the deworming efforts to be concentrated where the problem exists.

Annual parasite exams using the "Modified Wisconsin Sugar Flotation Method" should be conducted to determine whether a parasite infestation occurs within a particular facility. Once a parasite infection (such as the large roundworm – *A. suum*) becomes established in a facility, it is very hard to eradicate. Parasitism is considered a herd disease in cattle whereas with hogs, parasite infections often travel from one pen to another. If an infected pig contaminates the pen, other pigs within this pen will become infected. To determine whether a parasite infection is present in a facility requires sampling as many pens as possible. This will provide the best chance to find an infection if it exists. A single sample from an individual animal will most often determine whether an infection exists in a particular pen. Composite samples can be taken but they need to be blended to ensure good stratification.

MATERIALS AND METHODS FOR FECAL SAMPLING

For best results, samples should be collected fresh and then refrigerated. Samples can be taken rectally or picked up off the ground when freshly dropped. Refrigeration is important because heat causes worm eggs to develop and hatch while freezing can destroy some eggs; both will lead to incorrect diagnosis. For storing samples, samples can be refrigerated for long periods of time if need to be.

Sample size needs to be no larger than a teaspoon. Samples are best when placed in plastic bags such as "zip lock bags," baggies, or inverted rectal exam sleeves. Samples can be picked up easily by using the plastic baggie like a glove inverted over the hand; after the sample is taken, the baggie is reinverted, sealed, and marked with a pen to identify the sample.

Samples should be carefully marked to identify animal sampled by Group, pen number, or other location on the operation. Between 5% and 10% of the animals in a group or pen should be sampled. Where animals are held in a group or in a pen or pasture, taking samples from two to three animals are usually sufficient. It is important to take samples from different production levels such as nursery pigs, growers, finishers, gestating sows, lactating sows, etc.

In large operations, it is important to take from as many groups or pens of animals as possible. It is usually better to take one sample each from, say, 50 pens, than five samples from 10 pens since each pen has its own contamination level. One pen, for example, may show high levels of contamination levels while an adjacent pen may show little or no infection present.

SPECIFIC SAMPLE INSTRUCTIONS

1. **Sow farms:** Collect samples in late gestation. Sample by pen in group-housed sows, take 1 sample per pen, and 15–20 random samples per building depending upon the size of the sow units; with individually stalled sows, take 15–20 random samples per building.

2. **Wean to finish:** Collect fecals three to six weeks after arrival and again during the finishing period (>140–150 lb). Sample by pen, take one random sample per pen for a total of 15–20 samples per building.

3. **Grow-finish:** Collect fecals within two to three weeks after arrival onto grower floor (to determine patent infection in arrival pigs). Also, resample late finisher hogs to determine if finish floors are contaminated.

4. **Seed stock farms:** Sample sows as stated above. For young gilts, sample at the time gilts are being moved from finisher or developer facility. If samples are positive, resample during the growing phase to find the location or pens where the infections have come from.

5. **Sample methodology:** Collect freshly dropped sample:

   - Use a resealable sandwich-size bag for each sample.

   - Invert bag and collect a teaspoon size sample.

   - Reinvert bag, squeeze air out, and seal (check seal).

   - Identify sample by date collected and animal group/pen with permanent marker on the bag.
     - Put individual samples from each group in a large resealable bag and identify by date and animal group/pen, if testing more than one group.

   - Keep animal groups separate.
     - Individual samples only – not pooled samples from different pens or animals.
     - Refrigerate overnight to ensure each sample is sufficiently cooled – DO NOT FREEZE.

FECAL WORM EGG COUNT INTERPRETATION AND WHOLE HERD DEWORMING GUIDELINES

Often times, due to management considerations, whole herd deworming is the most convenient, easiest to manage, and can save labor, especially on large operations. Whole herd deworming works the best when parasite levels are not too high and environmental contamination is not the number one concern.

For herds with very low level of contamination where only occasional parasitism is found either through fecal exams, slaughter checks, or observing worms in the feces, a single whole herd deworming conducted once a year is adequate. Most whole herd deworming, however, is conducted twice a year approximately six months apart. Seasonal deworming is not as important in swine held in confinement as it is in with cattle on pasture; however, a late fall deworming is good because cool weather slows down egg development and retards contamination of the facilities. A second deworming in early summer helps reduce stress during hot summer months.

The goal of successful parasite control is to first determine the exact location where an infection is located within an operation. The first factor to determine is whether or not parasitism is present within an operation and, then second, to determine precisely where it is within the operation. If an infection is determined to be present, it is necessary to determine how the infection reached this particular phase of production or location within a facility or operation.

If an infection can be traced back to its original source, the ability to control the infection becomes much greater. For example, did the infection come from the sows or maybe the animals brought it from another location of the operation? Usually, an animal needs to be present at a particular location longer than six weeks for the infection to be endemic to that location. If the infection is present as an ongoing endemic infection to a particular location, clinical condition of the animals and fecal worm egg counts can help determine the intense or level of the contamination.

Controlling or reducing the contamination level of an infection is important because as the contamination levels increase, the chance for the contamination to spread to other parts of the operation also increases. Parasite levels and the subsequent damage caused by an infection are also often directly related to the production standards of an operation. Because of vast improvement in genetics, management, and nutrition over the past few years, the effects of parasites have become more pronounced as individual productions goals increase, and therefore, even low levels of infection can be very important in high-producing animals.

The efficient use of dewormers can be made in the swine industry if an operation can determine where an infection occurs through parasite diagnosis and then to devise individualized, preventative, strategic deworming strategies to control and eliminate this infection. The overall objective, of course, is for the producer to gain maximum treatment benefit for every dollar spent on control.

As swine confinement units have become increasingly more prevalent, the misconception has grown that roundworm parasites are eliminated because they cannot live indoors, and treatment pressure has declined in many operations. Fecal exams and slaughter checks have demonstrated over a period of years many of these confinement units, especially those which have been left untreated, have become contaminated (some heavily) with parasitic eggs and larvae.

What are suspected is that pockets of infection develop in a confinement situation and that this infection eventually spreads throughout a unit depending upon management and movement of pigs within the unit. It seems reasonable, therefore, that an infection, if left untreated, can work its way through an operation over time. Since the indoor environmental conditions with relatively high humidity and warm temperatures found in most confinement units are favorable for parasite development and survival, infection levels can often build to a high level before being detected.

The contamination of a facility begins with an infected animal that is moved into the facility and, thereby, contaminating the facility or the animals it is exposed to. An example of this is when a sow is moved into a farrowing crate after it has become infected during the gestation period. This sow becomes a source of infection for her baby pigs once they are born.

Once infected, the pigs then carry this infection until it reaches maturity when egg-laying adults are present, and the animals begin to shed worm eggs back into the environment. This process takes approximately six weeks post-infection, so by the time these animals are harboring patent infections they will be out of the nursery and on a grower floor. Here, they are often commingled with other pigs, so the infections can spread throughout this pen of animals continuing the contamination process of the facility.

TREATMENT TO CONTROL PARASITISM AND REDUCE PARASITE FUTURE CONTAMINATION IN A FACILITY

Based on results of fecal worm egg counts conducted within an operation, a preventative strategic control program can be designed. The results of the fecal lab should provide a basis on the type and intensity of the parasite infection ongoing in an operation.

If an operation, after numerous samples have been taken on all categories of hogs on the premise, proves to have a negative worm contamination level, a minimum preventative program can be set up and followed to keep the premises clean. All new animals entering the facilities need to be treated with Safe-Guard® for a thorough internal parasite control. Continued monitoring of the facility on an annual basis should be a part of the ongoing herd health program.

Where worm egg contamination is found, it is important to stop this contamination as soon as possible not only to stop the present infection but also to reduce or prevent future contamination problems. Timing the deworming around the worm life cycle in conjunction with management practices of the swine herd is key to the success of preventing parasite contamination.

Where a sow is dewormed prior to farrowing, the newborn pigs have little chance to receive an infection from their mothers. The first time these pigs can become infected is usually on the grower floor or when these animals encounter an infected facility. Keeping the sow parasite free is key to keeping an operation parasite-free.

For growing and finishing pigs, treatment should be given three to four weeks after transfer to the grower facility. A second treatment given to break the life cycle of any newly acquired worms is recommended four to five weeks later. If fecal counts are negative, and the facility is determined to be parasite-free, treatment is not necessary, but yearly fecal checks should be made. If parasite-damaged livers are observed in slaughter, treatment timing is important to stop this damage and, therefore, treatment should be given in the feed to finisher hogs approximately six weeks prior to finish. This treatment should be continued until liver checks become negative.

Conducting fecal worm egg counts throughout a swine operation is an excellent way that applies science to the deworming process. For the producer to treat only those animals, pens or facilities that need treating and then treating them at the right time is a very valuable service. Interpreting and recording the data is an important part of the process. This is especially important where heavy contamination rates are found, a treatment program needs to be instituted to clean-up this infection, and to keep future parasite losses from occurring.

DEVELOPING PARASITE DATA FOR SWINE CLIENTS

This fecal exam, therefore, is a necessary part of the process for developing individualized control strategies and for monitoring the treatment process. There are a number of options available for conducting fecal sample analysis for swine operations.

1. The consulting veterinarian or veterinary clinic can set up an "in house" fecal exam service for their clients.

2. Some Clinics set aside one day each week that fecal samples are run.

3. A special "parasite awareness lab day," i.e., once a month, once a quarter, etc., where clients bring in samples for analysis the day or a few days before the lab day.

Data collected from the fecal analysis serves as permanent data for a veterinary clinic or veterinary consultant about the type and level of parasitism found within each operation or location within the operation. The result can also help identify as to where on the operation parasite contamination is a problem. Once contamination levels are identified, a control strategy can be set up and monitored.

REFERENCES

1. Hale, O.M. and Stewart, T.B. (1987). Feed and maintenance costs of internal parasites in growing-finishing swine. *Agri-Pract.* 8 (4): 33–35.

2. Bliss, D.H. (1996). *Comprehensive Review of Internal and External Parasites in Swine – Current Strategies for Complete Control*. Hoechst-Roussel Agri-Vet.

3. Batte, E.G., McLamb, R.D., Muse, K.E. et al. (1977). Pathophysiology of swine trichuriasis. *AM. J. Vet. Res.* 38 (7): 1075–1079.

4. Biehl, L.G. (1984). Internal parasites of feeder pigs in Southern Illinois. *Agri-Practice* 5: 20–26.

5. Kennedy, T.J., Bruer, D.J., Marchiondo, A.A., and Williams, J.A. (1988). Prevalence of swine parasites in major hog producing areas of the United States. *Agri-Pract.* 9 (2): 25–32.

6. Todd, A.C. (1973). National Prevalence of swine parasites. Proceeding: Live and Learn Symposium. Section III Grand Bahamas, Shell Chemical Co.: 1–6.

Parasites in Small Ruminants   CHAPTER 7

Sheep have held an important place in the history of the United States, arriving in the United States as early as 1609. Sheep were first raised in small flocks primarily for their wool although older animals were often eaten as mutton. Looking at the US tax records for my ancestors dating back from 1840 to 1870 (in Mina, NY), they were recorded as having 286 acres of land with a flock of 30 sheep, 10 milk cows, 5 horses, and 2 mules (see Figure 7.1). Of course, as the western movement occurred following the Great Gold Rush of 1848, sheep production then moved westward through Montana toward California (see Figure 7.2). From the late 1880s until just after WWI, Big Timber, Montana was reportedly the Number #1 wool-producing area in the United States but, of course, that changed substantially as the demand for wool dropped and synthetics appeared soon after the war ended. Sheep ranchers would bring their wool to a warehouse on the railway in Big Timber where the wool was baled and shipped to the New England woolen mills (see Figure 7.3). The heyday for this shipping point for wool based on the graffiti found on the wall of this warehouse dated from early 1900 to the 1930s.

Furthermore, the common knowledge, that we were all told as kids, was that mutton was fed to the troops as a regular staple during WWII and most returning GIs said "no more mutton ever!" which significantly hurt the sheep industry. Many attempts have been made to revive the sheep industry. In the early 1950s, for example, a sheep project was created with the help of the University of Wisconsin to help introduce sheep raising to Northern Wisconsin but this project too was

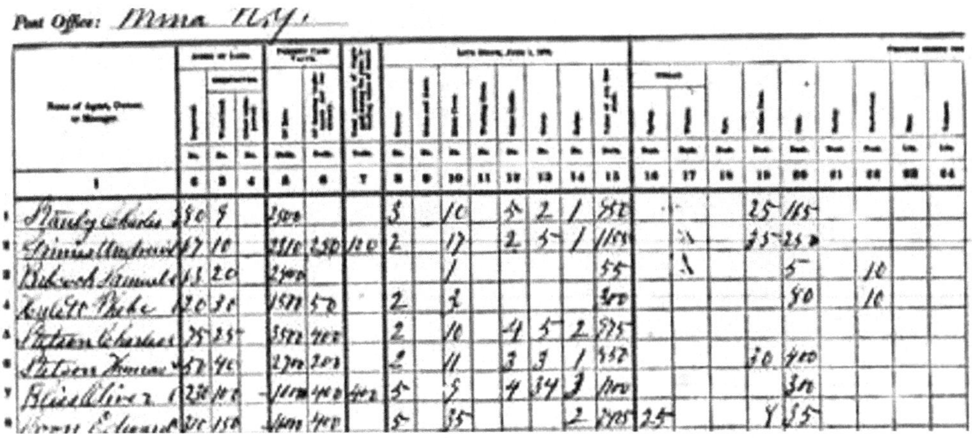

FIGURE 7.1   Tax records from the early 1800s.

Large Animal Parasitology Procedures for Veterinary Technicians, First Edition. Donald H. Bliss.
© 2024 John Wiley & Sons, Inc. Published 2024 by John Wiley & Sons, Inc.

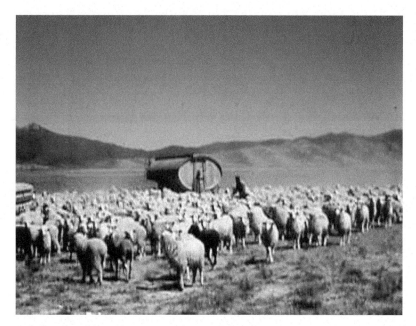

FIGURE 7.2   Sheep on Montana big range country.

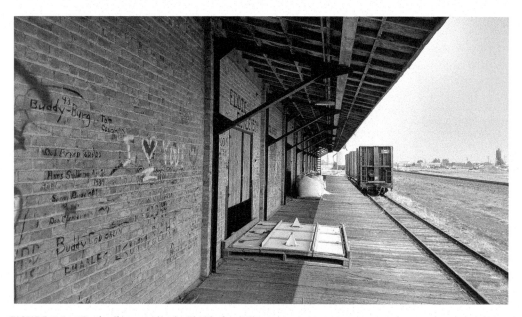

FIGURE 7.3   Wool railway station in Big Timber, MT.

soon halted when all the sheep began to die due to deer fluke infections (*Fascioloides magna*) [1]. Sheep production, however, is still very important in the United States but Texas (see Figure 7.4) and California are now the number one states for both sheep and goat production.

The demand for goat meat, on the other hand, has recently risen substantially over the past 30 years (see Figure 7.5). This demand for goat meat has expanded as immigrants from Hispanic,

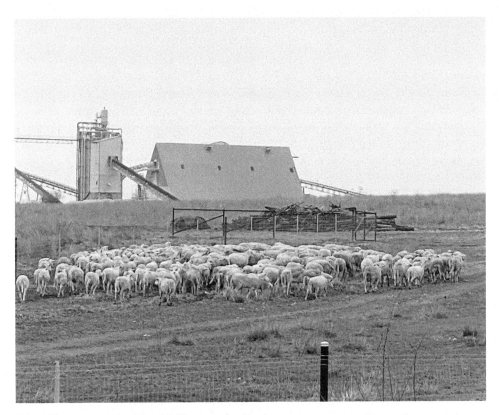

FIGURE 7.4   Large sheep herd in Texas on short pasture.

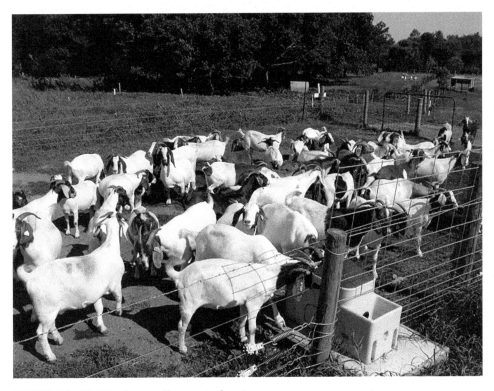

FIGURE 7.5   Goat herd on small overgrazed pastures.

Middle Eastern, Southeast Asian, and Caribbean countries have grown significantly in the United States and their desire for goat meat and goat milk products has caused goat production to expand. Small goat operations are now the norm and have become very prevalent throughout the Midwest and Southeast including Texas. Goat milk production used especially for cheese has also grown significantly during this time mostly in Northeast and the Midwest.

Llama and alpaca have also become popular (see Figures 7.6 and 7.7), first appeared in the United States in the late 1980s with breeding animals reaching very high prices during the 1990s into early 2000s. Once the markets settled, the United States has maintained a significant number of small alpaca and llama operations found all across the United States. A large alpaca operation

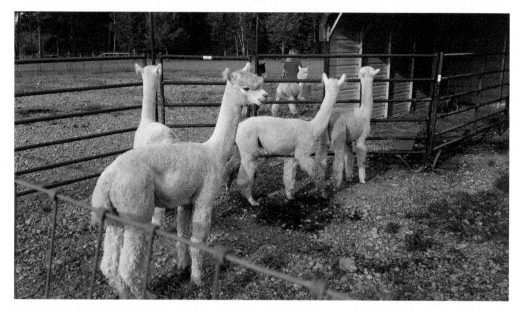

FIGURE 7.6   Small Alpaca farm in New York State.

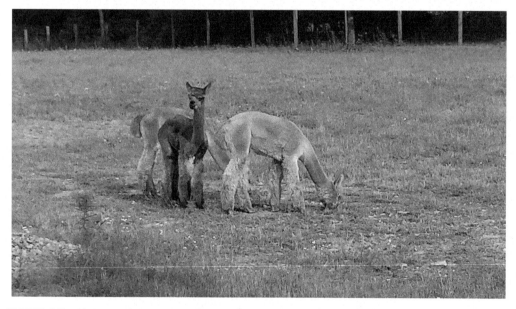

FIGURE 7.7   Alpaca grazing on poor unimproved pasture.

might have 50 animals while sheep or cattle operations may have hundreds and even thousands of animals in a single operation. *Camels*, on the other hand, are present in the United States in very small numbers with only a few thousands camels found across the United States, but what all these animals have in common with sheep, goats, and camelids is that controlling parasites, especially the barber's pole worm (*Haemonchus*) is a very big part of keeping all of these animals healthy and productive [2, 5].

Gastrointestinal nematode parasites are all very important to the health of all small ruminants. As with cattle, parasitism causes considerable production loss by interfering with the health and well-being of these animals. Parasites have been shown to adversely affect milk production, reduce breeding efficiency, reduce weight gains, decrease hair quality, reduce feed efficiency, and negatively affect the immune system by decreasing the animal's ability to fight off other disease problems [2–4, 9].

Small ruminants are affected by many different types of parasites. Each type of parasite has its own preferred location within an animal where it lives causing specific damage to the host animal. All parasites cause damage but the most prevalent and economically important nematode parasite of goat lives in the abomasum or fourth stomach and is called *Haemonchus contortus* (the barber's pole worm). Other common and economically important gastrointestinal and lung parasites found in goats are *Trichostrongylus* (the bankrupt worm), tapeworms, nodular worms, threadworms, *Nematodirus*, whipworms, *Dictyocaulus* (lungworms), and coccidia. All parasites can cause serious problems leading to death of small ruminants, but none are more prevalent and more important than *Haemonchus* commonly known as the barber's pole worm [5].

Parasitic gastroenteritis is more prevalent and often most serious in first, the camel, then comes goats, sheep, and then camelids in that order. Camels are native to desert and dry countries such as Egypt, Jordon, and the Middle East, so they have no innate immunity against parasites found in temperate country such as the United States. Once camels are exposed to parasites found in cattle or small ruminants, they often become very heavily parasitized and begin to suffer greatly. The same is true of goats since they are traditional browsers (see Figures 7.8 and 7.9) and when

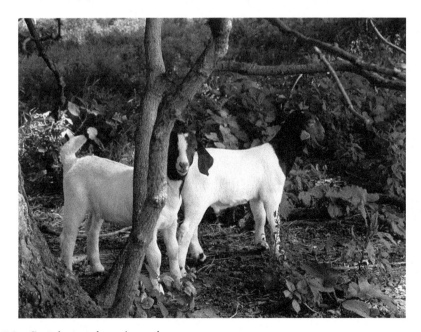

FIGURE 7.8   Goats by trees browsing on leaves.

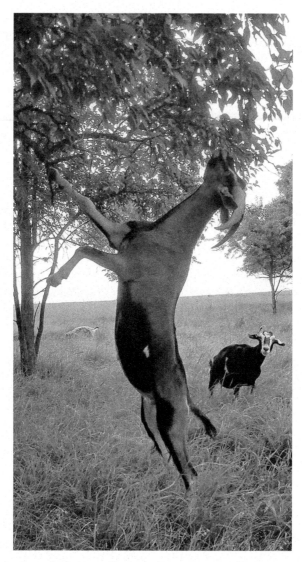

FIGURE 7.9 Single goat browsing on a small tree.

they are forced to graze overstocked pasture (see Figure 7.10), these animals will become heavily parasitized very quickly. Once goats are forced to graze intensively, they seem to develop high parasite burdens quicker than either sheep or cattle and are more susceptible to the ill effects caused by internal parasites. When placed in an intensive grazing situation, it is not uncommon, even for a small goat herd, to lose several animals a year to parasitism.

Sheep and camelids can also have severe parasite problems as well but both species have thousands of years of grazing experience and as long as stocking density is not too high and treatment is readily available, parasitism is usually controllable. I recently observed a sheep herd near Fredericksburg, Texas, using a donkey for protection. It is a clever idea since the sheep parasites will not pass on to the donkey (see Figure 7.11). Sheep that are overstocked with inadequate treatment protocol will certainly succumb to parasitism just like goats (see Figure 7.12).

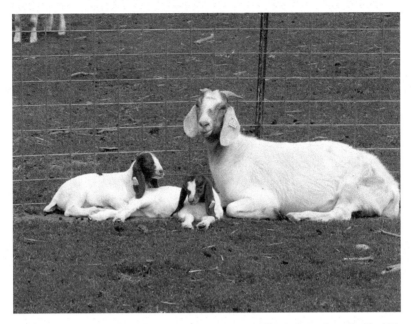

FIGURE 7.10   Nanny goat plus kids on pasture where parasite will soon be an issue for the kids.

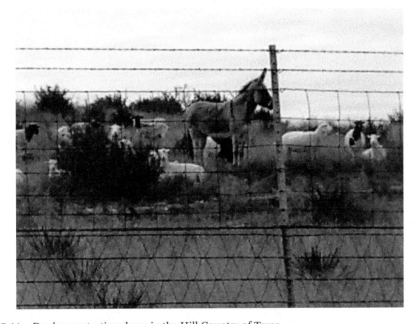

FIGURE 7.11   Donkey protecting sheep in the Hill Country of Texas.

One problem we find especially with camelids is that the meningeal worm (*Parelaphos-trongylus tenuis*) transmitted by deer (where little or no disease is apparent in white-tail deer) is lethal in sheep, moose, camelids, and sometimes goats and cattle. This parasite exists where ever deer are present (except in Texas, New Mexico, and Arizona, or extreme north western part of North America). Treatment for acute disease symptoms is recommended using fenbendazole

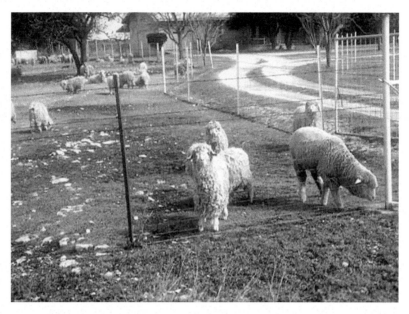

FIGURE 7.12   Sheep on overgrazed pasture.

(Safe-Guard®/Panacur® – Merck) at the rate of 10 mg/kg daily for five days [7]. Prevention of disease for camelids, sheep, and goats has traditionally been monthly treatment (30–40 days apart) with either ivermectin or doramectin [8].

Many small producers in the east and southeastern part of the United States, who owned or may have inherited a small farm, started a fad in the early 1990s turning to raising small ruminants, mainly meat goats, to meet the market demand coming from the large population centers on the East Coast. Almost 100% of these family farms had never seen goats or sheep previously, so it makes sense that if "parasite-free" goats were placed on goat parasite-free farms, these operations should remain parasite-free. Unfortunately, that is not what happened. Over a period of time, thousands of wormy goats were sold and moved to their new environment immediately contaminating their new home. For the most part, the first year the goats arrived to their new place everything was just great. The new owners were building fence and learning how to care for these new animals and the decision seemed pretty good. Then, in the second year, however, a few health problems began to appear while in the third year, things changed drastically. Most of these farms now struggle every year to keep their goats alive. My phone begins to ring every year starting in June, asking for help. We received almost daily reports at our lab concerning sheep and goats dying due to parasitism as parasite contamination of old cattle pastures now teem with new goat parasites, especially *Haemonchus* (barber's pole worm).

One of the biggest problems we observed immediately was that most of these operations were confining their animals to very small pastures and allowed the animals to overgraze the pastures. The closer the animals graze to the ground the more exposure to infective larvae they have and are able to consume. The extension personnel from the University of Georgia once told me that they monitored 22 herds for parasite resistance and that all herds except one were resistant. When I asked about the herd that showed no resistance, I was told it consisted of 75 goats on 20 acres. Nothing more needs to be said, because it was clear that these animals had plenty of room to roam and browse the brush which prevents the infective larvae from concentrating on one area to cause heavy reinfection (see Figures 7.13–7.16).

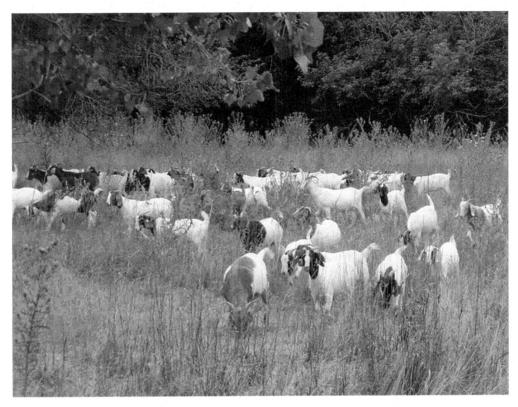

FIGURE 7.13   Goat herd a large pasture in Minnesota.

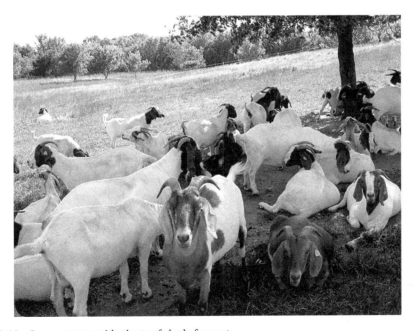

FIGURE 7.14   Large pasture with plenty of shade for goats.

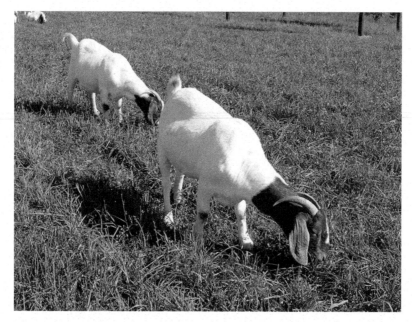

FIGURE 7.15   Goats grazing new parasite-free pasture.

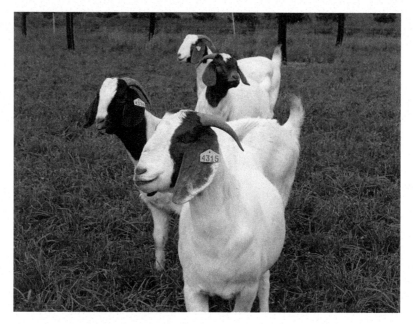

FIGURE 7.16   Four goats on a new parasite-free pasture.

The most severe problems usually occur around three months into the grazing season. In the Midwest and North Atlantic, animals start showing signs of severe parasitism in mid-summer or early autumn when forage is often in short supply and environmental contamination with parasitic larvae is at its highest level (see Figure 7.17). If the animals continue to shed worm eggs back on the pasture, pasture contamination will continue to climb reaching its peak about three months

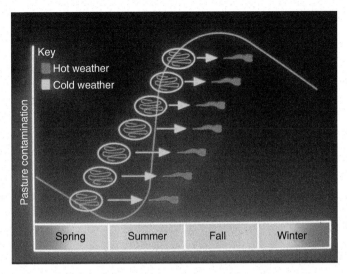

FIGURE 7.17   Seasonal parasite contamination pattern during summer grazing season.

into the season which can be as early as May in the south or as late as August under northern climate conditions, Unlike cattle, it is not uncommon to find small ruminants of all ages developing clinical parasitism. In many cases, therapeutic treatment is necessary just to save lives. Effective parasite control in small ruminants without preventing the buildup of high levels of environmental contamination with infective larvae is nearly impossible. In most cases, once clinical parasitism develops, the animals need to be removed from the infected pasture, just to save the animals from dying due to Haemonchosis.

Haemonchosis is the disease caused by a gastrointestinal parasite called *H. contortus* (see Figure 7.18). Infective larvae are consumed off the vegetation as the animals graze. The ingested larvae pass through the rumen losing their outer protective covering (sheath) and then moving into an existing gastric gland in the abomasum (fourth stomach) (see Figure 7.19). Once a larva has moved into the gastric gland, a mucus plug over the gland develops and the gland no longer produces the HCL acid needed for digestion. These encysted larvae can be seen upon necropsy

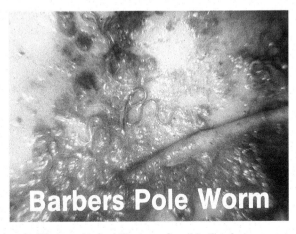

FIGURE 7.18   Barber's pole (*Haemonchus*) adult worms found in the abomasum at necropsy.

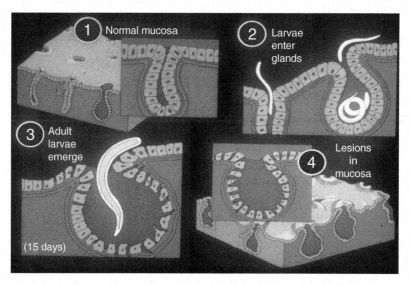

FIGURE 7.19   Diagram of Haemonchus larvae in the gastric glands in the abomasum.

with the naked eye (see Figure 7.20). The larva then begins development growing toward maturity, molting first into a fourth-stage larva and then to an early fifth-stage larva (growing larger each time) when it emerges into the lumen of the abomasa and attaches to the surface of the abomasa, sucking blood. Loss of blood causing anemia is the principal feature of Haemonchus. Both the adult and fourth stages of Haemonchus suck blood and, in addition, move and leave wounds which hemorrhage back into the abomasum. The projected average blood loss has been calculated at 0.05 ml/Haemonchus/day [4]. A high fecal worm egg count and pale eyelid are the best indicators of anemia development in a Haemonchus-infected animal(s) [5, 6].

Once out of the gland, these worms mature into adult worms, find a sexual mate, and then begin producing eggs to start the cycle over again. As the animals ingest more larvae, more gastric glands shut down due to larval invasion, the pH in the abomasa begins to rise and fiber digestion begins to fall and anorexia begins to develop. Several processes occur during larva development within a host animal that are noteworthy. Due to the destruction of the gastric glands by a larva,

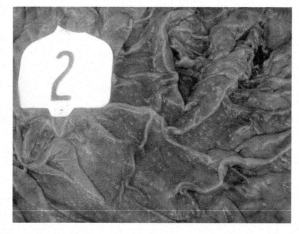

FIGURE 7.20   Inhibited Haemonchus larvae seen grossly on the abomasum.

acid production in the gut declines causing the pH to rise, reducing fiber digestion which can create a potbelly appearance in the animal. If this infection continues to grow, a bottle jaw appearance can often be seen. One of the noteworthy part of this whole process is that if the pH in the abomasa gets too high, it appears to become a triggering factor that tells the larvae that gut conditions have deteriorated and it is time to stop development (thus inhibition begins). It is not in the best interest of a parasite to kill its host since it too will die.

Once inhibition begins, the percentage of inhibition continues to climb until nearly all incoming larvae become inhibited. Only drought conditions, winter weather, or moving the animals off the infected pasture can stop this process. As winter or drought conditions approaches, larvae ingestions stop, the gut conditions begin to stabilize. If larvae ingestion stops for a period of time, the old worms die off and the inhibited begin redevelopment. As an indicator, worm egg counts will begin to climb. In the Midwest, fecal worm egg counts will often hit their peak in late winter or early spring (March). We often observe sheep and goats with over a 1000 eggs in 1 g sample which multiples out to 454,000 in a pound of manure. A high egg counts at this point means that the previous summer pasture was heavily contaminated and probably dangerous to use in the upcoming spring.

Haemonchosis is a fast-progressing disease with one of the very first signs to recognize is anemia. Fecal worm egg counts will quickly climb and then animals will soon start to die. Haemonchosis affects every animal slightly different depending on the number of larvae they consume, how heavy their current burden is, their age, their health status, and previous exposure to *Haemonchus*. One large sheep operation in Kansas reportedly was losing as many as 150 ewes every day. When I arrived at the operation, I witnessed over 3000 dead animals all due to Haemonchosis. The first step (and most important step) was to immediately move all animals to a parasite-free location. The best worm-free refuge can be created with a temporary fence around a hay meadow or to move them to concrete or dirt lots. The pastures with the heavy contamination cannot be used until late spring the following year.

Haemonchosis is a unique disease because it occurs around the same time every year and then some years can be worse than other years, causing considerable economic loss as well as a high death loss depending on the level of pasture contamination that has developed. Once worm burdens become high, it is extremely difficult to control Haemonchosis due to the high levels of parasite resistance that occurs to all dewormers on the market today.

This is where the problem begins as the owners, producers, and veterinarians' eye mucosal exams indicate anemia and possible parasite overload and therefore treatment is necessary; however, but by now successful treatment is nearly impossible to achieve because of huge population of larvae embedded in the gastric glands. Treatment failure is imminent. The adult worms are accessible for deworming but as they die off, a new population emerges immediately from the glands, and often the second state of the animal is worse than the first.

Some of the reasons that small ruminants become heavily infected during the summer grazing season:

1. Small ruminants graze closer to the ground than cattle which increases exposure to parasitic larvae. Pre-parasitic larvae (L_1) hatch from eggs passed in the fecal material; these larvae undergo several molts until they reach an infective stage (L_3). This infective stage is mobile and moves with moisture trails onto nearby vegetation to be eaten by its intended host. Pasture covered with morning dew or light rain provides an ideal time for parasite transmission to occur especially if the pasture is overgrazed and the vegetation is short.

2. Fecal material excreted by small ruminants is very concentrated and, therefore, worm egg counts can reach very high levels. Fecal worm egg counts from goats can be 10–50 times higher than those found in cattle. A small amount of goat's feces, therefore, can produce a very high level of parasite contamination.

3. Parasite control programs recommended for goats over the years have been more therapeutic than preventative. Treating goats after heavy parasite loads have developed has little impact on reducing future contamination of the environment and can lead to the development of parasite resistance. Furthermore, once high worm burdens are encountered, complete control is impossible to achieve.

4. One commonly recommended practice is to deworm small ruminants every eight weeks while on pasture. Since the time it takes for newly ingested larvae to develop into egg-laying adult parasite in goats is as short as two weeks, treatment every eight weeks allows goats to be clean for only two weeks out of each eight-week treatment period. For an efficient parasite control strategy to work for goats, the parasite treatment intervals needs to be significantly reduced.

FAMACHA is a selective treatment system for controlling Haemonchus in small ruminants: FAMACHA was developed in South Africa for classifying animals into categories based on levels of anemia [10, 11]. The FAMACHA treatment system is being currently being recommended and promoted by a number of universities and used by goat producers especially in the southeast. This FAMACHA system is designed to identify and treat only very ill animals after a heavy infection has been encountered. With this system, animals are exposed to high levels of infective larvae and then are individually treated only after they are identified to be suffering from high levels of infection and extensive production losses have already occurred. These animals following treatment are placed back on the same pasture where their heavy infections were generated.

To use FAMACHA, the color of ocular mucus membranes is observed and compared to a laminated card which has colored illustrations of eyes from sheep at different levels of anemia. FAMACHA, therefore, is a limited treatment system based on waiting and treating animals only after a heavy infection has occurred. It becomes a "Shotgun" approach to deworming when you wait until the pastures are highly contaminated and the animals are heavily parasitized before you institute selective treatment based on the level of anemia and return the anemic animal back to the highly contaminated pastures following treatment (see Figure 7.21). Since only animals with severe anemia are treated, the entire herd needs to be monitored every two to three weeks to monitor animals as they become anemic in order to treat, hoping to prevent death loss.

The following problems exist with the FAMACHA system:

1. It is designed for only one parasite: *Haemonchus*. It provides no control for the other economically important parasites such as whipworm, tapeworm, threadworm, *Nematodirus,* and nodular worm. The theory behind FAMACHA is to limit drug use to prevent the development of resistance.

2. Haemonchosis is not the only cause of anemia.

3. Treating animals after they are highly parasitized means production losses are already occurring before treatment is given and there is danger for the animals since it is not uncommon for animals to die despite treatment if the disease has progressed too far or if the dewormer is ineffective due to resistance.

4. It is impossible to achieve a high degree of efficacy in animals after a heavy worm burden has developed and pasture contamination is at a high level. This is a "shotgun" approach

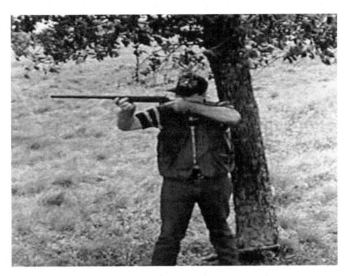

FIGURE 7.21   Shotgun approach to deworming small ruminants after the damage is already done.

to deworming animals rather than treating animals earlier in the season when burdens are much lower and pasture contamination is at its lowest level for the year. Deworming an animal harboring a heavy worm burden, for example, 300,000 parasites using a product achieving 95% efficacy means 15,000 worms will remain following treatment plus the animal immediately begins picking up infective larvae, developing a new infection just as soon as it begins to graze following treatment.

5. Scoring animals for anemia every two weeks is time consuming, labor intensive, hard on the animals, and is nearly impossible to accomplish in large herds. Haemonchosis is a severe problem found only in grazing animals. High levels of *Haemonchus* are seldom found in animals raised in total confinement.

To survive and be consumed by sheep or goats, *Haemonchus* needs a protective mircoenvironment provided by pasture vegetation and a mode of transmission to the animals provided by vegetation itself. Once the environment of grazing small ruminants is heavily contaminated with *Haemonchus* larvae, control is impossible to achieve because animals treated for haemonchosis are returned to the contaminated pasture and immediately become reinfected.

1. *Haemonchus* is a very prolific parasite. It appears that goats lack innate immunity against this parasite, allowing this species to develop rapidly into an adult parasite living within the gastrointestinal tract laying large numbers of eggs that pass back into the environment of the animals.

2. *Haemonchus* infections develop into egg-laying adults more rapidly in goats than cattle. In goats, developing larvae emerge from the gastric glands as a fourth-stage larva and develop into adult parasites on the surface of the abomasum on average, 15 days after infection. In cattle, the developing larvae emerge as fifth-stage larvae and develop into an adult parasite 25–30 days after infection. This rapid development of *Haemonchus* in goats provides a quick regeneration of this parasite and subsequently leads to very high levels of pasture contamination.

3. *Haemonchus* is a unique parasite in goats because this parasite can inhibit its development in the larval stage while in the gastric gland and remain dormant in the glands for months

before resuming normal development and becoming an egg-laying adult parasite. Furthermore, inhibited larval stages residing in the gland are protected and are very difficult to kill. If these inhibited larvae survive treatment, they can develop into egg-laying adults in just a few days.

Strategic parasite control designed to reduce environmental contamination by parasitic larvae for an entire grazing season. Prevention is the best method of controlling these parasites in the goat. Successful parasite control means reducing or eliminating environmental contamination and should include several key goals:

1. All small ruminants should be as free as possible of parasites during periods of low or reduced nutrition because of the high cost of feed. It is most important to have goats free of parasites during the wintertime so that the animals are not shedding eggs and immediately contaminating the pasture when spring grazing begins.

2. The doe should be confirmed parasite-free prior to kidding time.

3. Recontamination of spring pastures should be eliminated for the first two months of the grazing season.

4. Goats should never be moved to a new location without a confirmed parasite-free status.

STRATEGIC DEWORMING FOR SMALL RUMINANTS

PHASE I: "0–3–6–9" SPRING DEWORMINGS

Strategic timed dewormings in the spring are necessary to prevent high levels of parasitism from building up on the pastures and in the animals themselves later in the year. Strategic deworming is designed to prevent parasite build up on the pastures by creating "parasite safe grazing" through repeated dewormings given to prevent pasture contamination during the first 90 days (3 months) of the grazing season. This can be accomplished through repeated therapeutic dewormings given at three week intervals "0–3–6–9" strategic timed dewormings; parasite-safe grazing can be established for the rest of the year. Since the life cycle of *Haemonchus* is 21 days or less in small ruminants, the treatment interval should be no more than 3 weeks apart. Strategic timed deworming works for small ruminants as follows:

1. All animals grazing the same pasture must be free of parasites with a negative fecal worm egg count at the start of spring grazing (Day 0). The treatment clock starts ticking as soon as grass growth begins in the spring. Any worm eggs shed at this time will begin recontaminating the pasture for the current season.

2. Grazing animals will pick up infective larvae present on the pasture from the previous season but before the larvae can mature and beginning to shed worm eggs back on the pasture, the first strategic deworming eliminates these worms. The animals then pick up more larvae and then the second strategic treatment eliminates these worms before they contaminate the pasture, this process is repeated three weeks later for a third treatment. A fourth treatment is recommended in southern states because of a longer grazing season.

3. Depending upon location in the country, the animals treated in the fall or at kidding should still be parasite-free and may not need the initial treatment at the beginning of the spring. Because of inhibition of *Haemonchus*, fecal worm egg counts should be taken at least once during the winter months to confirm a negative count. Where year-around grazing or winter grazing takes place, all animals should be treated prior to extended spring grass growth to prevent recontamination of the pasture.

4. Strategic timed spring dewormings are effective and provide protection for the entire grazing season because parasitic larvae which survive the winter die off naturally due to exhausted stored food supply if they are not eaten by the animals grazing the pasture during the first two to three months of spring grazing. The strategic timed repeated dewormings keep the pastures from being recontaminated while the larvae not consumed by grazing animals die off and disappear from the pastures.

A strategic deworming protocol using Safe-Guard for the seasonal control of gastrointestinal parasites in traditional grazed breeding farms for deer and elk has been developed for use in sheep and goats. This is a unique protocol designed with strategically timed dewormings both to reduce parasitism in the animals themselves (especially encysted *Haemonchus*) as well as in the animal's environment for an entire grazing season (see Figure 7.22). It has been tested under field conditions at a number of locations across the country. Fecal monitoring is highly recommended.

1. **Fall deworming regime:** At the end of the grazing season (preferably after a hard frost), feed Safe-Guard Pellets or Flaked Meal during morning feed at the rate of 1.0 lb per 750 lb of body weight (Safe-Guard 0.5%) or 4 oz per 750 lb body weight (Safe-Guard 1.96%). Spread total dose over three days. On the fourth day, give Cydectin® (moxidectin) drench at the rate of 1 cc/20 lb or liquid sheep drench at the rate of 2.5× recommended dose. *Note*: Multiple days of Safe-Guard activates encysted larvae which are then killed by Cydectin. For animals that are severely debilitated or heavily pregnant, ivermectin can be substituted for moxidectin.

2. **Winter deworming:** Conduct a fecal exam in late February to early March. If positive: repeat fall treatment regime to make sure animals are not shedding worm eggs at the beginning of the grazing season.

3. **Spring–early summer strategic timed dewormings:** Begin treatment three weeks after turn-out or three weeks after first spring grass growth:
   First deworming = three-day Safe-Guard protocol given three weeks after beginning of grazing season.
   Second deworming = three-day Safe-Guard protocol given three weeks after the first treatment.
   Third deworming = three-day Safe-Guard protocol (plus Cydectin drench given orally on the fourth day) given three weeks after the second treatment.

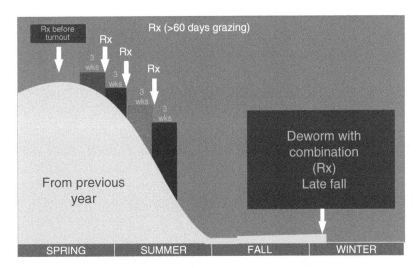

FIGURE 7.22   Strategic timed deworming (0–3–6–9) for small ruminants.

4. **Fall deworming:** Repeat fall program listed above in Number 1. (Fall deworming regime).*

The key to the success of strategic deworming, therefore, is that if the animals grazing spring pastures can be prevented from shedding parasite eggs on the pasture during the first two to three months of the season, parasite-safe grazing can be maintained and parasite burden developing in the animals over the summer grazing season can be significantly reduced. A treatment recommendation of "0–3–6–9" at a given location would be, for example, if grazing starts around the first of April and the animals are parasite-free to start (Day 0), the first spring treatment would be given the third week of April (Week 3), followed by a second deworming given the second week of May (Week 6) followed by a third treatment given the first week of June (Week 9) leaving the animals free from shedding worm eggs until approximately the last week of June or first week of July. No worm eggs would be shed during the months of May and June, and the larvae consumed by the animals during these months are removed by the repeated dewormings.

Strategic deworming works at the beginning of the grazing season by timing the treatment to kill the parasites after the infection process has begun in the animal but before the parasites have developed sufficiently to become adults and begin to lay worm eggs, which pass back on the pasture. The animals, therefore, work like vacuum cleaners eating the parasitic larvae present on the herbage, reducing pasture contamination while the "0–3–6–9" strategic timed treatments prevent further recontamination of the pastures, thus providing "parasite-safe pastures" for the entire grazing season.

PHASE II – FALL CLEANUP DEWORMING

A late fall deworming (given after the first of November or after the first hard frost) will reduce the chance of winter parasitism. Depending on location in the country, this treatment should also help ensure that the does are free of parasites at the time of kidding. A late fall or early winter treatment eliminates any parasites developed during the summer grazing season and ensures the animals are parasite-free to begin the grazing season in the spring. The late fall deworming also keeps animals' parasite-free during the winter when feeding cost are the highest.

SUMMARY

There is no single answer to preventing parasitism from interfering with raising goats for profit, either as breeding stock, milk, or meat. Using the two available FDA-approved dewormers in rotation with each other in a strategic timed program to prevent the buildup of infective larvae on pasture will eliminate any serious threat caused by *Haemonchus* as well as all other major worm parasites of goats. With strategic timed deworming, instead of animals being wormy all year around, they are parasite-free from the beginning of November through two weeks after the last spring treatment which may be as late as July in northern states. Furthermore, with strategic timed dewormings, the contamination level in the environment is greatly reduced throughout the summer grazing season.

FECAL MONITORING IS THE BEST WAY TO DETERMINE WHETHER TREATMENT IS EFFECTIVE

A. **The Modified Wisconsin Sugar Flotation Technique is a fecal exam (see** Figure 7.23**) that is conducted by floating worm eggs out of fecal material.** This technique is highly sensitive for use with small ruminants. Efficient use of a dewormer requires the knowledge of whether a particular dewormer is effective in a particular animal. Fecal worm egg counts, if conducted correctly, can determine the type of parasites present including tapeworms and coccidia (protozoan) (see Figure 7.24). A fecal worm egg count can also provide accurate

---

*Safe-Guard (fenbendazole) is a product of Merck Animal Health. Cydectin is a product of Bayer Animal Health. Ivermectin is a generic endecticide available through a number of companies.

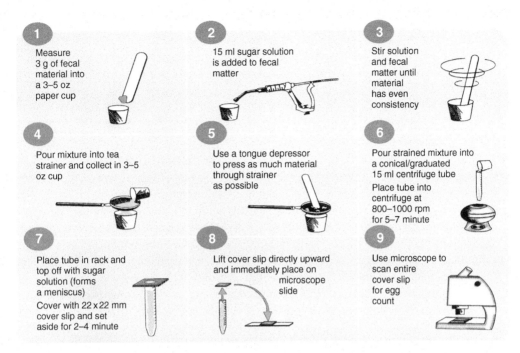

FIGURE 7.23 Modified Wisconsin Sugar Floatation Method.

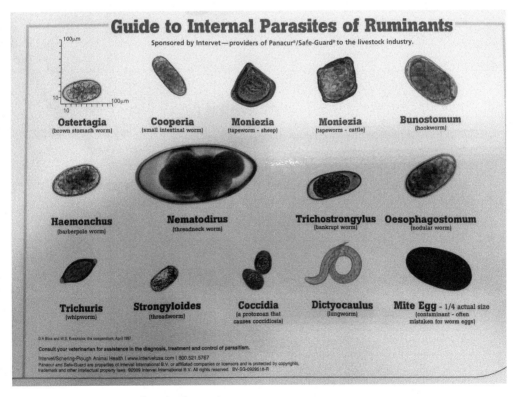

FIGURE 7.24 Worm egg color atlas for ruminants.

information on total numbers of worm eggs shed per pound of feces which determines the rate by which an animal is recontaminating its environment (see Figures 7.25 and 7.26). The Fecal Exam is a simple and effective way to check whether an animal is infected with gastro-intestinal parasites or whether parasite control has been successful is to conduct a fecal worm egg count analysis. Adult parasites living in the gastrointestinal tract lay eggs which pass out of the animals in the feces. Fecal worm egg counts conducted using the "Modified Wisconsin Sugar Flotation Technique" simply floats the worm eggs out of the fecal material, so they can be found and identified under a microscope.

B. **The best way to determine whether a dewormer is effective to conduct a Fecal Worm Egg Reduction Test (FECRT).** This test is accomplished by conducting a fecal exam before treatment and again 10 days following dewormer administration. Percent reduction in fecal worm egg counts due to treatment is calculated by subtracting the post-treatment egg count from the pre-treatment egg count divided by the pre-treatment egg count. If the percent reduction is not 90% or greater, "parasite resistance" is a possibility and the animals in question should be monitored regularly to make sure products used are working properly. Conducting a single fecal exam following treatment is also effective but knowing the level of egg shedding prior to treatment helps determine whether or not a dewormer is effective in the treated animal. Efficacy calculations are conducted by taking the pre-treatment count minus

FIGURE 7.25   Small ruminant parasite evaluation form.

Alpaca/Llama Parasite Evaluation Form

PEC ☐   Mail In ☐   Page____ of____

Collection Date: _____   Consultant: _____ Dr. Don Bliss _____

Name of Farm: _____   Sponsor: _____

Producer's Name: _____   Sponsor Contact: _____

Producer's Address: _____   Sponsor Address: _____

City _____ Phone _____   City _____ Phone _____

State _____ Zip _____ Fax _____   State _____ Zip _____ Fax _____

E-Mail: _____   Representative: _____

Lab ID	Animal ID (If testing specific animals please number sample bags in consecutive order)	Stomach Worm (Haemonchus)	Nematodirus	Cooperia	Hookworm	Threadworm	Whipworm	Tapeworm*	E. mac*	Coccidia*	Total Count (EPG)	Treatment Date month/day/year	Product Used
												Enter after test results recorded	

COMMENTS:

Donald H. Bliss, Ph.D.
MidAmerica Ag. Research
3705 Sequoia Trail
Verona, WI 53593

*(+ = 1-10) (++ = 11-50) (+++ =>51)
*Not reported in total egg count

Sponsor's E-mail:

For additional information and submission forms, visit: www.midamericaagresearch.net

FIGURE 7.26   Camelid parasite evaluation form.

the post-treatment count divided by the pre-treatment count. To be effective, the final calculations should show an efficacy value of 90% or greater.

C. **Taking Fecal worm egg counts should be an important part of the standard procedure for all small ruminant operations.** Monitoring fecals should be conducted at least semiannually to monitor treatment progress. One of the best time to take samples is during the winter months to make sure the animals are parasite-free when environmental contamination is at its lowest point and to make sure the animals are not recontaminating their environment immediately when grazing returns. The second best time to take fecals is in late summer or early fall in order to monitor whether the annual treatment program is successful. If average worm egg counts taken in late fall are greater than 100 eggs/3 g sample, adjustment in the treatment program should be made.

The Modified Wisconsin Sugar Fecal Exam: A 1-g fecal sample is mixed with a saturated sugar solution designed to float the eggs out of the fecal matter. The samples are strained to remove large debris, then poured into a 15 ml taper test tube, and centrifuged at a low RPM (<1000) for five minutes which increases the egg recover rate by a significant amount. After centrifuging, a few drops of sugar are added to form a meniscus on top of the tube. A cover slip is placed on the top of the tube for two minutes, removed, and examined under the microscope at 40× magnification. Eggs are identified to type and counted.

The collection process is conducted using a sealable bag or baggie, invert the bag like a glove, and pick up freshly dropped fecal material the size of a golf ball from each animal to check for parasites. Keep each individual sample separate. Seal each bag and write on the bag to identify the horse and date of collection. Keep samples cool after collection since heat causes the eggs to hatc and freezing distorts the eggs.

INTERPRETATION OF FECAL WORM EGG COUNTS IN SMALL RUMINANTS USING THE MODIFIED WISCONSIN SUGAR FLOTATION TECHNIQUE

Understanding the meaning of worm egg counts will provide veterinarians the necessary insight needed to help clients build a deworming strategy for a particular operation or operations. Factors that affect fecal worm egg shedding are numerous, so a number of these factors need to be considered every time an analysis is made and a fair assessment of the worm egg counts generated. The age of the animal, the season of the year, the amount of exposure to pasture, and the stocking rate of the animals on pasture all affect worm egg counts. The amount of rainfall or moisture on the pasture and the number of degree days with temperatures sufficient to promote parasite development on pasture are also very important to future infections. These factors directly affect egg count interpretation as infection levels build on the pasture and ingestion of these larvae increases and worm burdens rise in the animals themselves. Furthermore, the health of the animals, the stage of gestation, stage of lactation, and the numbers and type of parasites present at each examination must be considered. Post-lambing worm egg counts, for example, are almost always higher than pre-lambing counts.

The five most common types of internal nematode parasites in sheep and goats that are routinely diagnosed present in fecal exams are: Stomach worms (primarily the barber's pole worm – *Haemonchus* sp.), intestinal worms (*Cooperia* sp.), threadworms (*Strongyloides* sp.), whipworms (*Trichuris* sp.), and nodular worms (Oesophagostomum sp.). All eggs are counted and included in the worm egg count total, except for tapeworms and coccidia. Tapeworms and coccidia are commonly found but are listed on the worm egg count forms simply as positive at a low level (+) 1–10 eggs, medium level (++) 11–50 eggs, or high level (+++) 50 eggs or greater.

1 egg/g equals 454 eggs/lb of manure, i.e., a count of 500 equals 227,000 eggs/lb of feces, so 5.0 lb of feces per day would yield 1,135,000 eggs per day on the pasture per animal.

QUICK ASSESSMENT FOR SHEEP, GOATS, AND CAMELIDS BASED ON FECAL WORM EGG COUNTS

	Eggs/g Count	Estimated Parasite Level
Nematode egg counts	1–10 eggs	Low
Recorded on sheets	11–50 eggs	Moderate
	50+ eggs	High*
	300+ eggs	Very high*

*At this level, it appears that parasites begin to stop developing and undergo inhibition in tissues.

Positive worm egg counts for sheep and goats (other than very high counts) for the most part only indicate the presence or absence of parasites within a particular animal. It is impossible to determine how many parasites are present at any given time primarily because *Haemonchus* undergoes a phenomenon called inhibition or period of arrested development. This parasitic stage remains in the tissues for long periods of time and follow an annual development and inhibition cycle. The primary inhibition period begins about 45–60 days into a grazing period as the parasite contamination level on pastures buildup. These inhibited larvae can stage in the tissues through the beginning of the following grazing season.

The overall infection process begins when an infected animal grazes a pasture and sheds worm eggs on a daily basis that pass in the manure. These eggs hatch and the larval offspring develop into infective larvae which recontaminates the pasture thus exposing all animal grazing this pasture to new infections. If the pasture is already contaminated with infective larvae, the animals pick up new infections at the same time they shed eggs back on the pasture contributing future contamination levels. This process continues until the grazing season ends. Depending upon temperature and moisture these parasite eggs hatch, develop into infective larvae, and move away from the manure pats onto the vegetation where the reinfection process begins. The biggest and least understood issue with sheep and goats is that once *Haemonchus* infections reach a high level, the physiology of the gut changes. The parasites respond by stopping their development undergoing an arrested development period waiting for the physiology of the gut to return to normal. This why the simple guide (listed above) to predict parasite levels within an animal based on worm egg counts can be misleading.

The time of the year when the assessment is made can also have an impact on worm eggs as follows:

1. **Winter:** As winter progresses, animals are no longer ingesting infective larvae off pasture, existing worm burdens begin to mature and die off as they age, conditions in the gut then start to return to normal which, in turn, triggers inhibited parasites to become active. If counts come back following treatment, this means inhibited are present or if worm egg counts are high during the winter, these counts indicate that heavy worm challenge existed from the previous season.

2. **Spring:** When inhibited larvae are being released from the gastric glands, egg shedding can reach a high level which indicates the presence of high worm burdens carried over from the previous season. High egg shedding levels at this time is dangerous because egg shedding in the spring determine contamination levels for the rest of the year.

3. **Summer:** Once animals are on pasture and grazing begins, worm counts will begin to rise within three weeks. Once egg counts exceed 100 eggs/g (45,400/lb of manure), worm burdens have reached a point when incoming larvae undergo arrested development and become inhibited larvae in the gastric glands of the abomasum.

4. **Fall:** The quick assessment chart (listed above) is most accurate in the fall at the end of the grazing season. Low counts indicate successful control of worm burdens while high counts indicate economic loss may be occurring and trouble controlling these infections due to inhibited worm burdens may be occurring.

GASTROINTESTINAL AND LUNG PARASITE INFECTIONS FOUND IN SMALL RUMINANTS

Parasitism in small ruminants can be broken into three main categories: *Stomach worms, Intestinal worms,* and *Protozoa.* From a microscope standpoint, samples are scanned for worm eggs and then identified by shape and size, then counted and reported as eggs per gram of material used.

The following is an egg chart used to identify the species of worm the eggs are from:

STOMACH WORMS

Barber's pole worm (*H. contortus*) is a blood-sucking parasite that completes it life cycle from eggs passed in the manure, hatch and molt three times in the environment to become an infective L_3 larva which is infectious if eaten by sheep, goats, camelids, and camels. This parasite is a very economically damaging parasite in small ruminants but is especially damaging in sheep and goats becoming one of the most important causes of death in these animals. Larval stages have been found in the rumen and abomasal tissues and are extremely hard to kill. Eggs are easily identified in a fecal exam (see Figures 7.27–7.33).

Ostertagia (Brown Stomach Worm) is probably the most studied and most prevalent parasite of cattle but not so much for small ruminants. Larval stages invade and destroy the gastric glands. Large numbers of parasites can significantly reduce digestion efficiency. Larval stages can

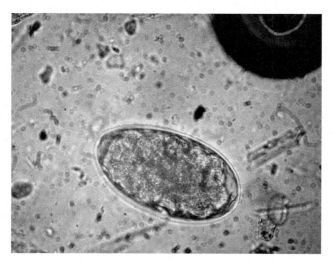

FIGURE 7.27   *Haemonchus* egg from a goat (40×).

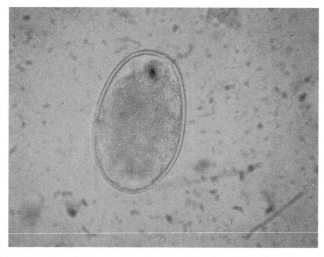

FIGURE 7.28   *Haemonchus* egg from an alpaca (40×).

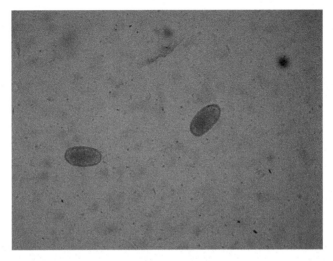

FIGURE 7.29   *Haemonchus longistipes* (camel) eggs (10×).

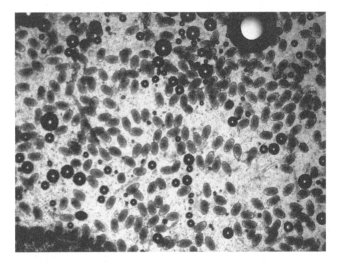

FIGURE 7.30   *Haemonchus* heavy shedding in sheep (4×).

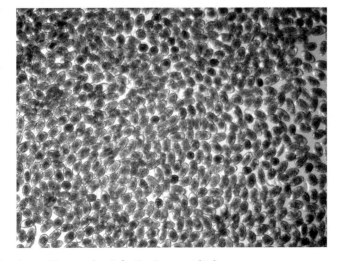

FIGURE 7.31   Very heavy *Haemonchus* infection in a goat (4×).

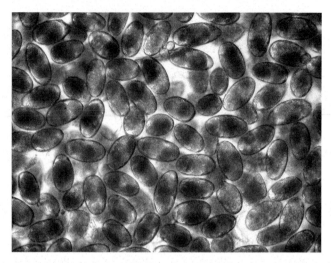

FIGURE 7.32   Very heavy *Haemonchus* (10×) infection in a goat.

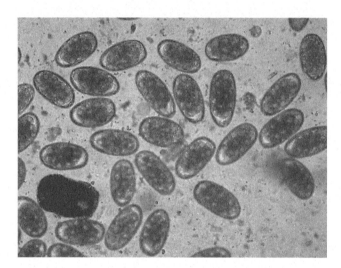

FIGURE 7.33   High number of *Haemonchus* eggs in sheep (10×).

undergo inhibition and remain in the glands for months before emerging into the lumen of the abomasum to develop into an adult worm. *Ostertagia* eggs are easily identified in a fecal exam since they are smaller than *Haemonchus* eggs (see Figures 7.34 and 7.35).

Trichostrongylus axei and *Trichostrongylus colubriformis* (bankrupt worm) are most often seen with *Haemonchus* infections. Most commonly occurs in the abomasum but also found in the upper part of the small intestine. These worms are associated with a chronic wasting disease when present in large numbers. Eggs are of similar size to Haemonchus but slightly bean shaped with clear area on each end of the egg (see Figures 7.36 and 7.37).

INTESTINAL NEMATODE PARASITES

Cooper's worm (*Cooperia curticei*) does not seem to be an important parasite of sheep as it is of cattle and bison. Cooperia disrupts digestive functions of the intestine and produces a strong immune reaction. This parasite is not as prevalent in small ruminants as in cattle. Eggs are easily found in a fecal exam and are distinct because of elongated parallel sides (see Figures 7.38 and 7.39).

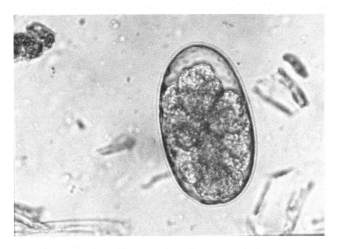

FIGURE 7.34   *Ostertagia* egg (40×).

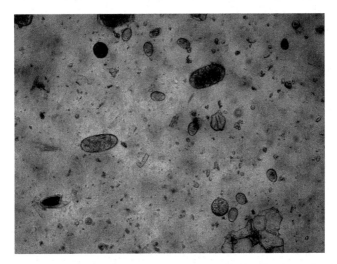

FIGURE 7.35   *Ostertagia* (smaller egg) and *Haemonchus* eggs with coccidia oocysts (10×).

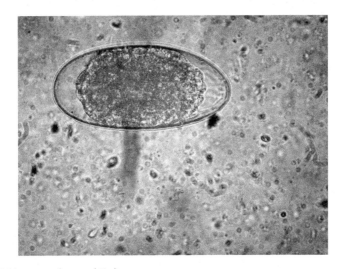

FIGURE 7.36   *Trichostrongylus* egg (40×).

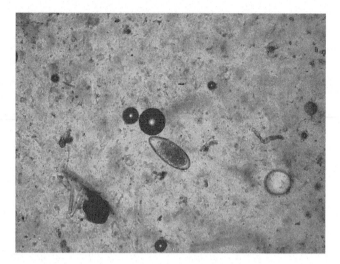

FIGURE 7.37   *Trichostrongylus* egg (10×).

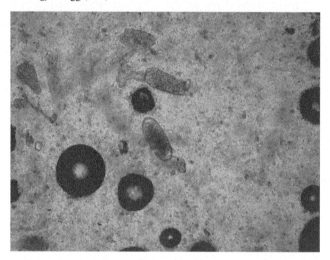

FIGURE 7.38   *Cooperia* spp. egg (10×).

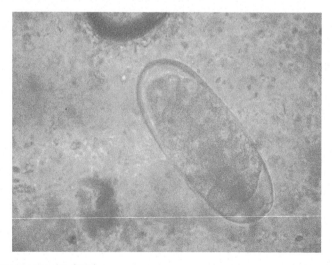

FIGURE 7.39   *Cooperia* spp. egg (40×).

Threadneck worm (*Nematodirus spathiger, Nematodirus filicollis*, and *Nematodirus battus*) is most commonly found in young animals. Larvae survive well in cold weather and can live for two years on pasture. This parasite is a common cause of diarrhea and oftentimes death in young and old small ruminants. Because it is very pathogenic, older animals acquired a strong immunity against this parasite. The egg is very large and is easily identified in a fecal exam (see Figures 7.40–7.43).

Threadworm (*Strongyloides papillosus*) infection is by skin penetration, by ingestion through mother's milk or through contaminated feed or bedding. Transmission is seldom found through grazing or pasture contamination. Threadworms can very harmful to baby lambs and kids but usually self-eliminate by two to three months of age. *Strongyloides* intact worms can be found in fecal samples as well as just in eggs (see Figures 7.44 and 7.45). *Strongyloides* infection

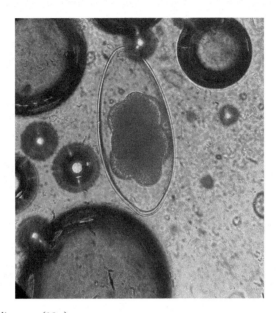

FIGURE 7.40   *Nematodirus* egg (10×).

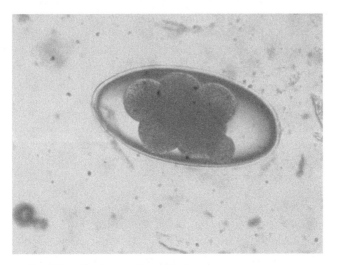

FIGURE 7.41   *Nematodirus* (threadneck worm) egg (40×).

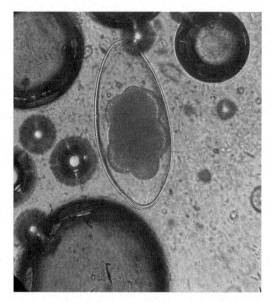

FIGURE 7.42   *Nematodirus* (40×) (goat).

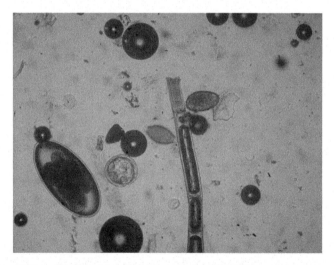

FIGURE 7.43   *Nematodirus, Haemonchus,* and whipworm eggs (camel).

is easily identified upon fecal exam by the presence of small thin-shelled embroynated eggs (see Figures 7.46 and 7.47).

   Whipworm (*Trichuris ovis*) lives in the cecum and is the organ that joins the small and large intestine. *Trichuris* is another very damaging parasite in young animals. Oftentimes symptoms are confused with coccidiosis because of the bloody diarrhea associated with this parasite. Several 100 worms can kill a young animal. The egg is very characteristic and looks like a football with polar caps on each end (see Figures 7.48–7.51). The female worm is not prolific and eggs are often missed in the fecal exam unless carefully conducted. The *Trichuris* egg remains in the egg until infective and can live 20–25 years in the soil. Cattle held in barnyards often become infected with *Trichuris*.

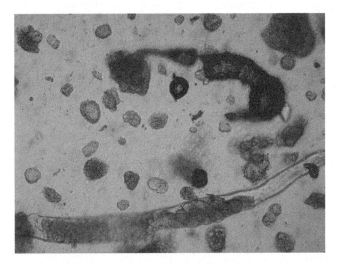

FIGURE 7.44   Gravid threadworm (*Strongyloides*) in fecal sample.

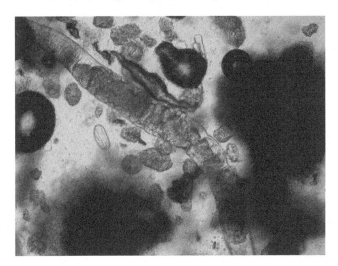

FIGURE 7.45   Gravid female threadworm (*Strongyloides*) plus *Strongyloides* egg in fecal sample.

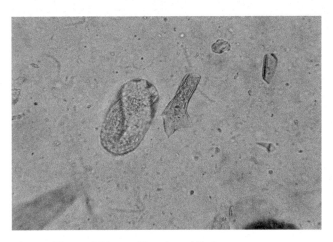

FIGURE 7.46   Threadworm (*Strongyloides papillosus*) egg (40×).

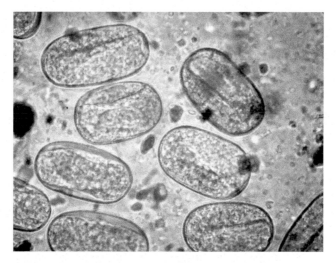

FIGURE 7.47 Heavy threadworm (*Strongyloides*) eggs found from dead calf (10×).

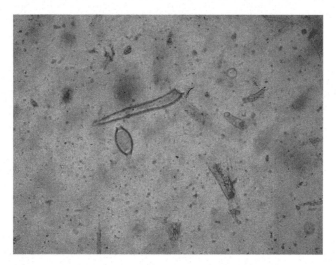

FIGURE 7.48 Whipworm found in Alpaca.

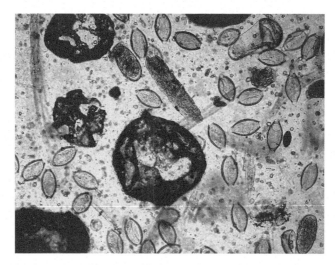

FIGURE 7.49 Heavy whipworm (*Trichuris*) infection.

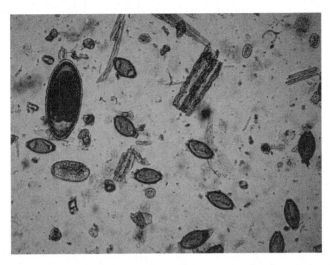

FIGURE 7.50   Heavy whipworm infection with *Nematodirus, Haemonchus* threadworm (upper left) eggs.

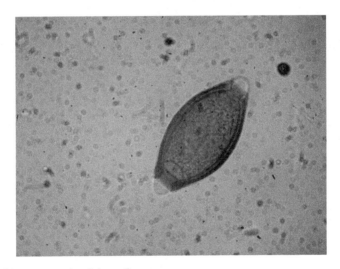

FIGURE 7.51   Whipworm egg (40×) (camel).

Capillaria (*Capillaria brevipes, Capillaria bovis*) infections in sheep and goats are of no veterinary importance and, therefore, its observance is only a simple matter of record. Capillaria are very thin filamentous worms and cannot be seen grossly in the gut contents. Capillaria eggs are similar to Whipworm eggs except they are smaller with non-protruding polar caps (see Figures 7.52–7.55).

Hookworm (*Bunostomum trigonocephalum*) occurs both in sheep and goats. Infections can occur by ingesting infective larvae or by skin penetration. If infection is through the skin, hookworm larvae pass through the lungs before being coughed up passing back to the small intestine where they attach to the intestinal wall, mate, and begin laying eggs back into the environment. Hookworm eggs are very large eggs (2× the size of Haemonchus) and show an 8-cell developmental stage with a thick rectangular-shaped cell wall (see Figures 7.56 and 7.57).

Skrjabinema ovis is a relatively unknown parasite but shows up occasionally, especially on the East Coast of the United States. No special studies have been made on the life cycle of the genus but no different pathogenesis attributable to *Skrjabinema* has been observed. It seems to be closely relative to the egg characteristics like those of pinworms in the horse (see Figures 7.58–7.60).

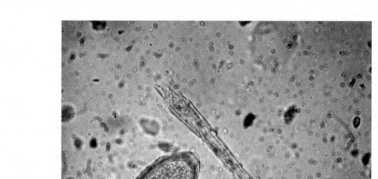

FIGURE 7.52   *Capillaria* egg (10×).

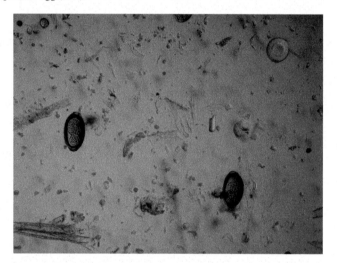

FIGURE 7.53   *Capillaria* eggs (4×).

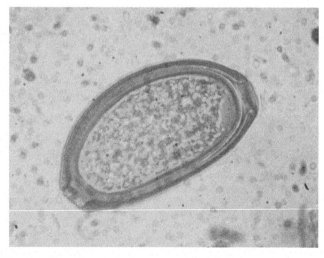

FIGURE 7.54   *Capillaria* egg (40×).

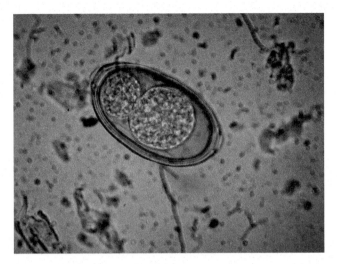

FIGURE 7.55   *Capillaria* spp. (40×).

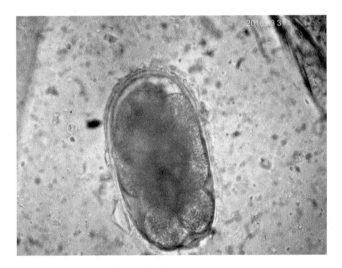

FIGURE 7.56   Hookworm (*Bunostomum*) eggs (40×).

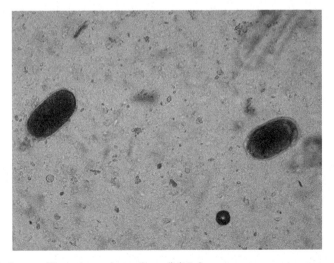

FIGURE 7.57   Hookworm (*Bunostomum*) eggs (camel) (10×).

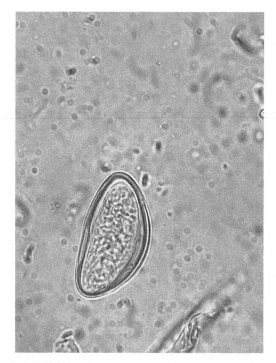

FIGURE 7.58   *Skrjabinema ovis* (40×).

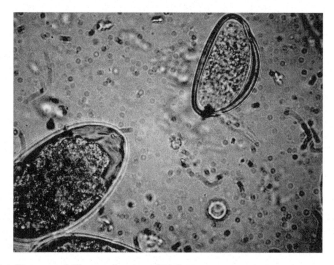

FIGURE 7.59   *Skrjabinema* and *Haemonchus* eggs (40×).

Nodular worm (*Oesophagostomum venulosum* and *Oesophagostomum columbianum*) is becoming more important in recent years because intestines are often condemned at slaughter if nodules caused by the nodular worms are found in large numbers. Parasites are associated with anorexia, depressed weight gain, and diarrhea. Most commonly found in adult animals. Nodular worm eggs are large eggs similar to Hookworm except they are usually in a 16–32 cell stage and oval-shaped eggs more similar to Haemonchus but a much larger egg (see Figures 7.61–7.63).

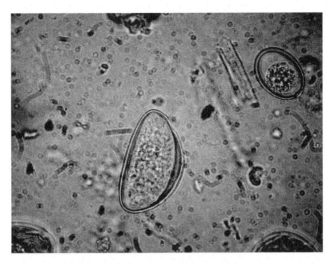

FIGURE 7.60   *Skrjabinema ovis* plus coccidia oocyst (40×).

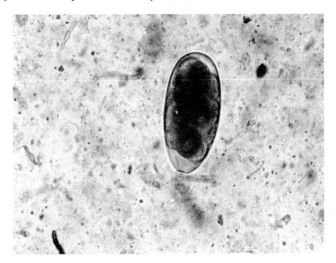

FIGURE 7.61   Nodular worm (*Oesophagostomum*) egg (40×).

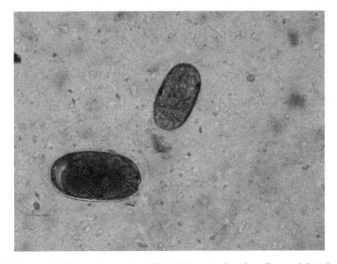

FIGURE 7.62   Nodular worm (*Oesophagostomum*) and *Haemonchus* (smaller egg) (10×).

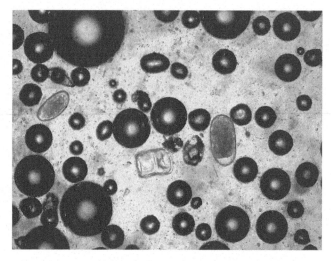

FIGURE 7.63   Nodular worm (larger egg), tapeworm, and *Haemonchus* eggs (10×).

INTESTINAL CESTODE (TAPEWORM) PARASITES (*MONIEZIA EXPANSA AND MONIEZIA BENEDENI*)

The small ruminant tapeworm develops in the soil mite, which is ingested by small ruminants. The development time to reach an adult after ingestion is reported to be from six to eight weeks. The adult tapeworm lives in the small intestine and can grow to be 1 in. wide and 6 ft long. They absorb nutrition through their cuticle. In high numbers, tapeworms can block the intestine. Tapeworm eggs are distinct and easily picked up in a fecal exam (see Figures 7.64–7.69).

TREMATODES PARASITES (LIVER FLUKES)

***Fascioloides magna* (deer fluke) and *Fasciola hepatica* (common fluke).** *Fascioloides magna* found in the Great Lakes region is relatively untreatable in sheep because it is so pathogenic. Diagnosis can only be done accurately upon necropsy since the larval stages migrate in the liver

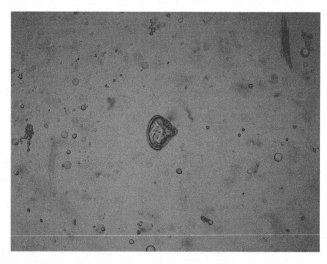

FIGURE 7.64   Tapeworm (*Moniezia benedeni*) egg (10×).

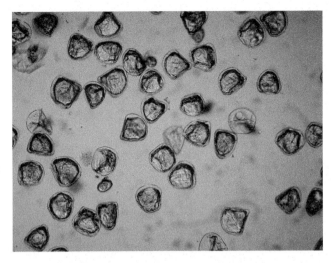

FIGURE 7.65   Tapeworm eggs with a coccidia oocyst in goats (10×).

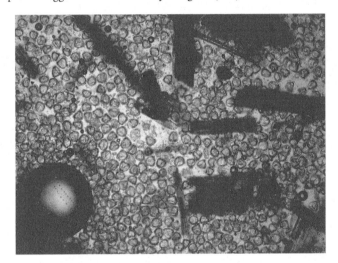

FIGURE 7.66   Heavy tapeworm (*Moniezia*) infection (4×).

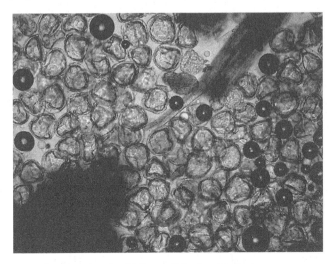

FIGURE 7.67   Tapeworm (*Moniezia*) eggs with heavy infection (10×).

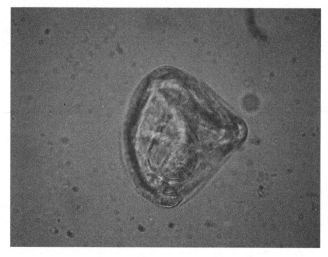

FIGURE 7.68   Tapeworm (*Moniezia benedeni*) egg (40×).

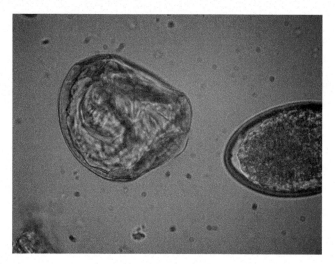

FIGURE 7.69   Tapeworm (*Moniezia*) and *Haemonchus* eggs (40×).

until it is destroyed. In cattle, the young flukes are eventually walled off and contained in the liver, where as in sheep, the young flukes continue to migrate throughout the liver until it is completely destroyed and the animals succumb. Keeping small ruminants away from wet areas and streams where deer congregate is currently the only method of control. One fluke egg which hatches is all that is needed to kill one sheep. *Fasciola hepatica* is rarely found in sheep but egg is easily recoverable and identifiable (see Figure 7.70).

  ***Dicrocoelium dendriticum* (lancet fluke)** is found mostly in the Northern Part of the country but can occur almost anywhere. The lancet fluke has a terrestrial life cycle involving two intermediate hosts including snails and ants. Once ingested by grazing sheep, the metecercariae from the ants when eaten by the sheep move to the liver where they mature to adult flukes. The Lancet fluke is considered to be relatively harmless to infected animals. This fluke egg is easy to identify with a singular polar cap on one end of the egg (see Figures 7.71 and 7.72).

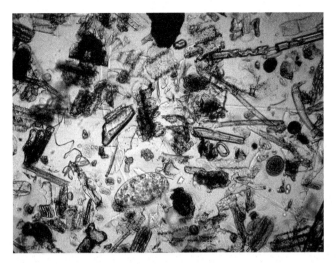

FIGURE 7.70   Fluke (*Fasciola hepatic*) egg (10×).

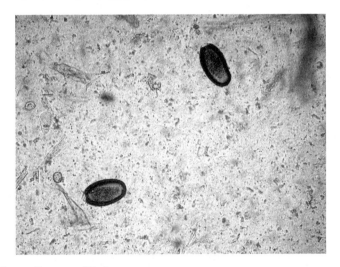

FIGURE 7.71   Dicrocoelium eggs (10×).

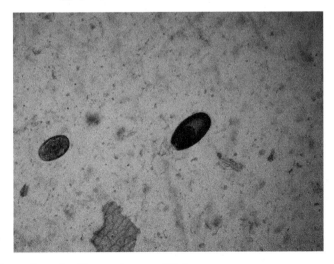

FIGURE 7.72   *Dicrocoelium* plus *Haemonchus* eggs (10×).

PROTOZOAN PARASITES OF SMALL RUMINANTS

Coccidia are single-celled protozoan parasites that all small ruminants are believed to be exposed to sometime in their life. Coccidia are very host-specific such that coccidia of swine, dogs, and chickens would not infect small ruminants. The reverse is also true. Coccidia are ingested through fecal-contaminated feedstuff. Wet muddy conditions usually increase infection levels (see Figure 7.73). Camelids do have a special pathogenic parasite not seen in other small ruminants called E. mac. (Eimeria Macusaniensis) (see Figures 7.74 and 7.75). Coccidia is a known pathogen that is opportunistic and thrives when the animal's immune system is under attack, for example, with high *Haemonchus* worm burden in the abomasum. In deworming a heavily infected animal that also shows a high coccidia count, the coccidia counts most often drop to a low level soon after the deworming is complete. It appears that once the worm burden is removed, the animal's immune system can suppress coccidian development. Some parasites like Stongyloides and coccidia are fairly common seen together (see Figure 7.76). Both of these parasites tend to favor the young with weak immune systems. It is very common to see a number of different coccidia species under one field (see Figures 7.77–7.79). Many times, however, we find heavy shedding of a single species of coccidia (see Figure 7.80).

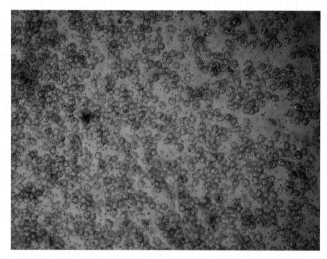

FIGURE 7.73   Heavy coccidia count from goats (10×).

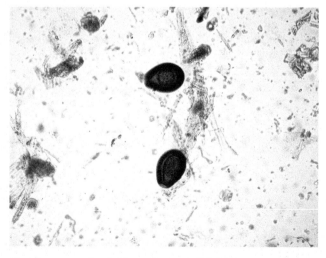

FIGURE 7.74   Two *Eimeria macusaniensis* (E. mac.) oocysts (10×).

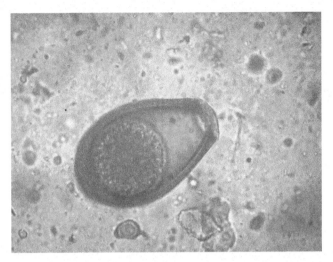

FIGURE 7.75 *Eimeria macusaniensis* (E. mac.) oocyst – Alpaca (40×).

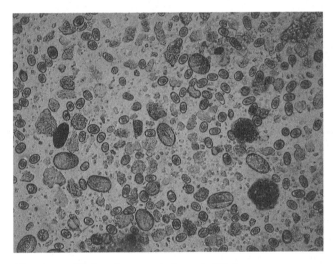

FIGURE 7.76 Coccidia oocyst with threadworm eggs in goats (10×).

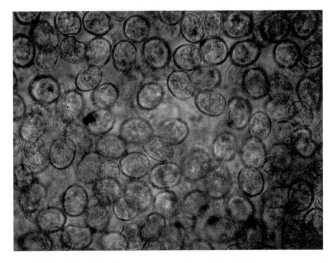

FIGURE 7.77 Heavy coccidia count (10×).

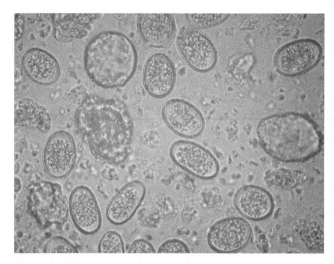

FIGURE 7.78   Coccidia oocysts in sheep (40×).

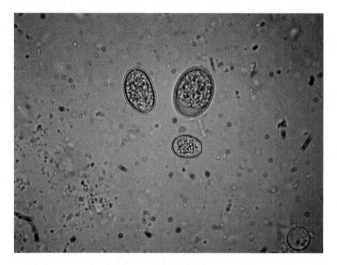

FIGURE 7.79   Three different coccidia species in sheep (40×).

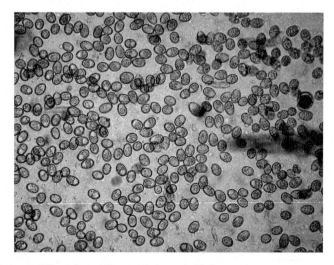

FIGURE 7.80   Heavy shedding of coccidia oocysts in goats (4×).

REFERENCES

1. Campbell, W.C. and Todd, A.C. (1954). Natural infections of *Fascioloides magna* infections in Wisconsin sheep. *J. Parasitol.* 40 (1): 94–100.

2. Thomas, R.J. (1973). Ovine parasitic gastroenteritis: epidemiology and control in hill sheep. Epidemiology and control in Lowground sheep. In: *Helminth Diseases of Cattle, Sheep and Horses in Europe* (ed. G.M. Urquhart and J. Amour), 411–449. Glasgow: Maclehose.

3. Shubber, A.H., Lloyd, S., and Soulsby, E.J. (1981). Infections with gastrointestinal helminths. Effect of lactation and maternal transfer of immunity. *Z. Parasitenk* 65: 181–189.

4. Clark, C.H., Kisel, G.K., and Goby, C.H. (1962). Measurements of blood loss caused by *Haemonchus contortus* infections in sheep. *Am. J. Vet. Res.* 23: 977–980.

5. Zajac, A.M. and Garza, J. (2019). Biology, epidemiology, and control of gastrointestinal nematodes of small ruminants. *Vet. Clin. North Am. Food Anim. Pract.* 36 (1): 73–87.

6. Wray, E.M., Tucker, C., and Powell, J. (2022). *Managing Haemonchus in Sheep and Goats.* Agriculture and Natural Resources, University of Arkansas Research and Extension.

7. Anderson, D.E. (2013). *"Brain Worm" (Meningeal Worm) Infestation in Llamas and Alpacas.* College of Veterinary Medicine, University of Tennessee, Tech Bulletin.

8. Pugh, D.G. (1995). Clinical paraelaphostrongylosis in llamas. *Compend. Cont. Ed. Pract. Vet.* 17: 600–606.

9. Malan, F.S., Van Wyk, J.A., and Wessels, C.D. (2001). Clinical evaluation of anemia in sheep: early trials. *Onderstepoort J. Vet. Res.* 68: 165–174.

10. Kaplan, R.M., Burke, J.M., and Terril, T.H. (2004). Validation of the FAMACH eye colour chart for detecting clinical anaemia in sheep and goats on farms in the southern states. *Vet. Parasitol.* 123 (1–2): 105–120.

11. Van Wyk, J.A. and Bath, G.F. (2002). The FACHAMA system for managing Haemonchosis in sheep and goats by clinically identifying individual animals for treatment. *Vet. Res.* 33: 509–529.

Parasites of Hoofed Wildlife CHAPTER 8

Parasitologists have long studied internal parasitic infections in the various hoofed wildlife species and have documented the existence of a wide variety of parasitic organisms. Parasites in hoofed wildlife are especially diverse and abundant. Among wild ruminants, 54 different species of worm parasites have been identified from the abomasum, 28 species from the small intestine, and 6 different species from the large intestine [1, 2]. The major internal parasites of hoofed wildlife are divided into four distinct groups: *nematodes* (stomach, intestinal, and lungworms), *cestodes* (tapeworms), *trematodes* (liver flukes), and *protozoa* (coccidian and giardia). The gastrointestinal parasitic *nematodes* are the primary concern for this discussion and have a characteristic life cycle similar to gastrointestinal parasites of cattle and small ruminants (see Figure 8.1). Hoofed wildlife become infected from ingesting infective larvae that were deposited as worm eggs in the feces of infected hoofed wildlife that deposited these eggs in the environment where they themselves or other deer might graze. Often, areas near a source of water is usually a prime contamination spot for hoofed wildlife to become infected (see Figure 8.2).

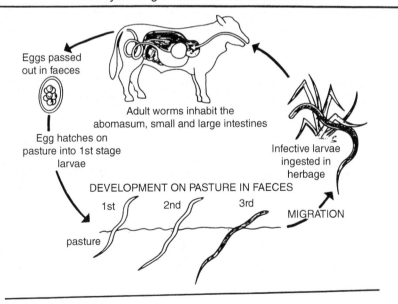

Life cycle of gut roundworms in ruminants

Eggs passed out in faeces

Adult worms inhabit the abomasum, small and large intestines

Egg hatches on pasture into 1st stage larvae

Infective larvae ingested in herbage

DEVELOPMENT ON PASTURE IN FAECES

1st   2nd   3rd   MIGRATION

pasture

FIGURE 8.1 Typical life cycle of gastrointestinal parasites in hoofed wildlife.

Large Animal Parasitology Procedures for Veterinary Technicians, First Edition. Donald H. Bliss.
© 2024 John Wiley & Sons, Inc. Published 2024 by John Wiley & Sons, Inc.

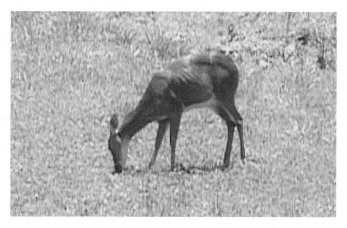

FIGURE 8.2   Deer grazing (where parasitic larvae are most likely to exist and are waiting to be consumed).

Treatment programs for deer and elk breeding farms are different than treatment under natural field conditions. Concentration of animals on breeding farms dramatically increases parasite transmission and associated problems with high parasite loads in pastured ruminants (see Figure 8.3).

A guideline for treatment falls under small ruminant (Chapter 7). A strategic deworming protocol using Safe-Guard® for the seasonal control of gastrointestinal parasites in traditional grazed breeding farms for deer and elk as developed for use in sheep and goats. This is a unique protocol designed with strategically timed dewormings both to reduce parasitism in the animals themselves (especially encysted *Haemonchus*) as well as in the animal's environment for an entire grazing season. It has been tested under field conditions at a number of locations across the country. Fecal monitoring is highly recommended.

1. **Fall deworming regime:** At the end of the grazing season (preferably after a hard frost), feed Safe-Guard pellets or flaked meal during morning feed at the rate of 1.0 lb per 750 lb of body weight (Safe-Guard 0.5%) or 4 oz per 750 lb body weight (Safe-Guard 1.96%). Spread

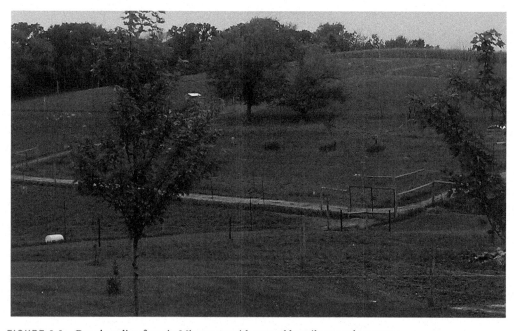

FIGURE 8.3   Deer breeding farm in Minnesota with several heavily grazed pastures.

total dose over three days. On the fourth day, give Cydectin® (moxidectin) pour-on at the rate of 1 cc/20 lb or liquid sheep drench at the rate of 2.5× recommended dose. *Note*: Multiple days of Safe-Guard activates encysted larvae which are then killed by Cydectin. For animals that are severely debilitated or heavily pregnant, ivermectin can be substituted for moxidectin.

2. **Winter deworming:** Conduct a fecal exam in late February to early March. If positive: repeat fall treatment regime to make sure animals are not shedding worm eggs at the beginning of the grazing season. Deworming wildlife, so they are worm-free during winter months, removes gastrointestinal parasites as additional source of danger to these animals when nutrition maybe lacking and severe weather maybe threatening (see Figure 8.4). Being parasite-free during the birthing process can also be extremely beneficial for the nutritional health of the mom and also for possible increased milk production for the baby (see Figure 8.5).

3. **Spring–early summer strategic timed dewormings (see** Figure 8.6**):** Begin treatment three weeks after turn-out or three weeks after first spring grass growth:
    first deworming = three-day Safe-Guard protocol given three weeks after beginning of grazing season.
    second deworming = three-day Safe-Guard protocol given three weeks after the first treatment.
    third deworming = three-day Safe-Guard protocol (plus Cydectin drench or given orally on the fourth day) given three weeks after the second treatment.

4. **Fall deworming:** Repeat fall program listed above as "Fall deworming regime":*

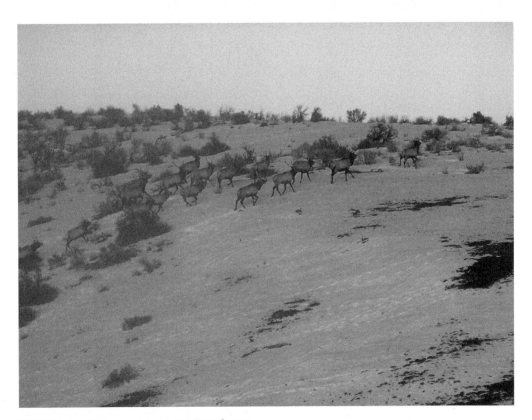

FIGURE 8.4   Elk herd surviving on winter forage.

---

* Safe-Guard (fenbendazole) is a product of Merck Animal Health. Cydectin is a product of Bayer Animal Health. Ivermectin is a generic endecticide available through a number of companies.

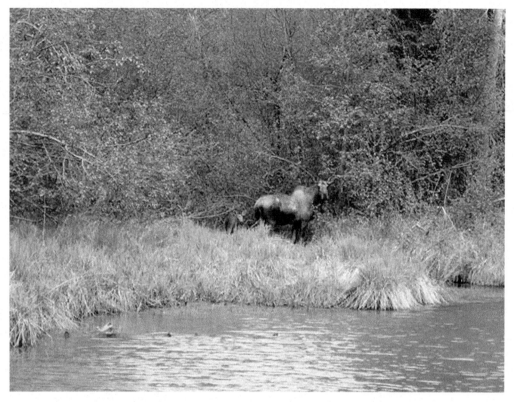

FIGURE 8.5   Moose with baby with plenty of summer forage.

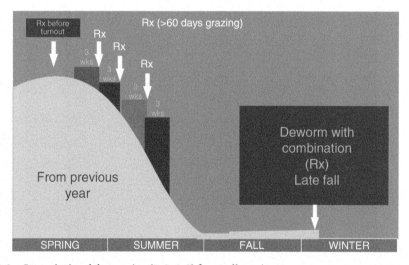

FIGURE 8.6   Strategic timed deworming (0–3–6–9) for small ruminants.

GASTROINTESTINAL NEMATODE PARASITES ARE IMPORTANT TO WILDLIFE

Parasites cause a multitude of problems for wildlife and although it often appears that wildlife have adapted to the presence of parasites, they have not adapted to the adverse effects of parasitism. Parasites have been shown to exist in wildlife both as a clinical and subclinical condition. Clinical parasitism is a condition where parasite numbers have reached a point that the negative effects of parasitism are visible with the naked eye. Animals with stunted horn growth and poor body condition are examples of problems due to clinical parasitism. Subclinical effects are harder to see and to measure (i.e., reduced growth rates, reduced reproductive rates, reduced milk production for the young, and a reduced ability of the infected animal's immune system to fight off other disease conditions). A remarkable difference is seen once the parasites are removed.

Research in wild ruminants has demonstrated that high worm burdens reduce forage intake with reduced feed efficiency and decreasing growth rates. Gastrointestinal parasites can also exacerbate the effects of malnutrition and food availability during periods of drought or severe winters. The synergism of food shortage and immuno-suppression by the parasites may result in pathogenic infections often resulting in death.

PARASITE LIFE CYCLES

Primarily, gastrointestinal nematode parasites of hoofed wildlife have a direct life cycle. The adult parasite lives in the gastrointestinal tract of the animal, lays eggs that pass out in the feces, the eggs then embryonate into infective larvae which reinfects the animals as they graze. The larval stage, to become infective, must undergo several molts before developing into an infective (L_3) larva. Once infective, these L_3 larvae are very mobile following moisture trails from the fecal pellets onto the vegetation in order to reinfect the wildlife. The key transmission times are in early morning or late evening when dew is on the vegetation and the animals are grazing.

Parasite development outside the animals is seasonal. The development of the egg and larvae only takes place during the time of the year when weather conditions are warm and moisture is present. Once the larvae reach the infective L_3 stage, these organisms can live from one to several years in the environment. The L_3 larvae as well as eggs are fairly weather resistant and can survive severe weather such as hot dry summers or freezing winter conditions.

TRANSMISSION OF PARASITES

In most parts of the country, parasite development and transmission to the animals takes place from early spring to late fall. As a general rule, when conditions are right for vegetation growth, conditions are also right for parasite development. Parasitic larvae that survive the winter become active in early spring as temperatures warm up and move onto the vegetation where they are consumed by grazing wildlife. Successful transmission depends on widespread parasite contamination of the environment. A key place for transmission to occur is around areas where wildlife find sources of water since moisture is important in parasite development and for movement onto the vegetation. Also, creeks, ponds, and other watering areas are often where wildlife congregate and parasite contamination is at a higher level compared to wide-open areas.

A dynamic link occurs between animal population density and parasite density. The greater the number of wildlife that exists in a given area, the greater the chance for increased parasite contamination of the environment. Several studies from Louisiana show that food plots provide increased nutritional input but also increase animal population. This in turn increases parasite contamination of the area because of increased animal density.

The key to having food plots that increase nutritional supplementation for wildlife successfully is to make sure the parasite effect is controlled and the value of the plot is not diminished by the increased parasite challenge.

CONTROL OF PARASITES IN THE WILD

Multi-millions of dollars are spent every year on deworming products for domestic animals including food animals, companion animals, and pets for the control of parasitism. The reason is clear, because the highly improved efficacy and high degree of safety of dewormers have provided animal owners the tools to significantly improve the health and well-being of their animals through controlling and preventing parasitic infections. Controlling parasites in wildlife is much more difficult because of the inability to handle the animals for treatment. Zoos, wildlife parks, and wildlife held in captivity, on the other hand, are routinely dewormed. Deworming free roaming and range wildlife is only in its infancy.

DEWORMER FOR HOOFED WILDLIFE

One of the most universally used deworming compounds in the United States for domestic animals over the past 20 years is a highly efficacious product called fenbendazole (Safe-Guard/Panacur® – Merck) [3, 4]. Fenbendazole is now approved as a medicated pellet for hoofed wildlife at the recommended rate of 7.5 mg/kg (3.4 mg/lb) to be fed over a period of three to five days. .Where feed bunks or deer feeders are permitted, hoofed wildlife can be dewormed using fenbendazole in deer supplement or with (Safe-Guard – Merck Animal Health) medicated blocks (see Figures 8.7 and 8.8). Being able to get a dewormer into hoofed wildlife often shows amazing results (see Figures 8.9 and 8.10).

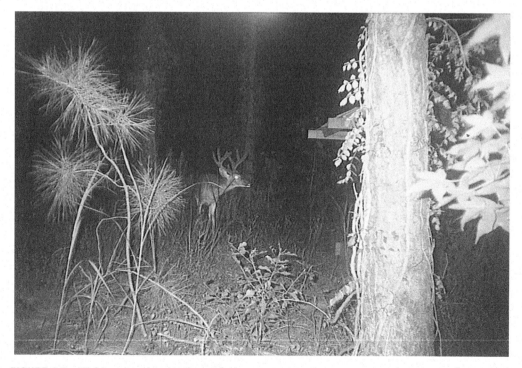

FIGURE 8.7   Night camera showing deer at feeder.

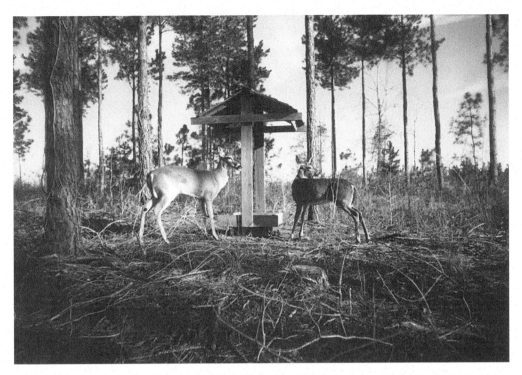

FIGURE 8.8   Deer at feeder where fenbendazole (Safe-Guard – Merck) can be administered free-choice with deer feed.

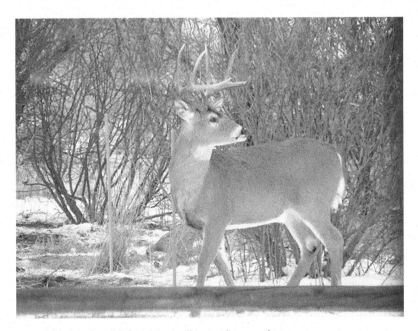

FIGURE 8.9   Healthy deer in wild showing excellent antler growth.

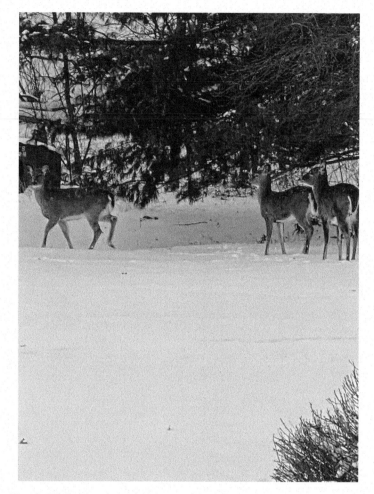

FIGURE 8.10   Deer in Wisconsin winter showing good health.

One of the most important characteristics of fenbendazole for wildlife is that it has a FDA safety rating of 100× which means one animal can consume 100 times the recommended dose with no noted adverse reaction. Since a dewormer is killing organisms living within another organism, having a product that can do this safely is paramount. Product safety is critical both for the target species and all other wildlife species such as wild turkeys, squirrels, and rodents that might consume the product incidentally.

Second, fenbendazole has a unique characteristic that allows a single dose to be fed over a varying period of time. This is also important because it is most often impossible to control or know when wildlife will visit a treatment area. Spreading the dose over an extended period of time ensures a large number of animals can receive their recommended dose. Fenbendazole is the only deworming product on the market with this FDA-approved label claim.

This cumulative dose effect is very important for the mass treatment of free-ranging animals or animals consuming product in a free-choice situation. The key to its success is that an individual animal does not need to consume its recommended dose all at one time. The animal can come to the treatment area, consume some product, leave and then come back a few days later, and consume more product. The product, once consumed, stays in the parasites until sufficient product is present to destroy the parasites all together.

DESCRIPTION AND DOSAGE RATE

Product to be fed at the recommended rate of 7.5 mg/kg (3.4 mg/lb) fed over a three to five days period. The product is a highly palatable water-repellent alfalfa wildlife pellet. These pellets can be administered in any open feeder (or spin cast feeder) or fed on the ground (in a clean area). To prevent further parasite contamination while feeding, it is recommended, if possible, to feed on a wooden plank or board off the ground or in a feeder to prevent ground contact.

ESTIMATING HERD SIZE AND REQUIRED DOSE

For effective treatment, two things are important to know about the herd: how many animals might frequent the treatment area and what their approximate weight is. Weight estimate will vary depending upon the time of the year since the weight of the fawns should be added to the overall approximate herd weight. The formula for calculating the amount of fenbendazole medicated pellets is simple: *Estimated number of animals × Average weight = Pounds of Wildlife to be Dewormed.*

STRATEGIC WILDLIFE DEWORMING PROGRAM

Successful deworming requires a seasonal program. A single deworming is important to reduce any parasite buildup in the animals; however, animals become reinfected as soon as they begin to graze again. A successful program is one that is designed to reduce the number of parasites in the animal as well as the parasite contamination in the environment. Recommendations for strategic deworming are as follows:

1. Hoofed wildlife should be dewormed with Safe-Guard in the winter when they group-up. This maximizes the number of animals within the herds that are treated. Winter deworming removes parasite burdens acquired during the previous summer grazing season. Deworming at this time helps winter survivability and maximizes available energy for spring horn growth. Winter deworming also helps reduce parasite contamination of the environment by preventing parasite eggs being passed during the winter and into early spring.

2. To reduce the overall parasite contamination of the environment, two spring dewormings should be given one month apart. This helps to reduce the contamination of parasite eggs in the environment. As animals pick up infective larvae in early spring, they are killed with the first treatment. They will then pick up more larvae, which are killed by the second treatment; this means it will be another month following the second treatment before they will shed eggs. Preventing the shedding of worm eggs for the first three months, beginning in early spring, helps to significantly reduce parasite contamination for the entire season.

3. An important Safe-Guard treatment should be given in late summer or early fall prior to the breeding season. This deworming keeps the immune system strong and provides the necessary energy for a successful breeding season.

THE MODIFIED WISCONSIN SUGAR FECAL EXAM (SEE FIGURE 8.11) PLUS A SUBMISSION FORM (SEE FIGURE 8.12) AND A PICTURE OF THE MOST COMMON EGGS FOUND WITH HOOFED WILDLIFE FECAL SAMPLES (SEE FIGURE 8.13)

A 1 g fecal sample is mixed with a saturated sugar solution designed to float the eggs out of the fecal matter. The samples are strained to remove large debris, then poured into a 15 ml taper test tube, and centrifuged at a low RPM (<1000) for five minutes which increases the egg recovery rate by a significant amount. After centrifuging, a few drops of sugar are added to form a meniscus on top of the tube. A cover slip is placed on the top of the tube for two minutes, removed, and examined under the microscope at 40× magnification. Eggs are identified to type and counted.

The collection process is conducted using a sealable bag or baggie, invert the bag like a glove, and pickup freshly dropped fecal material the size of a golf ball from each horse to check for parasites. Keep each individual sample separate. Seal each bag and write on the bag to identify the horse and date of collection. Keep samples cool after collection since heat causes the eggs to hatch and freezing distorts the eggs.

INTERPRETATION OF FECAL WORM EGG COUNTS IN HOOFED WILDLIFE USING THE MODIFIED WISCONSIN SUGAR FLOTATION TECHNIQUE

Understanding the meaning of worm egg counts will provide veterinarians the necessary insight needed to help clients build a deworming strategy for a particular operation or operations. Factors that affect fecal worm egg shedding are numerous, so a number of these factors need to be

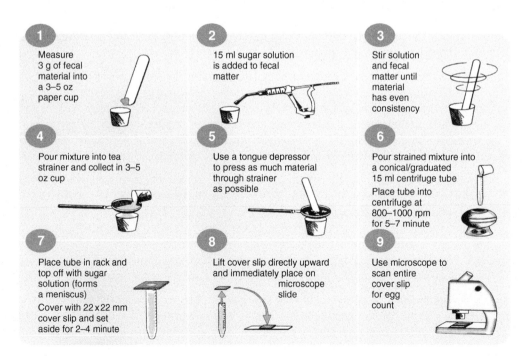

1
Measure 3 g of fecal material into a 3–5 oz paper cup

2
15 ml sugar solution is added to fecal matter

3
Stir solution and fecal matter until material has even consistency

4
Pour mixture into tea strainer and collect in 3–5 oz cup

5
Use a tongue depressor to press as much material through strainer as possible

6
Pour strained mixture into a conical/graduated 15 ml centrifuge tube

Place tube into centrifuge at 800–1000 rpm for 5–7 minute

7
Place tube in rack and top off with sugar solution (forms a meniscus)

Cover with 22 × 22 mm cover slip and set aside for 2–4 minute

8
Lift cover slip directly upward and immediately place on microscope slide

9
Use microscope to scan entire cover slip for egg count

FIGURE 8.11   Nine-step procedure for the Modified Wisconsin Sugar Flotation Method (see Chapter 2).

Small Ruminants & Wildlife Parasite Evaluation Form

PEC ☐   Mail In ☐   Page____ of____

Collection Date: _____   Consultant: _____ Dr. Don Bliss _____

Name of Farm: _____   Sponsor: _____

Producer's Name: _____   Sponsor Contact: _____

Producer's Address: _____   Sponsor Address: _____

City _____ Phone _____   City _____ Phone _____

State _____ Zip _____ Fax _____   State _____ Zip _____ Fax _____

E-Mail: _____   Representative: _____

Sample ID	Animal ID	Stomach Worm	Nematodirus	Cooperia	Hookworm	Threadworm	Whipworm	Nodular Worm	Tapeworm	Coccidia	Total Count* (EPG)	Treatment Date month/day/year	Product Used
												Enter after test results recorded	

COMMENTS:

Sponsor's E-mail:

For additional information and submission forms, visit: www.midamericaagresearch.net

Donald H. Bliss, Ph.D.
MidAmerica Ag. Research
3705 Sequoia Trail
Verona, WI 53593

*(+ = 1-10) (++ = 11-50) (+++ =>51)

FIGURE 8.12   Small ruminant and hoofed wildlife submission form.

considered every time an analysis is made and a fair assessment of the worm egg counts generated. The age of the animal, the season of the year, the amount of exposure to pasture, and the stocking rate of the animals on pasture all affect worm egg counts. The amount of rainfall or moisture on the pasture and the number of degree days with temperatures sufficient to promote parasite development on pasture are also very important to future infections. These factors directly affect egg count interpretation as infection levels build on the pasture and ingestion of these larvae increases and worm burdens rise in the animals themselves. Furthermore, the health of the animals, the stage of gestation, stage of lactation, and the numbers and types of parasites present at each examination must be considered. Post-birthing worm egg counts, for example, are almost always higher than pre-birthing counts.

The five most common types of internal nematode parasites in hoofed wildlife that are routinely diagnosed present in fecal exams are: Stomach worms (primarily the barber's pole worm – *Haemonchus* sp.), intestinal worms (*Cooperia* sp.), threadworms (*Strongyloides* sp.), whipworms (*Trichuris* sp.), and nodular worms (*Oesophagostomum* sp.). All eggs are counted and included in the worm egg count total, except for tapeworms and coccidia. Tapeworms and coccidia are commonly found but are listed on the worm egg count forms simply as positive at a low level (+) 1–10 eggs, medium level (++) 11–50 eggs, or high level (+++) 50 eggs or greater.

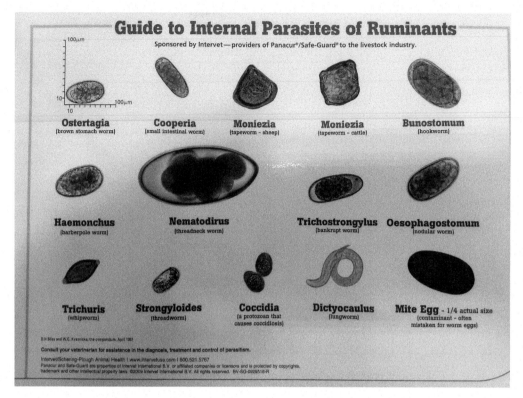

FIGURE 8.13 Color atlas of the most common worm egg found in small ruminants and hoofed wildlife.

One egg/g equals 454 eggs/lb of manure, i.e., a count of 500 equals 227,000 eggs/lb of feces, so 5.0 lb of feces per day would yield 1,100,000 eggs per day on the pasture per animal.

QUICK ASSESSMENT FOR HOOFED WILDLIFE BASED ON FECAL WORM EGG COUNTS

	Eggs/g Count	Estimated Parasite Level
Nematode egg counts	1–10 eggs	Low
Recorded on sheets	11–50 eggs	Moderate
	51–299 eggs	High*
	301+ eggs	Very High*

*At this level, it appears that parasites begin to stop developing and undergo inhibition in tissues.

Positive worm egg counts for hoofed wildlife (other than very high counts) for the most part only indicate the presence or absence of parasites within a particular animal. It is impossible to determine how many parasites are present at any given time primarily because *Haemonchus* undergoes a phenomenon called inhibition or period of arrested development. This parasitic stage remains in the tissues for long periods of time and follow an annual development and inhibition cycle. The primary inhibition period begins about 45–60 days into a grazing period as the parasite contamination level on pastures buildup. These inhibited larvae can stage in the tissues through the beginning of the following grazing season.

The overall infection process begins when an infected animal grazes a pasture and sheds worm eggs on a daily basis that pass in the manure. These eggs hatch and the larval offspring develop into infective larvae which recontaminate the pasture, thus exposing all animal grazing this pasture to new infections. If the pasture is already contaminated with infective larvae, the animals pick up new infections at the same time they shed eggs back on the pasture contributing future contamination levels. This process continues until the grazing season ends. Depending upon temperature and moisture, these parasite eggs hatch, develop into infective larvae, and move away from the manure pats onto the vegetation where the reinfection process begins. The biggest and least understood issue with hoofed wildlife is that once *Haemonchus* infections reach a high level, the physiology of the gut changes. The parasites respond by stopping their development undergoing an arrested development period waiting for the physiology of the gut to return to normal. This why the simple guide (listed above) to predict parasite levels within an animal based on worm egg counts can be misleading.

The time of the year when the assessment is made can also have an impact on worm eggs as follows:

1. **Winter:** As winter progresses, animals are no longer ingesting infective larvae off pasture, existing worm burdens begin to mature and die off as they age, conditions in the gut then start to return to normal which, in turn, triggers inhibited parasites to become active. If counts come back following treatment, this means inhibited larvae are present or if worm egg counts are high during the winter, these counts indicate that heavy worm challenge existed from the previous season.

2. **Spring:** When inhibited larvae are being released form the gastric glands, egg shedding can reach a high level which indicates the presence of high worm burdens carried over from the previous season. High egg shedding levels at this time is dangerous because egg shedding in the spring determines contamination levels for the rest of the year.

3. **Summer:** Once animals are on pasture and grazing begins, worm counts will begin to rise within three weeks. Once egg counts exceed 100 eggs/g (45,400/lb of manure), worm burdens have reached a point when incoming larvae undergo arrested development and become inhibited larvae in the gastric glands of the abomasum.

4. **Fall:** The quick assessment chart (listed above) is most accurate in the fall at the end of the grazing season. Low counts indicate successful control of worm burdens while high counts indicate economic loss may be occurring and trouble controlling these infections due to inhibited worm burdens may be occurring.

GASTROINTESTINAL AND LUNG PARASITE INFECTIONS FOUND IN SMALL RUMINANTS AND HOOFED WILDLIFE

Parasitism in small ruminants can be broken into three main categories: *Stomach worms*, *Intestinal worms*, and *Protozoa*. From a microscope standpoint, samples are scanned for worm eggs and then identified by shape and size, then counted and reported as eggs per gram of material used.

The following is an egg chart used to identify the species of worm the eggs are from:

STOMACH WORMS

Barber's pole worm (*Haemonchus contortus*) is a blood-sucking parasite that completes it life cycle from eggs passed in the manure, hatch, and molt three times in the environment to become an infective L_3 larva which is infectious if eaten by sheep, goats, camelids, and camels. This is a very economically damaging parasite in small ruminants but is especially damaging in sheep and goats becoming one of the most important causes of death in these animals. Larval stages have been found in the rumen and abomasal tissues and are extremely hard to kill. Eggs are easily identified in a fecal exam (see Figures 8.14 and 8.15).

Ostertagia (brown stomach worm) is probably the most studied and most prevalent parasite of cattle but not so much for small ruminants. Larval stages invade and destroy the gastric glands. Large numbers of parasites can significantly reduce digestion efficiency. Larval stages can undergo inhibition and remain in the glands for months before emerging into lumen of the abomasum to develop into an adult worm. *Ostertagia* eggs are easily identified in a fecal exam since they are smaller than *Haemonchus* eggs (see Figures 8.16 and 8.17).

Trichostrongylus axei and *Trichostrongylus colubriformis* (bankrupt worm) are most often seen with *Haemonchus* infections. Most commonly occurs in the abomasum but also found in the upper part of the small intestine. These worms are associated with a chronic wasting disease when present in large numbers. The eggs are oval shaped with fluid on each end similar in size to Haemonchus eggs but more shaped like a kidney bean (see Figures 8.18 and 8.19).

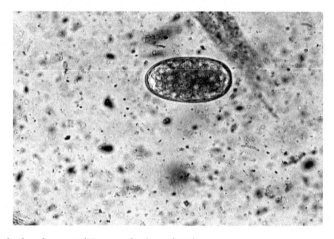

FIGURE 8.14   Barber's pole worm (*Haemonchus*) egg (10×).

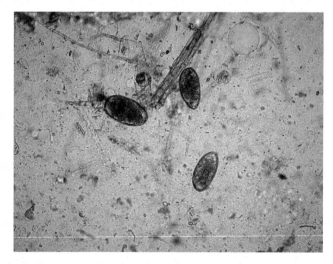

FIGURE 8.15   Barber's pole (*Haemonchus*) (larger) egg plus two brown stomach worm (*Ostertagia*) eggs.

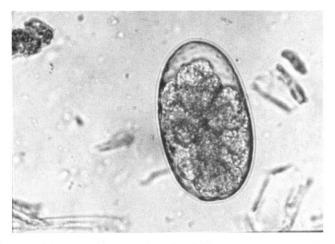

FIGURE 8.16   Brown stomach worm (*Ostertagia*) egg (10×).

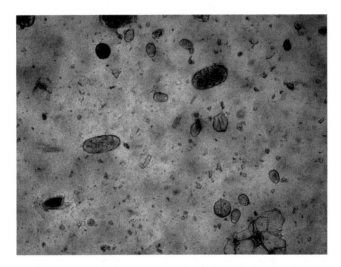

FIGURE 8.17   Brown stomach worm (*Ostertagia* – smaller egg) and barber's pole worm (*Haemonchus*) eggs with coccidia oocysts (10×).

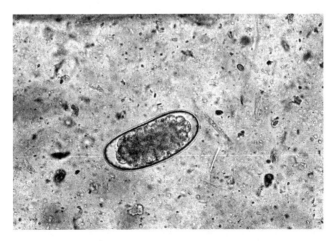

FIGURE 8.18   Bankrupt worm (*Trichostrongylus*) egg (40×).

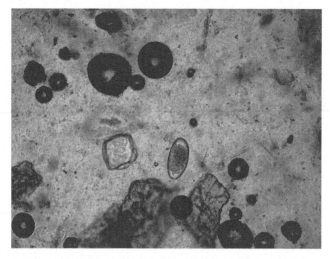

FIGURE 8.19 Bankrupt worm (*Trichostrongylus*) and tapeworm (*Moniezia*) eggs (10×).

INTESTINAL PARASITES

Cooper's worm (*Cooperia curticei*) does not seem to be an important parasite of sheep as it is off cattle and bison. *Cooperia* disrupts digestive functions of the intestine and produces a strong immune reaction. This parasite is not as prevalent in small ruminants as in cattle. Eggs are easily found in a fecal exam and are distinct because of elongated parallel sides (see Figures 8.20 and 8.21).

    Threadneck worm (*Nematodirus spathiger, Nematodirus filicollis,* and *Nematodirus battus*) is most commonly found in young animals. Larvae survive well in cold weather and can live for two years on pasture. This parasite is a common cause of diarrhea and oftentimes death in young and old small ruminants. Because it is very pathogenic, older animals acquired a strong immunity against this parasite. The egg is very large and is easily identified in a fecal exam (see Figures 8.22 and 8.23).

    Threadworm (*Strongyloides papillosus*) infection is by skin penetration, by ingestion through mother's milk, or through contaminated feed or bedding [5]. Transmission is seldom found through grazing or pasture contamination. Threadworms can very harmful to baby

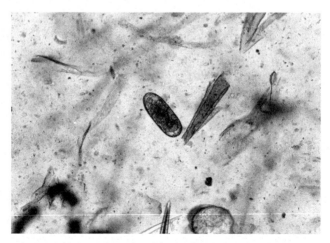

FIGURE 8.20 Cooper's worm (*Cooperia*) egg (10×) (Note: flat parallel sides).

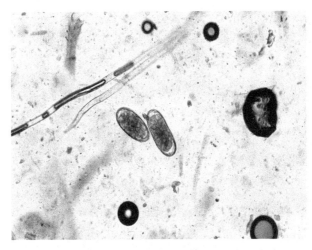

FIGURE 8.21   *Cooperia* egg (parallel sides) and *Ostertagia* egg.

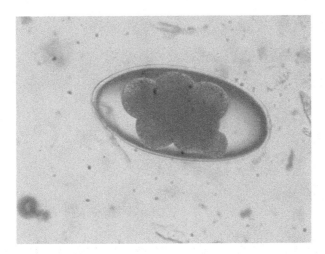

FIGURE 8.22   *Nematodirus* egg (40×).

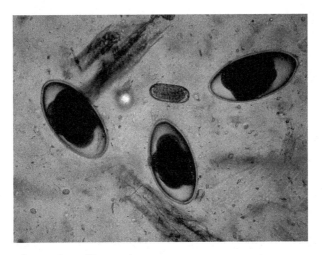

FIGURE 8.23   *Nematodirus* and two *Haemonchus* eggs.

lambs and kids but usually self-eliminate by two to three months of age. *Strongyloides* infection is easily identified upon fecal exam by the presence of small thin-shelled embryonated eggs (see Figures 8.24 and 8.25).

Whipworm (*Trichuris ovis*) lives in the cecum and is the organ that joins the small and large intestine. *Trichuris* is another very damaging parasite in young animals. Oftentimes, symptoms are confused with coccidiosis because of the bloody diarrhea associated with this parasite. Several hundred worms can kill a young animal. The egg is very characteristic and looks like a football with polar caps on each end (see Figures 8.26 and 8.27). The female worm is not prolific and eggs are often missed in the fecal exam unless carefully conducted. The *Trichuris* egg remains in the egg until infective and can live 20–25 years in the soil. Cattle held in barnyards often become infected with *Trichuris*.

Capillaria (*Capillaria brevipes, Capillaria bovis*) infections in sheep and goats are of no veterinary importance and, therefore, its observance is only a simple matter of record. Capillaria are very thin filamentous worms and cannot be seen grossly in the gut contents. Capillaria eggs are similar to whipworm eggs but smaller and with non-protruding polar caps (see Figure 8.28).

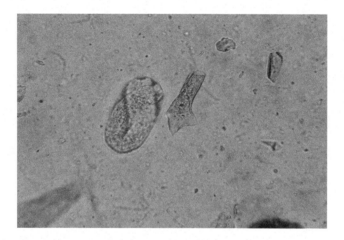

FIGURE 8.24   Threadworm (*Strongyloides papillosus*) egg (40×).

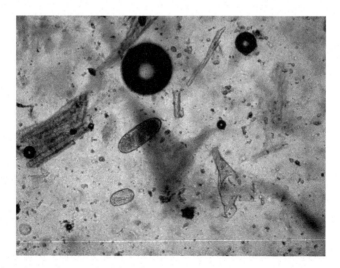

FIGURE 8.25   Threadworm (*Strongyloides*) and *Cooperia* eggs.

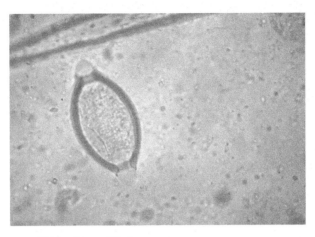

FIGURE 8.26   Whipworm (*Trichuris*) egg (10×).

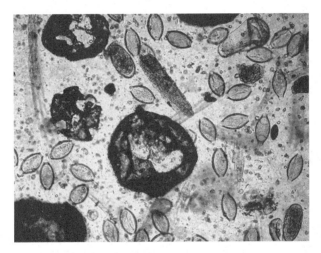

FIGURE 8.27   Heavy whipworm (*Trichuris*) infection.

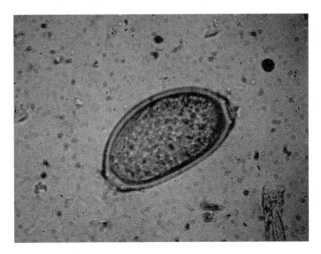

FIGURE 8.28   *Capillaria* egg (40×).

Hookworm (*Bunostomum trigonocephalum*) occurs both in sheep and goats. Infections can occur by ingesting infective larvae or by skin penetration. If infection is through the skin, hookworm larvae pass through the lungs before being coughed up passing back to the small intestine where they attach to the intestinal wall, mate, and begin laying eggs back into the environment. Hookworm eggs are large rectangular-shaped eggs with a thick outer shell and egg development in an 8-cell stage (see Figures 8.29 and 8.30).

Nodular worm (*Oesophagostomum venulosum* and *Oesophagostomum columbianum*) is becoming more important in recent years because intestines are often condemned at slaughter if nodules caused by the nodular worms are found in large numbers. Parasites are associated with anorexia, depressed weight gain, and diarrhea. Most commonly found in adult animals. Nodular worm eggs are much larger than Haemonchus eggs but slightly smaller than Hookworm eggs and are oval in shape with embryo in a 16–32 cell stage (see Figures 8.31 and 8.32).

Intestinal cestode (Tapeworm) parasites (*Moniezia expansa* and *Moniezia benedeni*): The small ruminant tapeworm develops in the soil mite, which is ingested by small ruminants. The development time to reach an adult after ingestion is reported to be from six to eight weeks. The

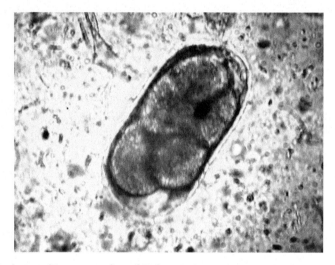

FIGURE 8.29   Hookworm (*Bunostomum*) egg (40×).

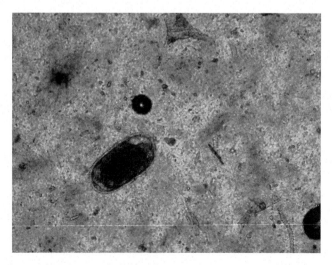

FIGURE 8.30   Hookworm (*Bunostomum*) egg (10×).

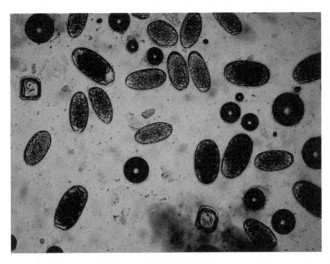

FIGURE 8.31   Nodular worm, *Ostertagia,* and Tapeworm eggs.

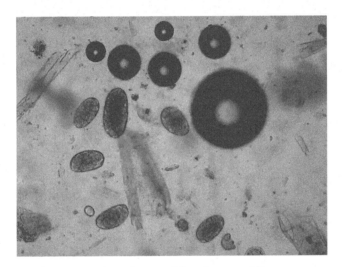

FIGURE 8.32   Nodular worm egg, *Haemonchus* eggs (5), and one coccidia oocyst.

adult tapeworm lives in the small intestine and can grow to be 1 in. wide and 6 ft long. They absorb nutrition through their cuticle. In high numbers, tapeworms can block the intestine. Tapeworm eggs are distinct and easily picked up in a fecal exam (see Figures 8.33 and 8.34).

    Fascioloides magna **(deer fluke) and** *Fasciola hepatica* **(common fluke).** *Fascioloides magna* found in the Great Lakes region is relatively untreatable in sheep because it is so pathogenic. Diagnosis can only be done accurately upon necropsy since the larval stages migrate in the liver until it is destroyed. In cattle, the young flukes are eventually walled off and contained in the liver, where as in sheep, the young flukes continue to migrate throughout the liver until they are completely destroyed and the animals succumb (13). Keeping small ruminants away from wet areas and streams where deer congregate is currently the only method of control. One fluke egg which hatches is all that is needed to kill one sheep. *Fasciola hepatica* is rarely found in sheep but egg is easily recoverable using a FlukeFinder kit (see Figure 8.35) and easily identifiable (see Figures 8.36 and 8.37). Instructions for using the FlukeFinder kit is given in Chapter 2.

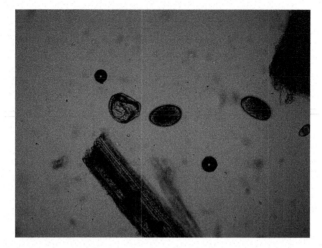

FIGURE 8.33   Tapeworm (*Moniezia)* egg with a threadworm (*Strongyloides*) egg.

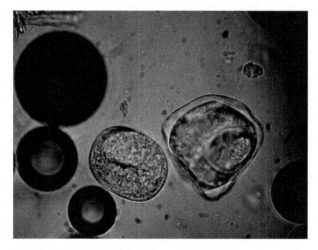

FIGURE 8.34   Tapeworm (*Moniezia*) egg and two *Haemonchus* eggs.

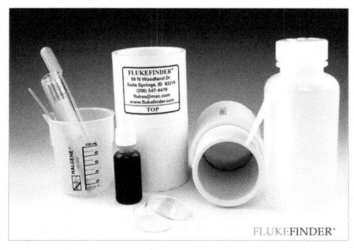

FIGURE 8.35   FlukeFinder kit.
Source: FLUKEFINDER.

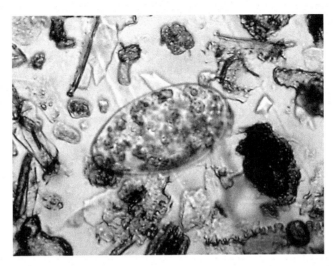

FIGURE 8.36 Liver fluke (*Fasciola hepatica*) egg.

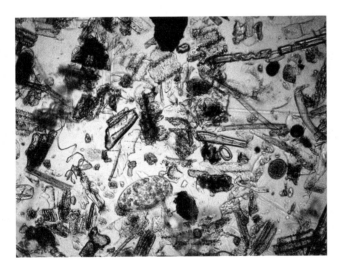

FIGURE 8.37 Liver fluke (*Fasciola hepatica*) egg.

Coccidia are single-celled protozoan parasites that all small ruminants are believed to be exposed to sometime in their life. Coccidia are very host-specific such that coccidia of swine, dogs, and chickens would not infect small ruminants. The reverse is also true. Coccidia are ingested through fecal-contaminated feedstuff. Wet muddy conditions usually increase infection levels. Camelids (alpaca and llamas) do have a special pathogenic parasite not seen in other small ruminants called E. mac. (Eimeria Macusaniensis) (see Chapter 7). Coccidia oocysts are easily identified. There are many different species of coccidia in hoofed wildlife and each species has its own characteristic size and shape but usually can be identified with a chart giving size measurements and shapes for each species. For general observation in a standard fecal sample, we list coccidia oocysts numbers seen as low (+0–10), medium (++11–50), or high (+++ >50) (see Figures 8.38–8.40). Coccidia is a known pathogen that is opportunistic and thrives when the animal's immune system is under attack, for example, with high *Haemonchus* worm burden in the abomasum. Deworming a heavily infected animal that also shows a high coccidia count, the coccidia counts most often drop to a low level soon after the deworming is complete. It appears that once the worm burden is removed, the animal's immune system can suppress coccidian development.

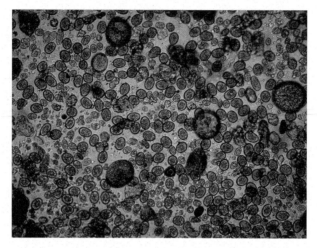

FIGURE 8.38 Heavy Coccidia infection found in Texas deer samples.

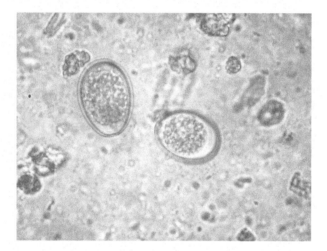

FIGURE 8.39 Coccidia oocysts found in Texas deer samples.

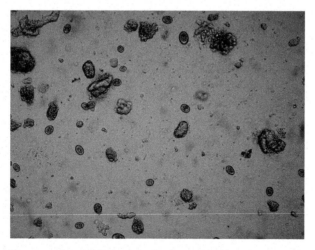

FIGURE 8.40 Coccidia oocysts found in Wisconsin deer samples.

REFERENCES

1. Davidson, W.R., Hayes, F.A., Nettles, V.F., and Kellog, F.E. (1981). *Diseases and parasites of white-tailed deer. Southeastern cooperative wildlife disease study*. Athens, Ga: Department of Parasitology, College of Veterinary Medicine University of Georgia.

2. Samuel, W.M., Pybus, M.J., and Kocan, A.A. (1971). *Parasitic Diseases of Wild Mammals*, 2e. Ames, IA: Iowa State University Press.

3. Schultz, S.R., Barry, R.X., Forbes, W.A., and Johnson, M.K. (1993). Efficacy of fenbendazole against gastrointestinal nematodes in white-tailed deer. *J. Range Manage.* 46: 240–244.

4. Janssen, D. (1985). Efficacy of fenbendazole for endoparasite control in large herds of nondomestic ruminants. *J. Am. Med. Assoc.* 187: 1189–1190.

5. Forrester, D.J., Taylor, W.J., and Nair, K.P.C. (1974). Strongyloides in captive white-tailed deer. *J. Wildl. Dis.* 10: 11–17.

Index

Note: *Italic* page numbers refer to figure and **Bold** page numbers reference to tables.

Large Animal Parasitology Procedures for Veterinary Technicians, First Edition. Donald H. Bliss.
© 2024 John Wiley & Sons, Inc. Published 2024 by John Wiley & Sons, Inc.